07288526

AF443218

Essentials of
Gynecology

Essentials of Gynecology

Editors

Sabaratnam Arulkumaran
DCH FRCS FRCOG FAMS MD PhD Hon: FACOG FSLCOG FSOGC
Professor and Head, Division of Obstetrics and Gynecology
St. George's Hospital Medical School, London, UK

V Sivanesaratnam
MBBS (S'pore) FRCOG FICS FACS FAMM
Professor, Department of Obstetrics and Gynecology
Faculty of Medicine, University of Malaya, Kuala Lumpur, Malaysia

Alokendu Chatterjee
FRCOG FICS
Formely, Professor and Head, Department of Obstetrics and Gynecology
NRS Medical College and Hospital, Calcutta
Salt Lake City, Kolkata

Pratap Kumar
MD DGO FICS FICOG FICMCH
Professor and Head, Department of Obstetrics and Gynecology
Kasturba Medical College, Manipal

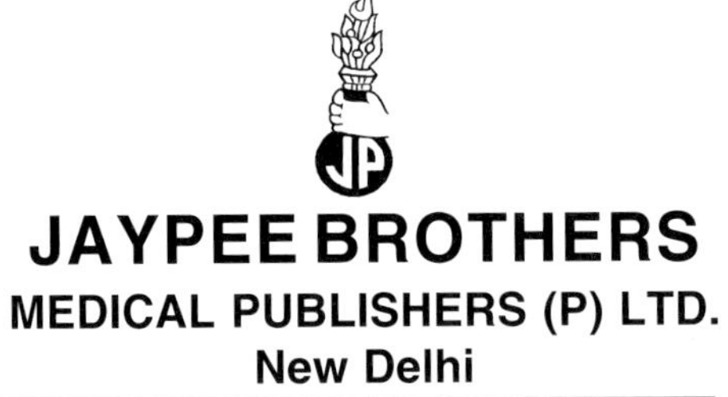

JAYPEE BROTHERS
MEDICAL PUBLISHERS (P) LTD.
New Delhi

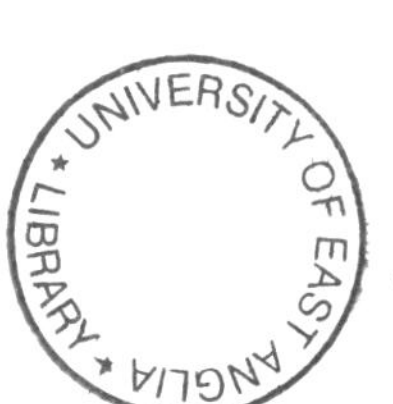

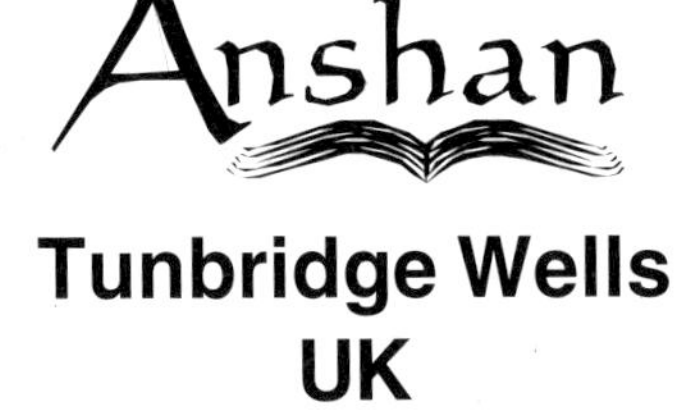

Tunbridge Wells
UK

First published in the UK by

Anshan Ltd
in 2005
6 Newlands Road
Tunbridge Wells
Kent TN4 9AT, UK

Tel/Fax: +44 (0)1892 557767
E-mail: info@anshan.co.uk
www.anshan.co.uk

ISBN 1 904798 292

British Library Cataloguing in Publication Data
A catalogue record for this book is available from the British Library

Printed in India by Gopsons Papers Ltd., A-14, Sector 60,Noida

Contributors

Noor Azmi bin Mat Adenan BSc (St. Andrews)
MB ChB (Glasg) M Med (Univ Mal)
Lecturer
Department of Obstetrics and Gynaecology
Faculty of Medicine, University of Malaya
50603 Kuala Lumpur, Malaysia
Tel: (60) 3 7950 2059
Fax: (60) 3 7955 1741
E mail: *azmi@ummc.edu.my*
Chapter: 16

Sapna Ahuja
Specialist Registrar
Department of Obstetrics and Gynaecology
Luton and Dunstable Hospital NHS Trust
Lewsey Road
LUTON, LU4 0EN
Chapters: 33, 36

Behram S Anklesaria MD DGO DFP FICOG ATMF (USA)
Professor and Head
Department of Obstetrics and Gynecology
LG Hospital and NHL Medical College
Ahmedabad, India
Chapter: 20

Sabaratnam Arulkumaran DCH FRCS FRCOG FAMS MD PhD
Hon: FACOG, FSLCOG, FSOGC
Professor and Head
Division of Obstetrics and Gynaecology
St George's Hospital Medical School
London, United Kingdom
e-mail: sarulkum@sghms.ac.uk
Chapters: 4, 10, 17, 33, 36, 37

Edwin Chandraharan MBBS MS (Obs and Gyn) DFFP (UK)
MRCOG
Clinical Lecturer
Division of Obstetrics and Gynaecology
St. George's Hospital Medical School
London SW 17 0RE
Chapter: 4

Premitha Damodaran MBBS MMed (O and G)
Kiara Gynaecology Centre
64-01, Jalan 27/70 A, Desa Sri Hartamas
50480-Kuala Lumpur
Tel: 6-03-23002351/52
Fax: 6-03-23001690
e-mail: premitha_prem@yahoo.com
Chapter: 29

Sheetal Dholakia MD DGO
9, Hemniketan, NS Road No. 5, JVPD Scheme
Vile Parle, Mumbai 400 056
Tel: 6206365, 6208623
E mail: drsheetal@spareage.com
Chapter: 7

Meenu S Handa MBBS DGO
Registrar
Department of Obstetrics and Gynecology
LG Hospital and NHL Medical College
Ahmedabad, India
Chapter: 20

Jayakrishnan MD DGO DIPNB
Director
KJK Hospital
Nalanchira, Thiruvanathapuram, Kerala
Phone: 0471-544080
Fax 0471-543926
e-mail: kjkhospital@vsnl.com
Chapter: 15

Lim Boon Kiong MBBS (Mal), MRCOG
Associate Professor and Consultant
University of Malaya Medical Centre
University of Malaya
50603 Kuala Lumpur
Fax No: 603-79551741
Phone No: 603-79502059
Chapter: 32

Pratap Kumar MD DGO
Professor and Head
Dept of Obstetrics and gynecology
Kasturba Medical College and Hospital
Manipal-576 119
Karnataka State, India
e-mail: drpratapkumar@hotmail.com
Phone: Hospital: 91-8252-71201-19 (19 lines), Ext-2211,
Residence: 91-8251-70999
Fax: 91-8252-70062
Chapters: 2, 3, 5, 6, 12, 13, 25

Pralhad Kushtagi
Department of Obstetrics and Gynecology
Kasturba Medical College and Hospital
Manipal - 576 119, India
e-mail: pralhadkushtagi@hotmail.com
pralhadkushtagi@indiainfo.com
Chapter: 18

AP Manjunath MD (principle correspondent)
Assistant professor
Department of Obstetrics and gynecology
Kasturba Medical College and Hospital
Manipal-576 119
Karnataka State, India
e-mail: manjunath@obgyn.net
Phone: 91-8252-71201-19(19 lines)
Ext-2211 (Hospital), 2081(Residence)
Fax: 91-8252-70061
Chapters: 3, 21

Dev Kumar Menon B Med Sci (Hons) BM BS MRCOG
Department of Obstetrics and Gynaecology
University Malaya Medical Centre
50603 Kuala Lumpur
Malaysia
e-mail: DrMenon2000@yahoo.co.uk
Tel: 603-79502473
Fax: 603-79551741
Chapter: 11

Krishnendu Mukherjee MS FRCS FRCS (Ed)
Consultant and Surgeon
Belle Vue Clinic
26, Beadon Street
Calcutta: 700 006
Phone No.: 0091-33-351-3991
e-mail: krishmukh@usa.net
Chapter: 22

Sambit Mukhopadhyay
Consultant
Department of Obstetrics and Gynaecology
Norfolk and Norwich University Hospital NHS Trust
Norwich
United Kingdom
Chapters: 10, 33, 36

Prashant Nadkarni FRCOG
Consultant Obstetrician and Gynaecologist
Infertility Specialist
Pantai Medical Centre
8 Jalan Bukit Pantai
59100 Kuala Lumpur
Malaysia
Tel: (+603) 4302351
Fax: (+603) 4301690
e-mail: prashantnadkarni@hotmail.com
Chapter: 28

Arun Nagrath
Retd Professor
Department of Obstetrics and Gynecology
Agra Medical College
Agra, India
Chapters: 5, 6

Jayaraman Nambiar MD DGO
Assistant Professor
Department of Obstetrics and Gynecology
Kasturba Medical College, Manipal- 576 119, India
Phone: 00-91-825 571201
Fax: 00-91-825 570061 and 570062
e-mail: drramnambiar@yahoo.co.in
Chapter: 21

Siti Zawiah Omar MBBS M Med (Obs and Gynae)
Lecturer
Department of Obstetrics and Gynaecology
Faculty of Medicine, University of Malaya
50603 Kuala Lumpur, Malaysia
Tel: 603-79502059
Fax: 603-70551741
Chapter: 14

Muralidhar V Pai
Associate Professor
Dept of Obstetrics and Gynaecology
Kasturba Medical College
Manipal 576 119
India
Tel: 91-8252-71201
Fax: 91-8252-70062
e-mail: mvpai@mahe.manipal.edu
Chapters: 26, 27

VP Paily MD FRCOG
(Former Professor of Obstetrics and Gynaecology,
Medical College, Thrissur)
Vakkanal, East Fort, Thrissur-5
Kerala, India
Pin - 680 005
Tele No.0487-336222
email-pailycom@vsnl.com
Chapter: 19

N Pandiyan
Chief Consultant in Andrology and Reproductive Sciences
Apollo Hospitals, 21, Greams Lane
Off Greams Road, Chennai-600 006
India
Phone: 91-44-8290200/8293333.
Fax: 91-44-8234429.
e-mail: gautham1@eth.net
Chapter: 9

Vani Ramkumar MD
Additional Professor of Ob and Gyn
Kasturba Medical College
Manipal 576 119, Karnataka
India
e-mail : ram54-vip@zetainfotech.com
Tel : (Res) 08252-70003
Chapter: 23

Rupinder Kaur Ruprai MD
Assistant Professor
Department of Obstetrics and Gynecology
Kasturba Medical College
Manipal, India
e-mail: rubyruprai@yahoo.com
Chapters: 5, 6

PK Sekharan MD
Former Professor and Head
Department of Obstetrics and Gynaecology
Institute of Maternal and Child health
Medical College, Calicut, Kerala, India
Tel: 91-495-356954
Tele Fax: 91-495-356954
e-mail sekharan@vsnl.com
Chapter: 8

PK Shah MD FICOG FCPS FICMU FICM CH DGO DFP
Professor and Unit Head
Department of Obstetrics and Gynaecology
LTM Medical College and LTMG Hospital Sion
Mumbai-400 022, India
Tel: 4076381, 4082504 to 4082515 Ext: 261, Fax: 4076100
Chapter: 7

Siya Sharan Sharma (Principal Author)
MD DNB DGO MICOG MNAMS
Assistant Professor
Department of Obstetrics and Gynaecology
Kasturba Medical College and Hospital
Manipal-576 119. India.
Tel: +91-8252-71201 Extn. 2211, Fax: + 91-8252-70061
e-mail: drsiya@yahoo.com
Chapters: 12, 13

Nozer Sheriar MD DNBE FCPS FICOG DGO
BDP Parsee General Hospital
Bomanji Petit Road
Cumballa Hill
Mumbai-400 026
India
Chapter: 1

Paul Tay Yee Siang MD MRCOG MB BCh
Department of Obstetrics and Gynaecology
University Malaya Medical Centre (UMMC)
Jalan University, 50630 Kuala Lumpur, Malaysia
e-mail: pystay@hotmail.com
Telephone: 03-79502473
Chapter: 24

V Sivanesaratnam MBBS FRCOG FICS FACS FAMM JSM
Head and Senior Consultant
Department of Obstetrics and Gynaecology
Faculty of Medicine
University of Malaya
50603 Kuala Lumpur
Malaysia.
Tel: 603-79502059
Fax: 603-70551741
e-mail: siva@medicine.med.um.edu.my
Chapters: 14, 30, 31, 32, 34, 35

O Tamizian
Specialist Registrar
Department of Obstetrics and Gynaecology
Kings Mill Hospital
Nottingham
United Kingdom
Chapters: 17, 37

Foreword

We are fortunate to have lived through a period of historic milestones, and the turn of the millennium. The last millennium saw dramatic technical advances in the field of medicine. The greatest single difference between women in rich countries and women in developing ones is in their reproductive health status, particularly the availability, affordability and access to the same.

The book *Essentials of Gynecology* is the work of leading experts in the field, detailing the methodology for clinical practice and modus operandi for appropriate treatment for the disease. The contributors are experienced professionals, who have distilled their wealth of expertise to provide invaluable guide for the problems faced in day-to-day practice and emphasize practical aspects. Utmost care has been taken to include essentials ranging from embryology to cancer detection, suited to all different geographical regions.

The substance as presented, invites readers to appreciate and engage themselves in a rational and logical approach to problems. The contents of this treatise will reiterate the importance of the art of clinical practice and the principles involved in scientific management. I hope it would become a springboard for some to rise to great heights in managing the selected subjects.

Shirish S Sheth
MD, FRCOG, FACS, FICS, FCPS, FICOG, FAMS, FSOGC
Consultant Gynaecologist
Breach Candy Hospital
Sir Hurkisondas Hospital
Past President, FIGO

Preface

Gynecology has always been a fascinating subject looking at the health issues of a female from birth to the menopause. This book takes the life cycle approach starting in sex differentiation, abnormal development of reproductive organs to pediatric and adolescent health. This is followed by menarche, menstruation and menstrual problems. The issues related to contraception and subfertility are dealt with in detail. Sexually transmitted diseases and pelvic inflammatory diseases are described followed by benign and malignant neoplasms of the reproductive tract. Menopause and cancer screening is discussed based on the current data and available evidence. There is little doubt that gynecological problems are increasingly managed medically and by minimally invasive surgery and where possible by outpatient procedures. Detailed descriptions of these are provided including the latest in technology.

The authors for each chapter have specially been selected based on their expertise and experience. A large number of figures have been included to make the subject easy to understand and to make an "imprint" in the reader's mind, so that the subject matter will remain for years to come. We have no doubt that this book will be of great value to those interested in the subject.

There are bound to be some overlap of subject matter due to the multi-author nature of the book and the need to repeat certain basic facts to provide a continuous flow of the subject matter. No book is perfect and ageless. With progress of time, there will be changes in practice and the editors and authors would provide this in the next edition. The readers are kindly requested to communicate any mistakes and omissions to the publishers or the editors, so that they can be incorporated in the next/reprint edition.

Sabaratnam Arulkumaran
V Sivanesaratnam
Alokendu Chatterjee
Pratap Kumar

Acknowledgements

The editors would like to sincerely thank the contributors to this book. It had a long conception period due to some chapters arriving late and the need to have an extensive editorial process to make the chapters uniform, avoid duplication and step down postgraduate into undergraduate knowledge. The latter process has made some chapters so different from the original submission by authors. We ask the authors for their understanding and acceptance of this process. The principal editor collated the chapters from the other editors to streamline the publication and would like to acknowledge the help and advice provided by Mrs. Sue Cunningham at St. George's Hospital Medical School, University of London. We are grateful to the authors and publishers for their patience in the production of this book. Mr. JP Vij, Chairman and Managing Director, Mr Tarun Duneja, General Manager (Publishing) and his team from Jaypee Brothers Medical Publishers (P) Ltd. need special commendation for the constant encouragement, in-house editorial work and production of the vast number of figures in the book. We would like to thank Dr. Shirish S Sheth, past President of FIGO and an internationally renowned Obstetrician and Gynecologist for writing the foreword for this book.

Contents

Part 1: General Gynecology

Part 2: Reproductive Endocrinology and Assisted Conception

Part 3: Gynecologic Oncology

1.
Embryology and Development of the Female Genital Tract

Nozer Sheriar

The reproductive organs in the female (as also in the male) consist of gonads, external genitalia and an internal duct system between the two. Since these three components originate from different primordia in close association with the urinary system and the hindgut, the embryological development is complex and developmental abnormalities are often interrelated.[1]

INDIFFERENT EMBRYO

The hindgut appears about the twentieth postovulatory day. The intermediate mesoderm develops adjacent to the midline dorsal mesentery of the gut, extending through the length of the body cavity (celom). A part of this intermediate cell mass medial to the mesonephros (primitive kidney), proliferates to form the *gonadal ridges.* These bilateral thickenings being recognizable in the 4 to 5 mm embryo (Fig. 1.1).

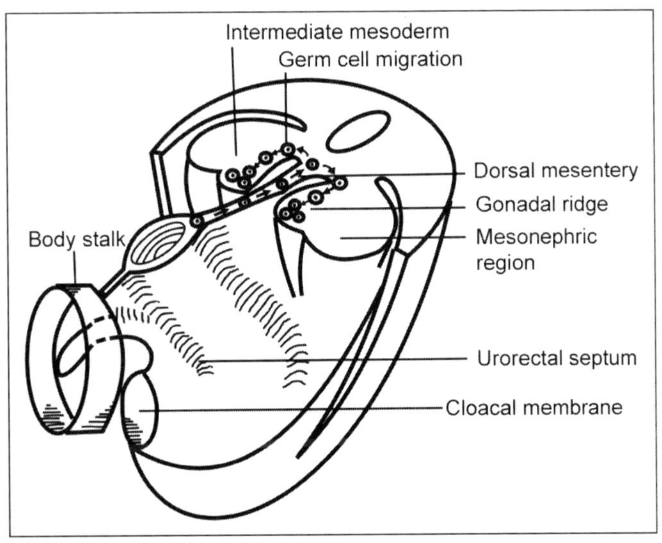

Figure 1.1: The caudal half of the embryo (30-35 days)

Indifferent Gonad

Primordial germ cells that are subsequently capable of meiosis, separate out from the pool of somatic cells that are capable only of mitosis. These *germ cells* are present in the allantoic diverticulum and the adjacent parts of the yolk sac in 17 to 20 day embryos. From here they migrate through the dorsal mesentery of the hindgut, reaching the *gonadal ridge* in the human embryo at 35 days (Fig. 1.1). The cause of this migration of the germ cells is yet unknown.

The area to which the germ cells migrate is referred to as the *indifferent gonad* until gonadal sex is established. At 35 days the indifferent gonad is formed by the primordial germ cells, cells from the overlying coelomic epithelium and the cells of the adjacent mesonephros. The germ cells now undergo rapid mitotic proliferation and are enclosed by extensions of the coelomic epithelium (sex cords) and the mesonephric ducts.

Mesonephric (Wolffian) Ducts

In 1759 Caspar Wolff studying the embryology of the chick described a symmetrical pair of paravertebral swellings as the precursors of the kidneys. The term *Wolffian* has been subsequently used to describe the mesonephric ducts and vesicles.

The first indication of the urinary system appears at 21 days when the mesonephric vesicles develop. These are associated with a solid cord of cells in the intermediate mesoderm, that acquire a lumen at 26 days, forming the *mesonephric ducts*. Skirting the hindgut the bilateral mesonephric ducts open into the urogenital sinus at 28 days (Fig. 1.2). At 32 days, the caudal end of each mesonephric duct gives rise to the ureteric bud and is incorporated into the posterior wall of the urogenital sinus, subsequently forming the trigone of the bladder and the posterior wall of the urethra. The mesonephros attains maximum size and function at 42 days, the metanephros taking over excretory function after 50 days.

Paramesonephric (Müllerian) Ducts

In 1830 Johannes Müller described a cord on the outer aspect of the Wolffian body, but thinner than the Wolffian

cord. These *müllerian cords* now referred to as the *paramesonephric ducts,* appear at about 40 days.

Each paramesonephric duct (müllerian duct) begins as a thickening and an invagination of the coelomic epithelium, on the lateral aspect of the intermediate mesoderm. It extends caudally as a solid rod of cells and is associated with and initially lateral to the mesonephric duct. The ducts are interdependent; the paramesonephric duct will not develop if the mesonephric duct is absent.[2]

As the paramesonephric cord of cells continues its descent, a lumen appears in its cranial portion in continuity with the intraembryonic body cavity. The lumen extends caudally, as the ducts pass ventral to the mesonephric ducts, come in close association with each other and reach the posterior aspect of the urogenital sinus (Fig. 1.2).

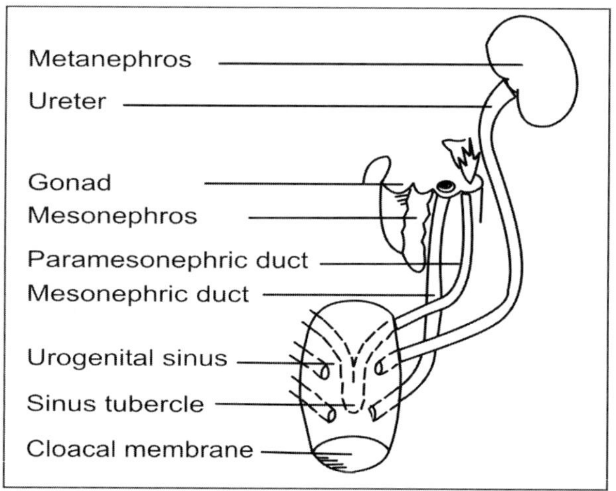

Figure 1.2: The embryo with urogenital ducts (after 40 days)

Urogenital Sinus

The hindgut and the cloaca are established by a process of flexion, as that part of the yolk sac enclosed within the tailfold of the embryo. At an early stage the hindgut and the urogenital ducts open into a common *cloaca* (Fig. 1.3A). The mesoderm between the allantoic diverticulum and the hindgut then extends caudally in line with the curvature of the tail fold as the urorectal septum. The urorectal septum reaches fuses with the cloacal membrane at 30 to 32 days, completely dividing the cloaca into the ventral *urogenital sinus* and the dorsal *rectum* (Fig. 1.3B).

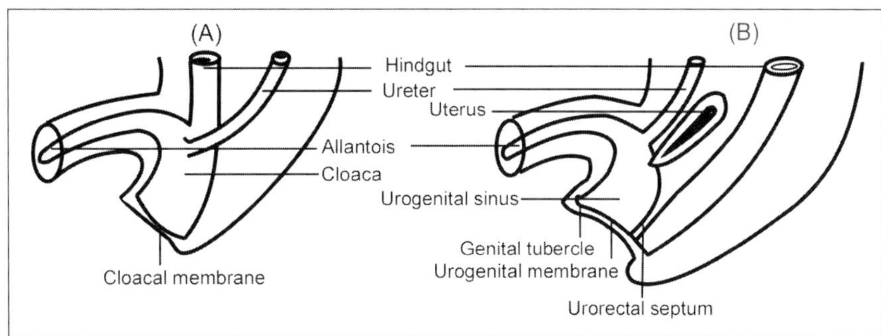

Figures 1.3A and B: (A) The hindgut and urogenital ducts opening into the cloaca,
(B) Fusion of the urorectal septum with the cloacal membrance

The functioning mesonephros now produces an increase in the pressure in the closed urogenital sinus, rupturing the ventral part of the cloacal membrane and allowing the urogenital sinus to communicate with the amniotic cavity.

FEMALE GONADAL DIFFERENTIATION

Male and female embryos are morphologically indistinguishable till 42 days when the transformation of the indifferent gonad into an embryonic testis begins to occur. The Leydig cells in the testes produce *testosterone* from 56 days onwards, while the Sertoli cells synthesise the *antimüllerian hormone*. The secretion of the antimüllerian hormone begins soon after testicular differentiation and continues into the prenatal period, though it is functional only for a short period during early gestation.

The transformation of the indifferent gonad into an *embryonic ovary* occurs gradually between 45 and 55 days.

Development of the Ovary

A gonad with the germ cells in meiosis is always an *ovary* since meiotic division does not occur in the testes until puberty. *Meiosis I* begins in the ovary in intrauterine life, only to be completed at ovulation some 15-45 years later. *Meiosis II* occurs at fertilization. During the early fetal stage, the ovaries contain five million germ cells, that along with the sex cords from the coelomic epithelium, remain in the superficial part of the ovary, the future cortex. The cords lose contact with the surface, forming small groups of cells each with a germ cell, a *primitive follicle*.

Meanwhile the ovary descends extraperitoneally, its descent controlled by the *suspensory ligament* that connects it to its site of origin on the genital ridge, and the *gubernaculum*. The gubernaculum is the inferior continuation of the genital mesentery, that becomes attached to the uterine cornu forming the proximal ovarian ligament and continues as the distal round ligament passing through the inguinal canal and ending in the labium majus[3] (Fig. 1.4).

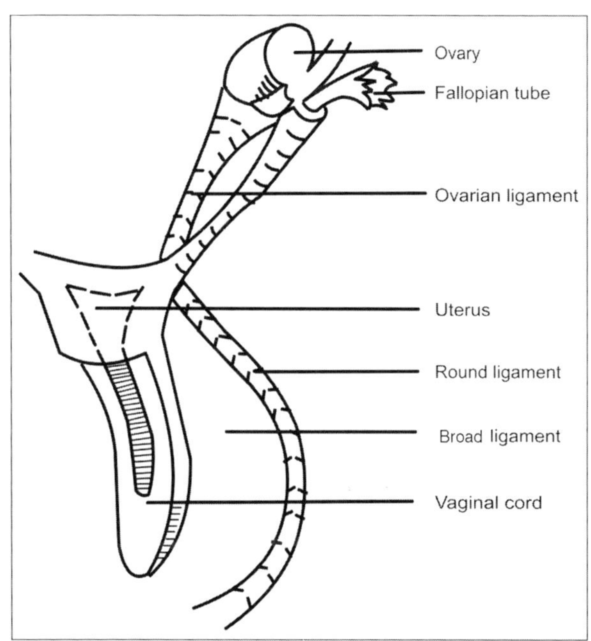

Figure 1.4: Descent of the ovary into the pelvis

The total number of germ cells in the ovary decline to about two million at birth and only 4,00,000 oocytes at the onset of puberty. Of these 400 will be ovulated during reproductive life, the remaining 99.9% undergoing atresia.

FEMALE GENITAL DUCT DIFFERENTIATION

At the end of the embryonic period the fetus has *gonads* recognizable as either testes or ovaries, but possesses both the *mesonephric ducts* and the *paramesonephric ducts*. The subsequent differentiation of the ducts is governed by fetal testicular hormones. In the male fetus müllerian duct regression begins under the influence of the *antimüllerian hormone* at 50 to 60 days,[4] while the mesonephric ducts are stabilized under the influence of testosterone between 56 and 70 days. In contrast, the absence of testicular hormones in the female fetus allows the stabilization of the müllerian ducts and a regression of the mesonephric ducts to take place.

The basic sequence of change from the bipotential state is directed by chromosomal sex determined gonad formation, which then favors the development of male or female duct systems and external genitalia. In final analysis this depends on endocrine effects and not chromosomal sex.[5]

The development of the female genitourinary tract is nearly complete at the end of the first trimester, with some changes such as the final canalization of the vagina and repositioning of the gonads taking place later.

Development of the Uterus

The paired müllerian ducts meet in the midline, fusing within the urorectal septum at the end of the embryonic period. The müllerian ducts fuse, forming the uterus around 63 days, the median septum being completely reabsorbed by 80 days, forming a single uterovaginal canal. While the complete failure of fusion between the ducts results in a *didelphic uterus*, a partial failure results in an *arcuate* or a *bicornuate uterus* and a failure of septal resorption results in variants ranging from a *subseptate* to a *septate uterus.*[5,6]

In the fetus the cervix forms two-thirds of the uterus. The corpus differentiates into the *serosal, muscular* and *mucosal layers* at 19 weeks, the *endometrial glands* forming a week later. The uterus at birth and during childhood is devoid of flexion and version, these characteristics developing at puberty.

Development of the Fallopian Tubes

The separated upper part of each müllerian duct retains its identity to from the fallopian tube, the open cranial segment of the duct developing fimbriae. The transverse lie of the tubes is established by the descent of the ovaries.

Development of the Vagina

There is general agreement that the vagina originates as a composite formed partly from the müllerian ducts and partly from the urogenital sinus.

The *müllerian tubercle* is the point of contact between the müllerian ducts and the urogential sinus. The tip of the fused müllerian ducts proliferates to form the solid vaginal cord that elongates to meet bilateral evaginations from the urogenital sinus (sinovaginal bulbs). The sinovaginal bulbs fuse with the vaginal cord to form the vaginal plate. Canalization of the vaginal cord occurs, followed by epithelialization, mostly with cells from the urogenital sinus.

According to current hypothesis only the upper third of the vagina is formed from the müllerian ducts, with the lower vagina developing from the vaginal plate of the urogenital sinus below.

Development of the External Genitalia

The external genitalia develop in the area bound by the body stalk above and the tail below, the sex of the external genitalia being unrecognizable till the twelfth week.

Five swellings appear around the *urogenital sinus* on the surface of the embryo. The *genital tubercle* is the midline swelling at the cephalic end formed by the fourth week. The paired *genital or labial swellings* develop on either side of the urogenital membrane, with the paired *genital folds* appearing medial to them (Fig. 1.5A). The genital tubercle will become the *clitoris*, the genital swellings developing into the *labia*

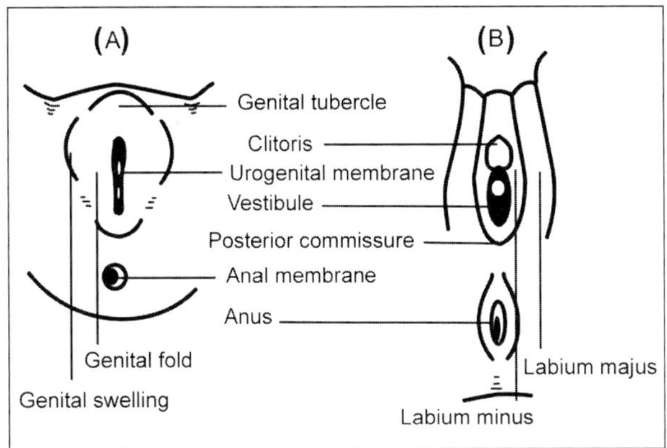

Figures 1.5A and B: (A) The indifferent external genitalia, (B) Feminization of the external genitalia

majora and the genital folds into the *labia minora* (Fig. 1.5B).

The Bartholin's glands and the Skene's glands develop from outgrowths from the urogenital sinus. The urorectal septum will finally form the perineal body.

REFERENCES

1. Boyd ME, Daniels E. Development of the female genital tract and external genitalia. In Gidwani G, Falcone T (Eds): Congenital Malformations of the Female Genital Tract. Lippincott Williams & Wilkins: Philadelphia 1999; 1-20.
2. Lytle W. The deep inguinal ring: Development, function and repair. Br J Surg 1970; 57:531-37.
3. Terruhn V. A study of impression moulds of the genital tract of female fetuses. Arch Gynecol 1980; 229:207-17.
4. Josso N, Picard JY, Tran D. The antimüllerian hormone. Recent Prog Horm Res 1977; 37:117-20.
5. Duncan S. Embryology of the female genital tract: Its genetic defects and congenital anomalies. In Shaw R, Soutter W, Stanton S (Eds): Gynecology. New York: Churchill Livingstone, 1997, 1-22.
6. Rock J, Schlaff W. The obstetric consequences of uterovaginal anomalies. Fertil Steril 1985; 43:681-92.

Pratap Kumar

2.
Disorders of the Development of Müllerian System

ANOMALIES OF THE FEMALE REPRODUCTIVE TRACT

Anomalies of the female reproductive tract can result from agenesis or hypoplasia, fusion and/or canalization defects, duplication abnormalities, or failure of resorption, resulting in septa.

Arrest in the normal development of the müllerian ducts can cause several anomalies:

1. *Aplasia:* in which the organs fail to develop.
2. *Hypoplasia:* in which the organs are rudimentary.
3. *Atresia:* in which there is partial or complete failure of canalization of these ducts leading to varying degrees of gynatresia.
4. *Müllerian duct anomalies* like:
   a. Unicornuate uterus (asymmetrical development) (Fig. 2.1) with or without rudimentary horn.

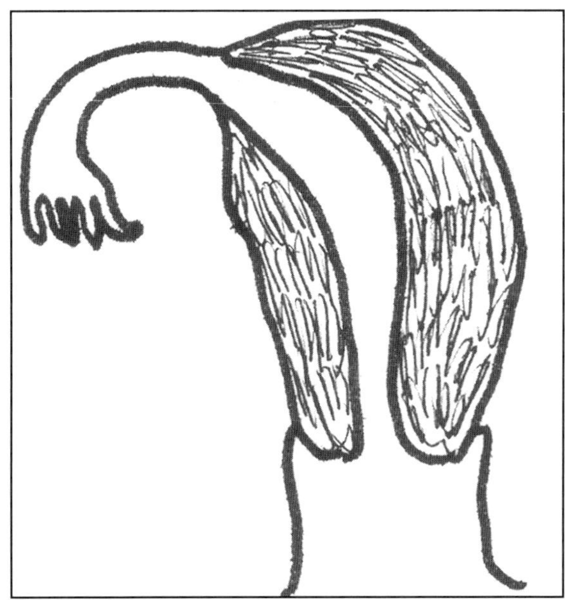

Figure 2.1: Unicornuate uterus

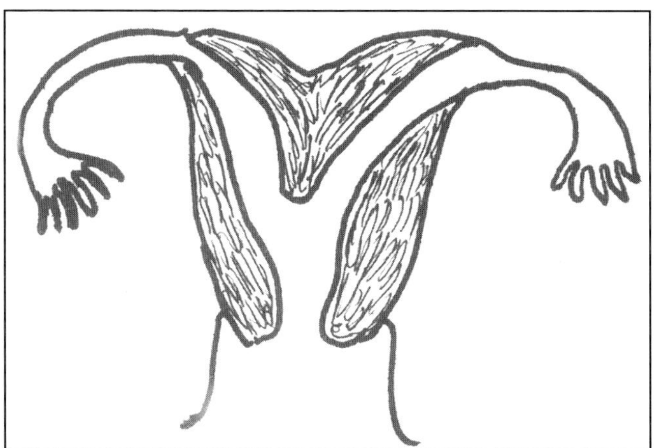

Figure 2.2: Bicornuate uterus

b. Failure of fusion in part or whole may lead to duplication of the genital tract—Uterus didelphys (two separate uterus, two cervix; or a bicornuate uterus (Fig. 2.2). When the müllerian ducts incompletely fuse at the level of the uterine fundus, a bicornuate uterus is formed. In this anomaly, the lower uterus and cervix are completely fused, resulting in 2 separate but communicating endometrial cavities with a single-chamber cervix and vagina. Failure of disappearance of the intervening septum leads to septate or subseptate uterus (Fig. 2.3).

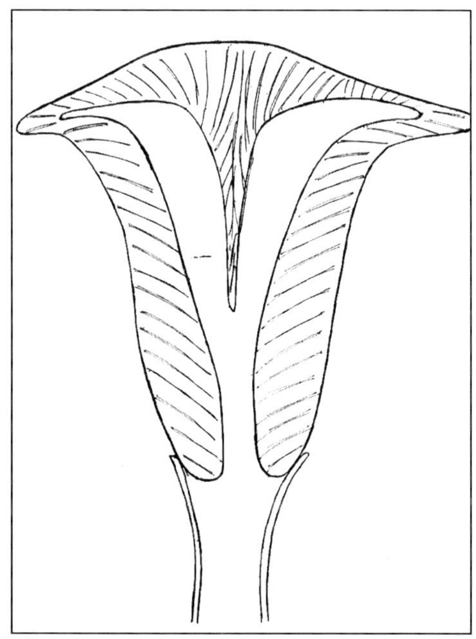

Figure 2.3: Uterus subseptus

c. Failure of vaginal recanalization of vagina leads to absence of vagina/imperforate hymen.

Clinical Problems

1. *Ovary:* Ovarian absence is called as ovarian agenesis/dysgenesis and this leads to Turner's syndrome (chromosomes will be 45XO) and this will present a primary amenorrhea and has special characters like short stature, web neck.
2. *Uterus:* Uterine anomalies described above usually does not cause problems. However in obstetrics it may cause increased incidence of abortions, preterm labors, malpresentations.
3. *Vagina:* Noncanalization of vagina leads to cryptomenorrhea (hidden menses) and may present during adolescent age as primary amenorrhea. There will be cyclical pain (because of menses which is collected above the noncanalized vagina). If there is only imperforate hymen then the bulge is at the exterior. At this stage there can be retention of urine also along with primary amenorrhea.

Diagnosis in Infancy or Childhood

Occasionally, diagnosis can occur in infancy. The patient presents with a bulging yellow-gray mass at or beyond the introitus. The presence of an abdominal mass has been described in association with urinary obstruction.

Diagnosis has been made *in utero* with obstetrical ultrasonography. Ultrasonography is an essential first step in diagnosis.

Hymenal Obstruction

Usually the problems are seen only at puberty when they present with primary amenorrhea. Unfortunately, the typical findings at diagnosis include a large collection of blood within the uterus (hematometra) and an even larger collection of blood within the distensible vagina (hematocolpos) (Fig. 2.4). Additional findings may include blood-filled fallopian tubes (hematosalpinges) and signs of retrograde menses, occasionally to the point of the development of intra-abdominal endometriosis and severe adhesions. An imperforate hymen must be corrected surgically. Surgical decision-making should focus on appropriate diagnosis and timing of surgical repair.

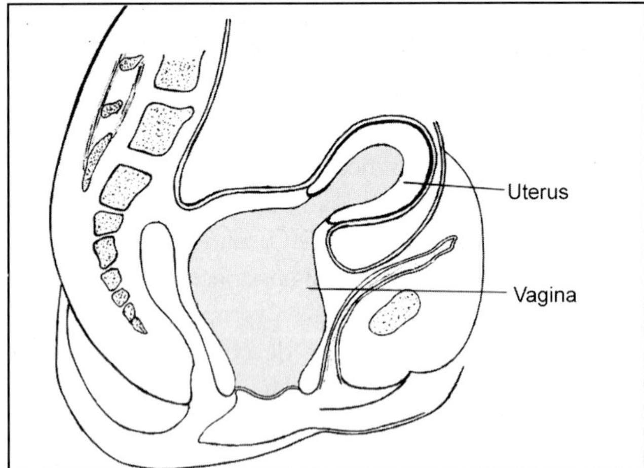

Figure 2.4: Hematocolpos (distended vagina filled with blood)

- Pelvic and abdominal ultrasound/MRI
  - A pelvic ultrasound is the essential initial diagnostic test to confirm, and a transabdominal route is needed. Renal anomalies should be ruled out when other müllerian defects of the uterus and vagina are suspected.
  - Pelvic and abdominal MRI: If the diagnosis of imperforate hymen is not absolutely certain based on physical examination or pelvic ultrasound findings, MRI is indicated to clearly define the anatomy prior to any planned surgical procedure.

Surgical Procedure for Imperforate Hymen

A cruciate incision along the diagonal diameters of the hymen, rather than anterior to posterior, avoids injury to the urethra directly anteriorly and can be enlarged by removal of excess hymenal tissue. In either approach, the vaginal epithelium then is sutured to the hymenal ring using interrupted stitches with fine absorbable suture (e.g. 4-0 polyglycolic acid suture). The application of 2% lidocaine jelly to the suture line to provide postoperative analgesia is suggested.

Aspiration or puncture of the mucocolpos or hematocolpos without definitive enlargement of the vaginal orifice should be avoided because a pyocolpos or ascending infection may develop. Pelvic examination should not be done since it will cause ascending infection.

Surgical Management of Vaginal Agenesis

Surgical and nonsurgical methods of treatment have been utilized. The nonsurgical approach relies on the use of graduated dilators and may take several months or a few years before a functional vagina is formed. Surgery remains the most effective method of treatment for vaginal agenesis.

Choosing the proper time to perform a vaginoplasty is of paramount importance. Surgical treatment should be considered only when the patient wishes to become sexually active and is highly motivated to use a vaginal prosthesis for several months postoperatively.[1]

Preoperative Evaluation

Routine preoperative evaluation should include an intravenous pyelogram (IVP) and renal ultrasound to exclude urinary tract anomalies. Discovery of a pelvic kidney is important in planning corrective surgery since its presence may limit the amount of potential space.

Surgical Techniques for Vaginal Agenesis

McIndoe's operation: The aim of surgical treatment is to create a neovagina. The modified McIndoe procedure remains the most common surgical approach to vaginoplasty for vaginal agenesis. Obtaining a satisfactory split-thickness graft is one of the most important steps in performing the modified McIndoe procedure. A space is created between the bladder and the rectum.

  i. *Prosthesis assembly:* The stent should be made from material that can maintain patency of the vaginal cavity. A foam rubber form measuring 10 cm by 2 cm works well. The prosthetic device is sterilized, and the size is customized to fit the patient's vagina. The prosthetic material is cut to twice the desired size of the vagina, folded in half, and compressed by the placement of 2 condoms over the surface. The condoms are tied at the open end.

  ii. *Graft attachment to prosthesis:* The skin graft is placed over the stent, dermal aspect out, and sutured over the form using 5-0 synthetic absorbable sutures. The graft-covered prosthesis is carefully inserted into the vaginal canal. The edges of the graft are sutured to the previously cut edges of the mucosal margins of the vaginal introitus. This contact is often adequate, rendering sutures unnecessary. If the contact between the graft and the vaginal space is too tight, serum may collect and compromise the engraftment. The labia minora are sutured around the stent using non-reactive sutures.

Patient education regarding the importance of continuous, prolonged dilatation as well as stent care during the healing phase is important. The foam is worn continuously for 6 weeks and is removed only for urination and defecation. Low-pressure douches with warm water are performed daily. At the same time, the form is cleaned with a povidone-iodine solution, covered with a fresh condom, lubricated, and reintroduced into the neovagina. After 6 weeks, a silicone form that is inserted nightly for the next 12 months replaces the original stent. In most cases, the vagina is functional 6-10 weeks postoperatively.[2,3]

Williams vulvovaginoplasty is an alternative to the McIndoe procedure: This procedure is particularly useful for patients with previously failed vaginoplasty. It utilizes full-thickness skin flaps from the labia majora to create a vaginal pouch. Unlike the McIndoe procedure, vaginal dilation is required for only 3-4 weeks. The vagina created by this approach is not anatomically similar to a normal vagina or the neovagina created by the McIndoe procedure. Instead, the vaginal pouch axis is directly posterior and horizontal to the perineum; however, the vagina is functional and well-received by patients. Fistula formation, which can occur with the McIndoe procedure, is rare.[4]

Uterus Didelphys, Non-obstructed (Fig. 2.5)

Women with non-obstructed didelphys uterus usually are not candidates for surgical unification. The decision to perform metroplasty should be individualized, and only selected patients may benefit from surgical reconstruction. Metroplasty using the Strassman procedure[5] deals with the method of unification of the uterine cavities at the fundus while the cervices are left intact. This is not done in modern gynecology, since unification was causing higher incidence of rupture of uterus during subsequent pregnancy. Rarely they can present with double uterus and double vagina (Fig. 2.6).

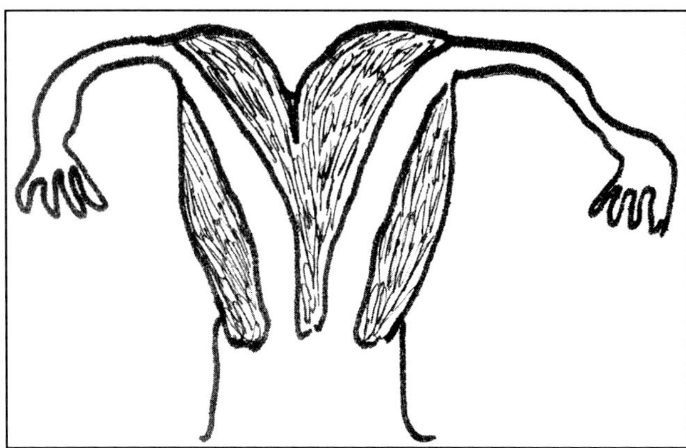

Figure 2.5: Double uterus with single vagina

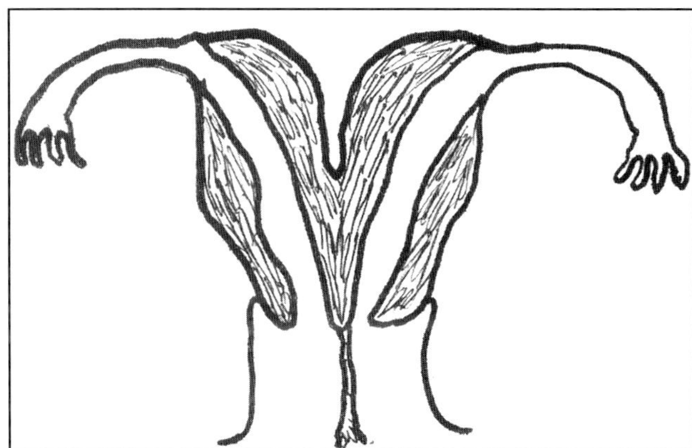

Figure 2.6: Double uterus with double vagina

Bicornuate Uterus

Bicornuate uterus is considered an incidental finding. Patients usually have no difficulty becoming pregnant and usually do not have much of obstetrical problem except rarely it may be the cause of preterm labor. At times they have one rudimentary horn (Fig. 2.7)

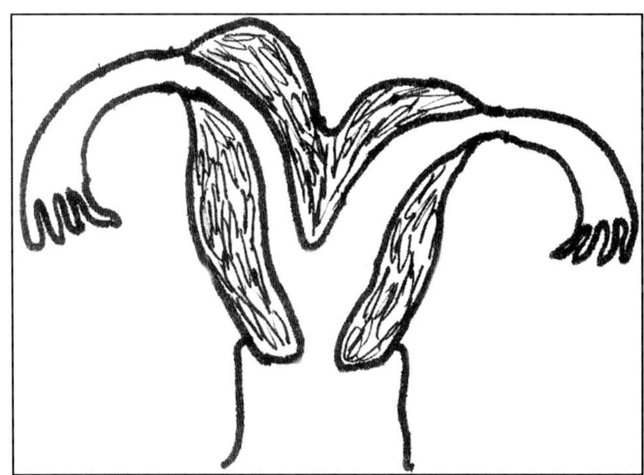

Figure 2.7: Bicornuate uterus with rudimentary left horn

Surgical Techniques for Bicornuate Uterus

Although a number of metroplasty procedures are available, the Strassman procedure was the surgical treatment of choice for bicornuate uterus and didelphys uterus. This approach involves the removal of the septum by wedge resection with subsequent unification of the 2 cavities. Since it causes a weak uterus this procedure is not recommended in recent times.

Septate Uterus (Fig. 2.3)

The septum is considered complete if it extends to the internal os, thus dividing the endometrial cavity, and partial if it does not. In addition, septa may be segmental, which results in partial communication between the endometrial cavities . Although fertility does not appear to be significantly compromised its presence alone is not an indication for surgery.

Transvaginal ultrasound is a useful aid in diagnosing septate uterus, with one study demonstrating a sensitivity of 100% and a specificity of 80%.[6]

Surgical Management of Septate Uterus

Surgical techniques: As the surgical procedure of choice, transabdominal Tompkin's metroplasty has been replaced by operative hysteroscopy. Currently, surgical correction of septate uterus is rendered through hysteroscopic division of the septum.[7-9] The surgical approach utilizes concurrent laparoscopy and hysteroscopy. Laparoscopy is essential to the success of the surgery; it helps confirm the diagnosis of septate uterus as opposed to bicornuate uterus, and it helps reduce the risk of uterine perforation during septal incision.[8,9]

Postoperative Management

Postoperative placement of a Lippes loop intrauterine device for a month is controversial.[9] Some think that it may prevent intrauterine adhesion formation, while others maintain that this procedure is unnecessary and may provoke local inflammation with subsequent synechiae.[10] Currently, no unanimity exists for this practice.

Conjugated estrogens (1.25 mg/d for 25 d) and progesterone (10 mg/d added on days 21-25) are frequently prescribed postoperatively to assist epithelialization. At present, there is no consensus on this practice. Some experts believe that hormonal therapy has not been proven necessary and can often be withheld.[11]

A 1 month postoperative follow-up examination is recommended. Either hysteroscopy or hysterosalpingography can be performed to assess the uterine cavity. Ultrasound can also be performed.

The risk of pelvic adhesions is limited, and recovery is rapid with no prolonged postoperative delay in conception. Hysteroscopic metroplasty allows vaginal delivery, obviating the need for subsequent cesarean section as was recommended using the transabdominal approach.

CONCLUSION

Müllerian duct anomalies are a morphologically diverse group of congenital disorders involving the female reproductive tract. Establishing an accurate diagnosis is essential for patient management and planning treatment strategies. Uterine shape or anomalies do not require active measures of surgery most often, except for the wide uterine septum. Vaginal reconstruction operations have a place in those whose vagina is absent.

REFERENCES

1. Coney P. Effect of vaginal agenesis on the adolescent: Prognosis for normal sexual and psychological adjustment. Adolesc Pediatr Gynecol 1992; 5: 8.
2. Rock JA. Surgery for anomalies of the müllerian ducts. In Thompson JD, Rock JA (Eds): Telinde's Operative Gynecology, 7th ed. Philadelphia: JB Lippincott 1992: 603-46.
3. Mc Indoe. The treatment of congenital absence and obliterative condition of the vagina. Br J Plast Surg 1950; 2:254-67.
4. Williams EA. Congenital absence of the vagina—a simple operation for its relief. J Obstet Gynecol Br Commonwealth 1964; 71: 511.
5. Strassman EO. Fertility and unification of the pregnant uterus. Fertil Steril 1966; 17: 165.
6. Pellerito JS, McCarthy SM, Doyle MB. Diagnosis of uterine anomalies: Relative accuracy of MR imaging, endovaginal sonography, and hysterosalpingography. Radiology 1992; 183(3): 795-800.

7. DeCherney AH, Russell JB, Graebe RA. Resectoscopic management of mullerian fusion defects. Fertil Steril 1986; 45(5): 726-28.
8. Donnez J, Nisolle M. Hysteroscopic surgery. Curr Opin Obstet Gynecol 1992 4(3): 439-46
9. Israel R, March CM. Hysteroscopic incision of the septate uterus. Am J Obstet Gynecol 1984; 149(1): 66-73.
10. Vercellini P, Fedele L, Arcaini L. Value of intrauterine device insertion and estrogen administration after hysteroscopic metroplasty. J Reprod Med 1989;34(7): 447-50.
11. Propst AM, Hill JA 3rd. Anatomic factors associated with recurrent pregnancy loss. Semin Reprod Med 2000; 18(4): 341-50.

3.
Ovulation and Menstruation

AP Manjunath
Pratap Kumar

INTRODUCTION

Menstrual problems are one of the commonest presentations to the physicians. The understanding of the physiological spectrum of menstruation is essential to tackle such problems. We hope to provide a fundamental basis for better understanding of normal ovarian physiologic process relevant to the pathophysiology of ovarian dysfunction, as well as clinical intervention to treat infertility or to achieve contraception.

OVULATION AND MENSTRUATION

Menstruation is the periodic and cyclical discharge of blood, mucus and cellular debris from the uterine mucosa, which occurs due to progesterone withdrawal after ovulation in non-fertile cycles. It is initiated in response to changes in the hormonal production by the ovaries which themselves are controlled by the pituitary and hypothalamus. It takes place at approximately 28-day intervals between menarche (onset of menstruation) and menopause (cessation of menstruation).

Ovarian Cycle

The ovary has two functional roles. First gametogenesis and second hormonogenesis. During fetal life gonads contain 6-7 million oogonia at 16-20 weeks of gestation. Only 1-2 million survive to reach neonatal life. At puberty this number has depleted to only 300,000-500,000. Less than 500 of the original 6 million ovarian follicles will be selected to ovulate in the reproductive years.

The ovary contains thousands of primordial follicles. They are in a continuous state of development and atresia from birth through menopause. Ovarian follicles may be found in four basic conditions: at rest, growing, atretic or ready to ovulate as shown in Figure 3.1. In the process of oogenesis formation and maturation of the oocyte takes place. It is initiated with the growth of primordial follicle through the stages of prenatal, antral and preovulatory follicle (Fig. 3.2) Approximately 85 days are required for primordial follicle to grow and become a preantral stage. From preantral to preovulatory stage it takes 14 days, which occurs during follicular phase of ovarian cycle. The initial stage of follicular development is independent of hormonal stimulation. Development beyond preantral stage is stimulated by pituitary gonadotrophins [FSH (Follicular stimulating hormone) and LH (luteinizing hormone)] which orchestrate the whole events of ovarian and menstrual cycle. In the absence

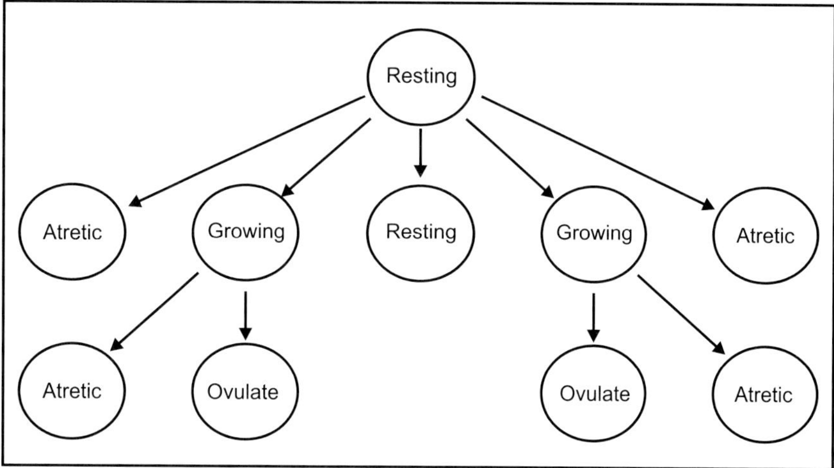

Figure 3.1: Different types of follicles

of correct hormonal milieu the follicles undergo atresia. Even though anatomically there are two ovaries, it functions as a single unit.

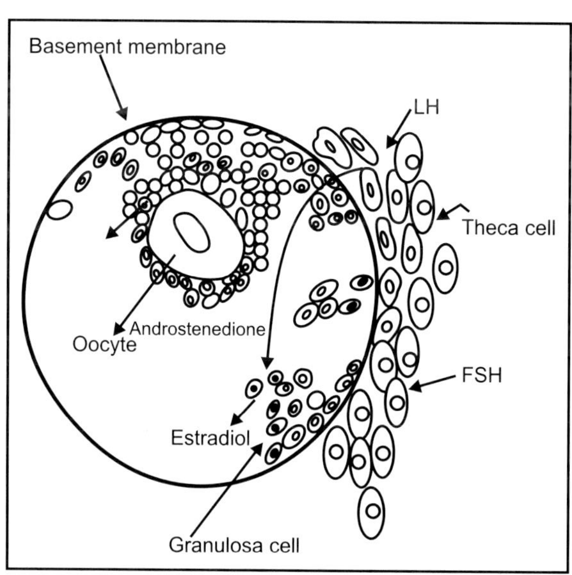

Figure 3.3: FSH and granulosa cells; LH and theca cells—two cell, two gonadotropin system

Figure 3.2: Growth and different stages of follicle

The hormonogenesis is functionally compartmentalized within the follicle as "two cell two-gonadotrophin system" as shown in Figure 3.3. In the preantral and antral follicles, LH receptors are present only on the theca cells and FSH receptors only on granulosa cells. In response to LH, the thecal cells are stimulated to produce androgens. The FSH induces aromatization in the granulosa cells, which converts the thecally-derived androgens into estrogen.

Androgen production within the follicle may also regulate the development of the preantral follicle. Low level of androgen enhances aromatization and increases estrogen production. In contrast high androgen production inhibits aromatization and produces follicular atresia. A delicate balance of FSH and LH is required for early follicular development. The ideal situation for the initial stage of follicular development is, low LH level and high FSH level as seen in the early menstrual cycle.

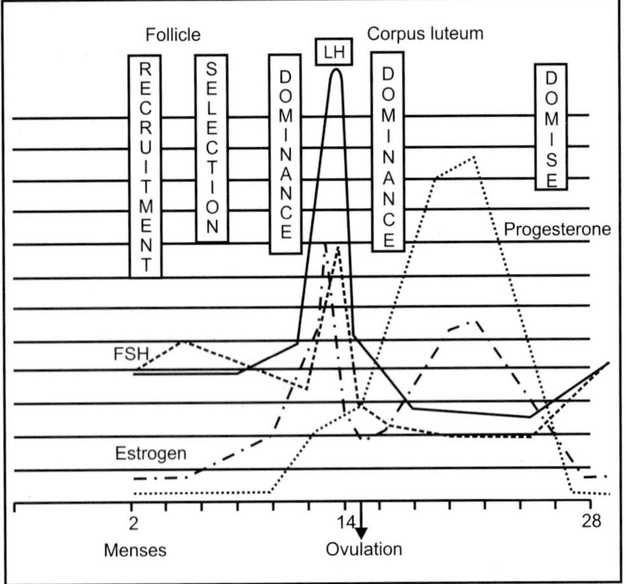

Figure 3.4: LH, FSH, progesterone and estrogen levels in relation to growth of follicle

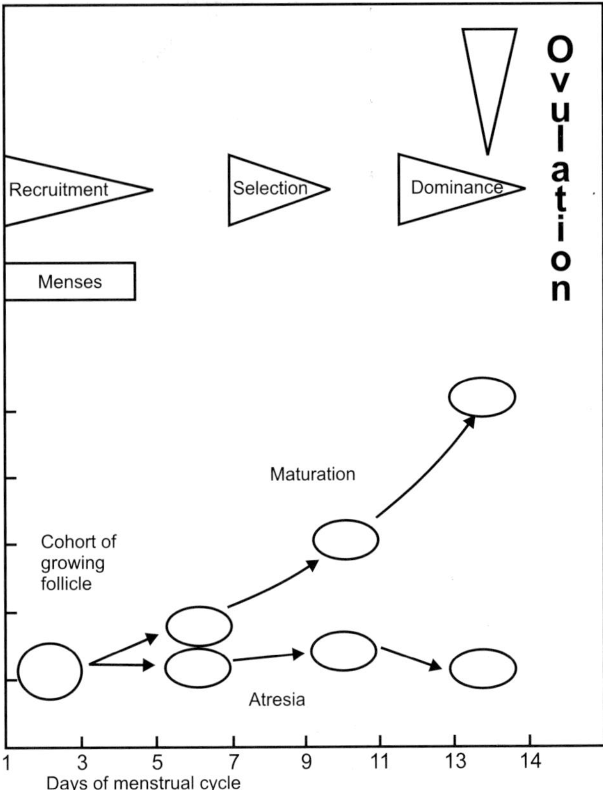

Figure 3.5: The dynamics of folliculogenesis

The pelvic clock in the ovary, regulated by endocrine messages from hypothalamus-pituitary, is essential for successful reproduction and for generating a 28-day menstrual cycle. In a normal ovarian cycle typically only a single follicle containing a single oocyte usually reaches maturity. The hormonal milieu created and controlled by this follicle induce timed and specific changes within the cervix, fallopian tube, endometrium and hypothalamic-pituitary axis.

The ovarian cycle essentially consists of two phases: follicular phase and luteal phase.

Follicular Phase

During the follicular phase an orderly sequence of events takes place, the end results of which is one surviving mature follicle. The process occurs over a period of 10-14 days.

The understanding of the endocrine dynamics of the folliculogenesis is essential for meaningful clinical intervention. The dynamics of this process have been characterized and divided into four phases (Figs 3.4 and 3.5).

- Recruitment
- Selection
- Dominance
- Ovulation.

Recruitment: The process of recruitment begins at the end of the luteal phase of the previous cycle from the onset of menses to approximately day 5 to 7 of the current cycle. During recruitment multiple follicles are present that possess the ability to proceed to ovulation. But eventually only a single follicle will be able to utilize its hormonal milieu efficiently enough to sustain development until the interval of recruitment is completed. During recruitment, follicles in both ovaries actively grow and secrete estrogen.

Selection: Between day 5 and 7 of the current cycle, a single follicle becomes destined to ovulate. This is termed as selection of the dominant follicle. Selection of a dominant follicle creates an environment in which only it can adequately mature and reach ovulation.

Dominance: The interval of growth preceding ovulation but following selection is called dominance. The dominant follicle controls the endocrine milieu as it prepares itself, the reproductive tract, and hypothalamic-pituitary axis for ovulation.

Ovulation: One of the paramount events at the mid cycle is the LH surge which stimulates three major events.

1. Resumption of meiosis.
2. Luteinization of the granulosa and theca cells with increased production of progesterone.
3. Extrusion of the mature oocyte about 36 hours after the beginning of the LH surge.

Mechanism of ovulation: This involves proteolytic digestion of follicular wall (mediated by prostaglandins) leading to follicular rupture and extrusion of oocyte.

Unless fertilized the ovum survives only 12- 24 hours and then disintegrates in the tube without leaving any trace.

Luteal Phase

After expulsion of oocyte, the granulosa and theca cells within the follicle convert from the production of estrogen and follicular peptides to the production of estrogen and progesterone. This process termed luteinization, actually begins prior to ovulation, but requires LH surge for completion.

The luteal function depends both qualitatively and quantitatively on normal development of the granulosa and theca cells during the preceding follicular phase. Inadequate proliferation of gonadal stromal cells during the follicular phase or incomplete luteinization during the early luteal phase results in decreased secretion of estrogen and progesterone. This in turn may cause altered function of the fallopian tube and endometrium, possibly resulting in abnormal gamete or embryo transport and decreased opportunities for implantation.

The lifespan of corpus luteum is fixed being around 14 days. At the end of the luteal phase the corpus luteum regresses unless rescued by human chorionic gonadotropin (hCG) from the implanting embryo. This is known as luteolysis.

Endometrial Cycle

The most obvious manifestation of a normal menstrual cycle is the presence of regular menstrual periods. Every month the uterus prepares for a pregnancy by generating a thick bed of secretory endometrium for the implantation. Due to failure of fertilization of the oocyte or implantation, the menses starts. Hence menstruation is described as "weeping of a disappointed uterus for a baby."

The endometrium is the superficial epithelium, which lines the uterine cavity. It has two principle components, the glandular epithelium and supporting stromal cells. During the menstrual cycle the epithelium differentiates to form three functional zones. The basalis, spongiosum and stratum compactum.

The endometrial events can be divided into three phases (Fig. 3.6).

1. Menstrual phase.
2. Proliferative phase.
3. Secretory phase.

Menstrual Phase

The beginning of each endometrial cycle is characterized by complete shedding of the spongiosum and stratum compactum layers (Day 1) during menstruation which lasts for 3-5 days. The fall in plasma progesterone and estrogen levels due to degeneration of corpus luteum leads to withdrawal of hormonal support of the endometrium, which causes menstruation. The first event is profound vasoconstriction of uterine blood vessels, which leads to decreased supply of oxygen and nutrients to endometrium. Disintegration starts in the entire lining except the basalis layer that will regenerate the endometrium in the next cycle. After the initial period of vasoconstriction, the endometrial arteriole dilates resulting in hemorrhage through vascular capillary walls. The menstrual flow consists of blood mixed with endometrial debris and mucus.

Proliferative Phase

Menstrual flow ceases and endometrium begins to thicken as it regenerates from the basalis layer. The period of growth lasts for 10 days or so between cessation of menstruation and occurrence of ovulation. The ovarian follicular phase corresponds to menstrual proliferative phase of endometrial cycle. The uterine changes during the menstrual cycle are caused by the changes in plasma concentration of estrogen and progesterone. During proliferative phase a rising plasma estrogen level will lead to reconstruction and growth of

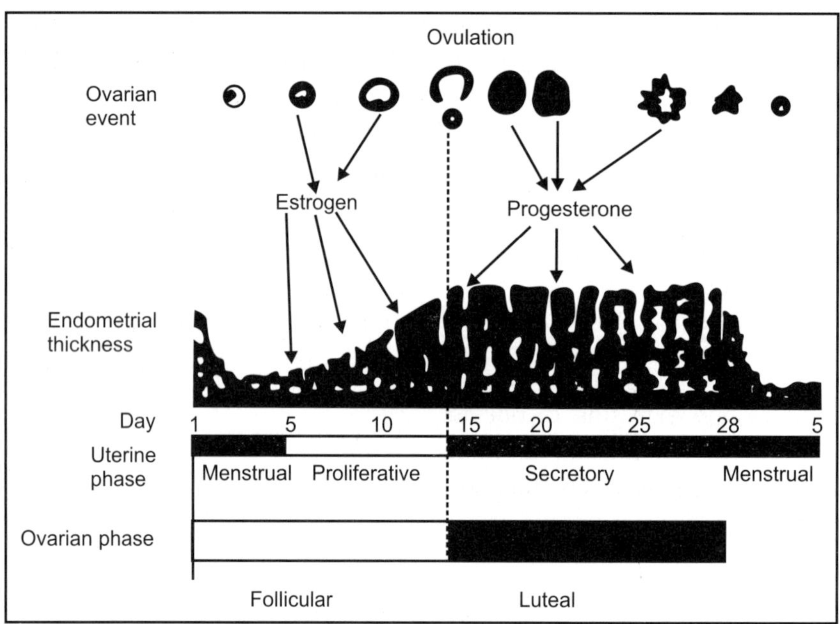

Figure 3.6: Growth and atretion of follicle related to the endometrial growth in menstrual cycle

endometrium. Both glandular and stromal component achieve proliferation which peaks at 8-10 days of cycle and corresponds to peak estrogen level. During this phase, the endometrium grows from approximately 0.5 mm to 3-5 mm in height.

Secretory Phase

Soon after ovulation the endometrium begins to secrete various substances and the part of the menstrual cycle between ovulation and the onset of next menstruation is called secretory phase. The circulating progesterone which is secreted by the corpus luteum after ovulation acts upon the estrogen primed endometrium to convert it to actively secreting tissue. Its glands become coiled and filled with glycogen. The blood vessels become more numerous and densely coiled. Various enzymes are secreted in the glands and connective tissue. These changes are essential to make the endometrium a hospitable environment for an embryo.

FEEDBACK OSCILLATION OF THE HYPOTHALAMO-PITUITARY OVARIAN SYSTEM

The intermittent pulsatile secretion of gonadotrophin releasing hormone (GnRH) produced by the hypo-thalamus is transported to the pituitary gland in the portal circulation. This pulsatile secretion of GnRH stimulates the pituitary gonadotrophin (FSH and LH) secretion. These pituitary gonadotrophins orchestrate the interplay of hormones from the pelvic clock.

The feedback oscillation that controls the rhythm of the menstrual cycle is better understood with the following sequence of three successive events.

Follicular Growth Phase

Two to three days before menstruation the corpus luteum has regressed to almost total involution and the corpus luteum secretion of estrogen and progesterone decreases to the lowest level. This releases the hypo-thalamus and anterior pituitary from negative feedback effect of these hormones. Therefore, just before menstruation pituitary secretion of FSH begins to increase again and LH also increases slightly. These hormones recruit new ovarian follicles. There is progressive increase in secretion of estrogen from these follicles especially after the selection of the dominant follicle on day 5-7. During the first 11-12 days pituitary secretion of FSH and LH decreases slightly because of the negative feedback effect of the estrogen on anterior

Table 3.1: Summary of ovarian events in menstrual cycle and its hormonal dynamics

Days	Ovarian events	Endometrial events	Hormonal events
1-4	Recruitment: Cohort of follicles will start growing	Endometrial lining sloughs	E and P are low FSH and LH are released from inhibition
5-7	Selection: A single follicle is destined to ovulate. No surrogate follicle	Endometrium proliferates	Plasma E rises because of secretion from selected dominant follicle
8-12	Dominance: • Atresia of all other follicles except dominant follicle • Dominant follicle thrives uniquely, despite the suppressive milieu	Increased E will stimulate the growth of glands and stroma	Increased E and inhibin will inhibit FSH
13-15	Ovulation: • mediated by follicular enzymes and prostaglandins • Oocyte is induced to complete its first meiotic division	Transition from proliferative to secretory endometrium	LH surge induced by high plasma E (positive feedback)
15-25	Corpus luteum forms	Secretory endometrium develops	P and E are secreted and FSH and LH secretion is inhibited, so no new follicle develops
25-28	Luteolysis: • Corpus luteum degenerates • Recruitment of new ovarian follicle for next cycle begins	Endometrium begin to slough due to withdrawal of progesterone support	Plasma E and P decreases, release of hypothalamus and pituitary from negative feedback effect. FSH begins to rise.

Key: E= estrogen, P= progesterone

pituitary. This leads to withdrawal of FSH support from the other less developed follicle leading to atresia. The dominant follicle is capable of continued development in the face of falling FSH level. The increasing estrogen level is thought to trigger a marked increase in secretion of LH and to a lesser extent of FSH, which is followed by ovulation.

Preovulatory Surge of LH and FSH Causes Ovulation

At about 11-12 days after the onset of monthly cycle decline in the secretion of FSH and LH comes to an abrupt halt. It is believed that the high level of estrogen at this time (or beginning secretion of progesterone from follicle) causes peculiar positive feedback stimulatory effect on the anterior pituitary, which leads to terrific surge of secretion of LH and to a lesser extent of FSH surge. The great excess of LH leads to ovulation

and subsequent development of corpus luteum. Thus the hormone system also begins its new round of secretion until next cycle.

Postovulatory Secretions of Ovarian Hormones and Depression of Pituitary Gonadotropins

After ovulation corpus luteum secretes large quantities of both progesterone and estrogen. These hormones have a combined negative feedback effect on the anterior pituitary gland and hypothalamus to cause suppression of both FSH and LH secretion, decreasing them to the lowest level at about 3-4 days before menstruation.

The ovarian events, uterine events and the hormonal dynamics in normal menstruation is summarized in Table 3.1.

PRACTICE POINTS

Clinical Features of Normal Menstruation

The physiologic spectrum of normal menses are as follows. The amount of flow is 30 ml. Duration of flow is 2-7 days. The cycle length can vary from 21 days to 35 days. In healthy menstruation the blood which is discharged does not coagulate. Because normally the blood is coagulated as it is shed from the endometrium, but thereafter it is liquefied by fibrinolytic activity (plasminogen activator). Hence history of passing clots during menses indicates abnormally excessive bleeding (more than 80 ml). For all practical purposes, during reproductive age, regular menstruation means regular ovulation.

Clinical Correlation for Ovulation Induction

Ovulation induction with clomiphene citrate and injectable gonadotrophins is used for management of infertility. Coordinating the onset and duration of these treatments with the status of developing cohort of follicles is necessary while managing patients with infertility.

Physiologic Basis for Use of Combined Oral Contraceptive Pills

The selection of the dominant follicle on day 5 is crucial time in the cycle. Exogenous estrogen administered even after the selection of the dominant follicle, disrupts the preovulatory development and induces atresia by decreasing the FSH level below the sustaining level. The combined oral contraceptive pills take the advantage of this physiologic mechanism for ovulation inhibition. Thus the estrogen component suppresses FSH secretion and prevents the selection and emergence of a dominant follicle. The progestational component suppresses LH secretion thus preventing ovulation.

FURTHER READING

1. Franscisco I, Gary DH. Mechanism of ovulation. Reproductive endocrinology: Endocrinology and Metabolism Clinics of North America 1992;21:19-38.
2. Speroff L, Glass RH, Kase NG. Clinical gynecologic endocrinology and infertility. 6th edn. Lippincott Williams and Wilkins. 1999; 201-46.

Edwin Chandraharan
Sabaratnam Arulkumaran

4.

Gynecological History and Examination

INTRODUCTION

It is often said that patients are poor historians. However, the onus of eliciting a good, relevant and informative history lies on the clinician. This is especially so in gynecology, whereby one needs to explore and inquire into personal and often intimate problems. Hence, developing a good rapport with the patient and winning her confidence are of paramount importance. The need for greeting the patient, proper introduction, creating a friendly and relaxed atmosphere and privacy cannot be overemphasized.

HISTORY TAKING

There is no ideal model of history taking. However, it is best to have an outline, which will enable us to elicit the relevant information to reach a differential diagnosis at the end of our history taking. Such an approach will guide us through the clinical examination and may also help us to plan our investigations. A suggested outline is given below but sometimes one has to be flexible, innovative and sensitive to the patient's feelings. It may not be a wise idea to ask about sexual promiscuity or the number of sexual partners a woman has had over the past two months, in the presence of her husband, even though her symptoms may be suggestive of an acute pelvic inflammatory disease! This history may be elicited at a different setting.

Name, Age, Parity and the Place of Residence

These may help us to know of the patient's background and to identify some of the risk factors. Abnormal bleeding in a postmenopausal woman may lead us to consider a totally different set of differential diagnosis as compared to a teenager presenting with the same symptom. Likewise parity may help us to understand the etiopathology for her symptoms as in genital prolapse.

Presenting Symptom

This may help us to understand the underlying problem and to organise our thoughts to probe further. One needs to be always aware that all patients don't have classical clinical presentations as described in textbooks and that more than one pathology or disorder may be present in the same patient. A patient who presents with peri-menopausal symptoms may in fact have hyperthyroidism in addition to her estrogen deficiency. Therefore, it is essential to have an open mind with regard to the presenting symptoms.

History of Presenting Complaint

We need to expand on the presenting complaint by considering the nature of the problem, the possible etiological or predisposing factors that may have contributed to the problem as well as the complications, if any that may have occurred. We should also look for any other associated or co-existing problems. A few examples relevant to gynecology are given below:

Abnormal Menstrual Bleeding

We need to elicit what is or was normal for the patient prior to her developing the problem. An attempt to quantify the amount of loss by means of the number of sanitary pads she uses, the passage of blood clots or flooding (staining the underwear) as well as symptoms of anemia may help. Associated symptoms like dysmenorrhea or dyspareunia may help us formulate a differential diagnosis. We also need to elicit the degree to which the problem affects her quality of life, in terms of absence from work, social life and household duties.

Abdomino-pelvic Mass

We need to ask when it was noticed, the duration, the rapidity of growth, the presence of pressure symptoms and features of malignancy, which include cachexia and weight loss.

Pelvic Pain

This is a very common presenting symptom and it is important to take a good history to plan the appropriate management. Details about the site, onset, duration, progression, character, radiation, aggravating and relieving factors are important and its relationship to the menstrual cycle. An acute pelvic pain associated with vaginal bleeding after a period of amenorrhea

(POA) may indicate an ectopic pregnancy, whereas a chronic pelvic pain associated with dyspareunia and dysmenorrhea without POA may indicate a chronic pelvic inflammatory disease (PID). It is quite obvious that a proper history may help us to differentiate between these two conditions, which will make a big difference to the ultimate wellbeing of the patient.

Lump at the Vulva

It is important to identify nature of the lump and any associated conditions. A woman who has a utero-vaginal prolapse on inquiry, may reveal pre-disposing factors like chronic cough and constipation. Appropriate management of these conditions may help to control her symptoms and for her treatment to be more successful. Due to the close anatomical proximity, disturbances of the functions of the urinary tract may be present and need to be noted, as this will help in formulating the overall management plan.

Vaginal Discharge

It is essential to establish whether it is physiological or pathological. If it is pathological, it is vital to determine the possible cause based on the history. The amount, odor, color, itchiness and the presence of blood etc. may help in identifying a cause. From the management point of view, a vaginal discharge caused by fungal infection may not require urgent attention as compared to one caused by a genital tract malignancy, i.e. indicated by a white discharge with pruritus compared with a blood stained discharge.

Menstrual History

It is the cornerstone of any gynecological history and it must be remembered that in certain instances, it may have to be elicited immediately after the presenting complaint. For example, if a woman presents with menorrhagia, it may be prudent to understand her menstrual history before going to the history of presenting complaint. The age of menarche (age of commencement of periods), regularity of the menstrual cycles and the duration of blood flow are important. Associated features like mid-cycle pain or spotting, primary dysmenorrhea and the presence of premenstrual symptoms may indicate 'ovulatory' menstrual cycles.

Contraceptive History

It is important to know if the patient is using any contraceptive method or she has done so in the past. Irregular periods or amenorrhea may be secondary to hormonal contraceptives and a woman who has missed her pills and presents with a lump in the abdomen may in fact be pregnant!

Past Obstetric History

It is important to ask about the details of previous pregnancies and their outcome in a chronological order. A previous history of termination of pregnancy, traumatic delivery, prolonged labor or ectopic pregnancy may be relevant to planning management.

Past Gynecological History

Some of the gynecological disorders have a long history and patients may have been treated earlier for the same disorder. Conversely, a past gynecological disorder or condition may have predisposed to the current problem. Classic examples include Ashermann's syndrome following a vigorous curettage leading to amenorrhea or subfertility; recurrent miscarriage following previous surgery on the cervix.

Past Medical/Surgical History

Many an occasion a diagnosis is missed due to the failure to ask about a patient's previous medical or surgical history. Disorders of the thyroid gland may have contributed to the menstrual disturbances and diabetes mellitus may be the cause of her vaginal discharge. Taking a relevant medical history is also vital for planning management, as a multi-disciplinary input may be required. Patients with cardiovascular or respiratory disorders may require referral to an anesthetist prior to any surgical procedures.

Drug History/Allergies

Knowledge of drug history is essential not only to identify a cause-effect relationship (e.g. patients on anti-coagulants presenting with menorrhagia) but also to avoid drug interactions (patients on anti-epileptic drugs may have a higher failure rate with the combined oral contraceptive). It is important to avoid drug induced anaphylactic reactions that could be fatal.

Social History

This not only includes the living conditions, the diet, employment and access to transport and healthcare but also her family support and level of education. Certain gynecological disorders may be related to the patient's socio-economic status and her present problem may have an impact on her social life. At times, the proposed plan of management may not be feasible due to the patient's social status. In certain countries, it may not be appropriate to discuss the use of Danazole for the management of endometriosis, if the patient cannot afford it.

Sexual History

It is placed last not because it is least important but it requires the establishment of certain rapport and trust between the patient and the clinician due to its intimate nature. Patient should feel confident and free to discuss matters relating to her sex life. The onus is on the clinician to win her trust during history taking to keep her at ease. However, in certain circumstance like a woman presenting with infertility or requesting emergency contraception, sexual history may need to be included in the history of presenting complaint. The age of first coitus, frequency of intercourse, presence of pain (dyspareunia) and the number of partners and awareness of safe sex may need to be inquired, depending on the presenting complaint.

At the end of taking a relevant and comprehensive history, it is important to arrive at a differential diagnosis, prior to embarking on physical examination. A friendly advice on presentation of a good history that is often given by senior colleagues to students sitting for examinations in clinical medicine is that it should be long enough to cover the relevant areas but short enough to maintain interest. It is by constant practice that the art of history taking can be perfected.

GENERAL EXAMINATION

It is an important aspect of the physical examination, which may reveal some of the systemic signs of a primary problem as well as the severity of the problem. The general condition of the patient, her mental status and disposition may give a clue to the underlying pathology. In modern gynecological practice, we need to be aware of the role of stress, anxiety and body weight on menstrual function. One needs to look for pallor, icterus, lymphadenopathy, oedema as well as the normality of the thyroid gland and the breasts. This should be followed by a systemic examination of the cardiovascular and respiratory system. It is not very rare to find evidence of respiratory disease in a patient with stress incontinence. Neurological examination may not be routinely indicated. However, if a patient complains of incontinence or there is any evidence to suggest a neurological problem in the history, a complete neurological examination is warranted. Referral to a neurologist may be appropriate in certain situation. Similarly, if a pituitary neoplasm is suspected to cause her menstrual irregularity, a visual field examination is mandatory.

Abdominal Examination

Pelvic organs become abdomino-pelvic when they enlarge. Hence, abdominal examination is an integral part of a gynecological examination.

- *On inspection*, any evidence of distension, hernia and the pattern of distribution of the pubic hair should be noted. Surgical scars, including laparoscopy scars should be noted and any evidence of incisional hernia should be elicited by asking the patient to cough.
- *Palpation* should be performed in a systematic manner, after finding out any areas of tenderness or pain, which should be palpated last.
- *Superficial palpation* should be done first and any masses or areas of tenderness should be identified. Bilateral tenderness may indicate pelvic inflammatory disease whereas tenderness over the supra-pubic region may denote a bladder or uterine pathology. If tenderness is present, then it is important to exclude the presence of guarding, rigidity and rebound tenderness all of which are features of peritoneal irritation.

- *On deep palpation*, it is essential to describe any mass that is felt in terms of its site, size, margins, shape, surface, consistency, tenderness and mobility. Generally, uterine masses have a horizontal mobility and limited vertical mobility and ovarian masses have free horizontal and vertical mobility. However, a pedunculated fibroid may have horizontal and vertical mobility.

  Conversely, a fixed ovarian mass may have a restricted mobility. Palpation is made complete by the examination for the enlargement of the liver, spleen and the kidneys.

- *Percussion* is an important physical sign not only to differentiate between a solid abdomino-pelvic mass from distended bowel, but also to define the margins of an ill-defined mass. It can also be used to elicit the presence of free fluid inside the peritoneal cavity. In gynecological practice, presence of hemo-peritoneum from a ruptured ectopic pregnancy and ascitic fluid in ovarian neoplasms should be looked for. It is worthwhile to recollect the signs one has learnt during the early years of clinical medicine. The 'Puddle sign', 'Shifting dullness', 'Horse-shoe dullness' and 'Fluid thrill' will be helpful in identifying the presence of minimal, mild, moderate and large amount of free fluid, respectively.

- *Puddle sign* is elicited in the knee-elbow position, which causes the ascitic fluid to collect around a peri-umbilical area. Percussion from lateral to medial side (or auscultating while moving a coin from lateral to medial side) would reveal a change in the resonance from tympanic to dullness, suggesting the presence of free fluid.

- *Shifting dullness* is a sign that is useful when there is about 500 ml of fluid. Percussion is carried out from the midline (from about a finger breadth above the bladder dullness) laterally towards the right paracolic gutter (flank). If the percussion note changes from resonance to dullness, it may indicate free fluid. This can be confirmed by asking the patient to lie on her left side for about 30 seconds, which will shift the fluid from the right to the left paracolic gutter due to gravity. Hence, the character of resonance will change from dullness to resonance in the right flank, whereas it will de dull on the left flank.

If a patient has more fluid (about a liter or more), the fluid will fill the paracolic gutters and the pelvis, allowing the loops of bowel to float in it. This will result in resonance in the peri-umbilical region of the abdomen due to the air contained in the bowels and dullness all around due to the presence of the fluid. Hence, the name *Horse-shoe dullness* to denote the presence of dullness on both sides as well as inferiorly, which gives an appearance of a U-shaped horse-shoe.

- *Fluid thrill* is a physical sign that is elicited when there is a large amount of free fluid in the abdomen (over 2 liters), which makes it very tense. A gentle tap on the flank while keeping the palm of the other hand on the opposite flank would make the clinician feel a 'thrill' due to the transmission of the pressure wave created secondary to the tap on the flank, through the fluid to reach the opposite side. In order to minimise the thrill felt as a result of transmission of the pressure wave through the structures of the anterior abdominal wall, one needs to ask an assistant to apply a gentle pressure with his or her ulnar border of the hand in the midline, to cut off such waves transmitted through the anterior abdominal wall and hence, to reduce a false positive test.
- *Auscultation* is not quite useful in routine gynecological practice but may sometimes help in differentiating whether the acute abdomen is due to a bowel pathology. Moreover, it may be helpful post-operatively to determine whether oral feeds could be started.

Bimanual Examination

This is the most crucial and challenging part of gynecological examination though it may be omitted in patients with virgo intacta. It is a very embarrassing, stressful and unpleasant experience for most women and therefore it is important to be sensitive and supportive. A full explanation for the reason for the examination and what it entails should be given. The use of diagrams and models may help to illustrate the need for the examination. Presence of a chaperone, quite relaxing environment, utmost privacy as well as an empathetic and understanding clinician would go a long way to allay anxiety and fear. It is wise to keep in mind a well-relaxed patient would enable the clinician to extract optimum information possible during a pelvic examination within a short period of time. A tense, uncomfortable patient may contract her vaginal and abdominal muscles leading to an unproductive bimanual examination.

Position

Most commonly in the clinical setting, patients are examined in the 'dorsal position', whereby they lie on their back with the legs flexed at the knee joint. This will give a good exposure of the perineum and the introitus and facilitates use of Cusco's speculum easily. However, patients may feel too 'exposed', unless the abdomen and up to the knees are covered by a clean cloth. An alternative is the *lateral position* which may be acceptable to some patients. As the name suggests, the patient lies on her side (left) with both knees flexed. *Sim's position* is a variant of the lateral position, in which the inner (left) leg is kept extended whereas the outer (right) leg is flexed. Moreover, the left arm is flexed with the palms resting under the head and the patient's neck is flexed forwards. This position enables the visualization of the anterior vaginal wall and was initially used by Sim's for the repair of vesico-vaginal fistulae. It is also useful in the demonstration of enterocoele and uterovaginal prolapse. *Lithotomy position* with its various modifications is used especially when various procedures are carried out. This is a modified 'dorsal' position in which the feet are held in stirrups, with the thighs abducted and flexed to increase space and exposure. This position is rarely made use of in a gynecological clinic.

Technique of Bimanual Examination

This is essentially composed of three steps:
1. Inspection of the external genitalia
2. Visualisation of the vagina and cervix with a speculum

3. Bimanual examination of the uterus and the adnexa.

i. *Inspection of the external genitalia*

It is prudent to be systematic in describing the external genitalia. One useful suggestion is to start with labia majora and move inwards, commenting on the appearance of each structure. Hence, it is important to describe the appearance of pubic hair distribution, labia majora, minora, clitoris, urethral orifice, vestibule, the peri-anal region and the anal verge. This should be followed by opening the introitus with the thumb and the index finger of the left hand, placed at the junction of the upper two thirds and lower third of the labia, to comment on the presence of any abnormal vaginal discharge or bleeding. At this stage a rectocele or urethrocele may be visible. This should be followed by asking the patient to cough and strain. These maneuvres may unmask the presence of stress incontinence or utero-vaginal prolapse, respectively.

ii. *Visualization of the vagina and cervix using a speculum*

Two common types of specula are available: Cusco's and Sim's (Fig. 4.1), out of which the former is routinely used in clinical practice. However, there are numerous other specula, which are beyond the scope of this chapter. Modifications of *Cusco's bivalve speculum* have resulted in various sizes, including a speculum to examine a vagina with an intact hymen and disposable forms. *Sims' speculum* on the other hand is used in the Sims' position especially in the examination of an enterocele. It is also used in the examination of the utero-vaginal prolapse and in vaginal surgery, where more access and space is required. Insertion of the Cusco's speculum (Fig. 4.2) is described below:

After parting the labia, it is helpful to ask the patient to strain when inserting the speculum as this may aid the opening of the vaginal introitus as well as help to relax the patient by diverting her attention. The labia are parted by two fingers of the one hand near the junction of the upper two thirds and the lower third of the labia and a well lubricated and warm bivalve speculum is held in the right hand with the blades projecting between the index and middle fingers, while

the main body of the speculum with the handle and the locking mechanism, rests on the palm. It is important to keep both blades closed during insertion to avoid discomfort to the patient. The handle was originally designed to face downwards as the speculum was designed to be used in the lithotomy position. However, if special gynecology 'detachable' examination beds are not available in the clinic setting, it is best to keep the handle superior, taking due care not to traumatise the urethra or the clitoris. The angle of insertion should be along the axis of the vagina (45 degrees downwards) and the speculum should be advanced with gentle pressure on the posterior wall of the vagina, to open the vagina until it is not possible to advance it any further. The blades could be now opened to visualise the cervix.

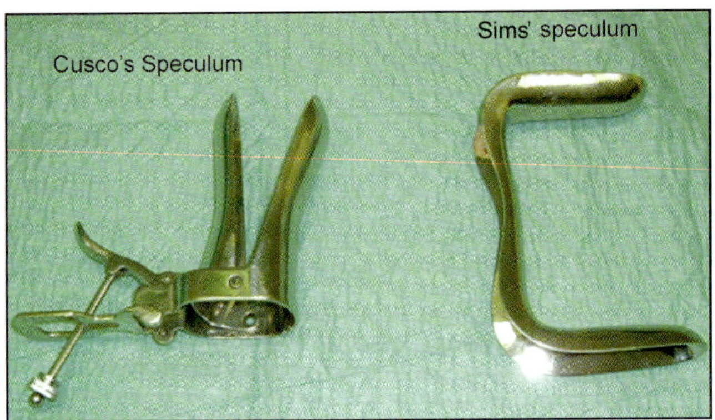

Figure 4.1: Cusco's and Sims' speculum displayed on the left and right respectively

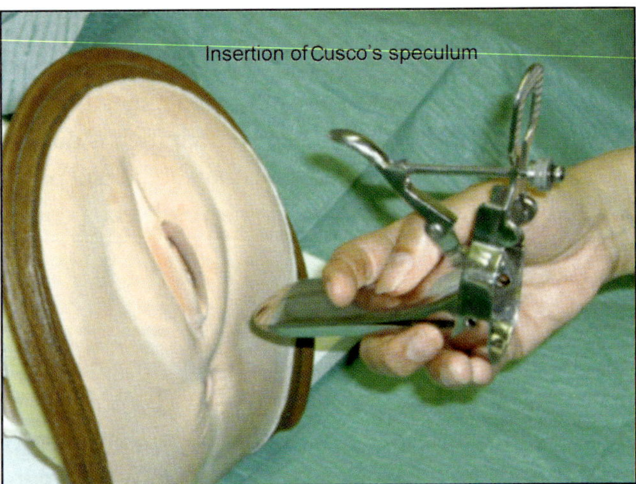

Figure 4.2: Insertion of Cusco's speculum—should be done with the bivalves together and the lock in position

Non-visualization of the cervix is often due to the mal positioning of the speculum and it may help to 'pull-back' a few centimetres prior to attempting to open it again. The rugosity of the vagina as opposed to the smooth surface of the cervix, the appearance of more mucus on the upper or lower blade of the speculum and partial visualisation of the cervix should help to re-direct the speculum to visualize the cervix. Care should be taken in postmenopausal women with genital tract atrophy as the cervix may be sometimes flushed with the vaginal wall.

It is important to describe the appearance of the cervix and if required, a cervical smear may be taken at this stage. High vaginal swabs (HVS) and endo-cervical swabs may also be taken under direct vision. During the removal of the speculum, it is important to observe the vaginal walls for any pathology as the speculum is withdrawn. If the blades are closed very early, they may cause entrapment of the cervix causing pain and discomfort. Hence, it should be removed gently under direct vision. The blades should be closed once the cervix disappears from the view and care should be taken to prevent the trapping of the vaginal mucosa between the blades.

iii. *Bimanual examination of the uterus and the adnexa*

Patient should preferably have an empty bladder prior to the procedure. After separating the labia with the thumb and index finger of the left hand, two fingers of the right hand are introduced into the vagina with the palmer surface facing up (Fig. 4.3). As with speculum examination, asking the patient to strain may facilitate entry. Throughout the whole examination, the clinician should observe the patients face to notice any sign of pain or discomfort.

The position and consistency of the cervix are felt. The left hand is placed on the abdomen and the bimanual examination commenced. As the name suggests, the pelvic organs are examined between the abdominal and vaginal fingers. The vaginal hand is often termed 'passive' and the abdominal hand 'active' because the vaginal fingers are inserted, they should be kept stationary. The pelvic organs are 'pushed' with the

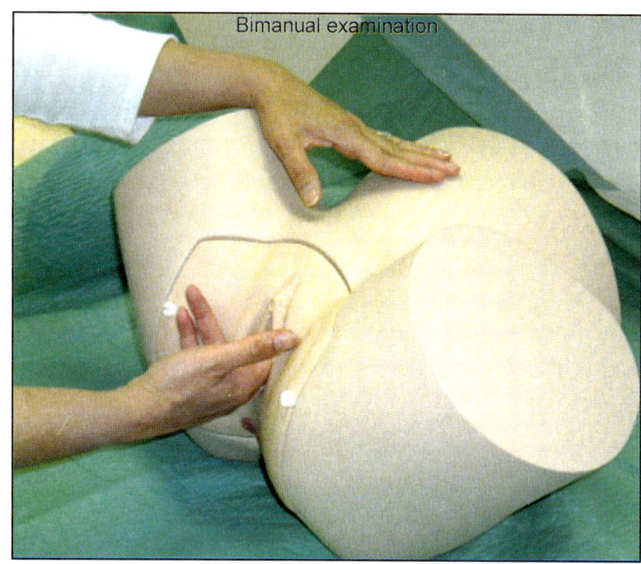

Figure 4.3: Bimanual examination on a model. Hands should be gloved in patients and thumb kept away from clitoral area

abdominal hand towards the vaginal hand, so that they could be felt. At times, when faced with an obese patient, the cervix and uterus may have to be 'pushed up' by the fingers in the vagina to help palpate them. Once the uterus is felt, the vaginal fingers are moved to the right fornix of the vagina and the abdominal hand is moved to the right iliac fossa to feel the right adnexa. The same procedure is repeated on the left side. The contents of the pouch of Douglas is examined by sweeping the vaginal fingers across the posterior fornix and lifting any contents to be palpated by the hand on the abdomen. If the uterus is not felt, it may be retroverted. Therefore, it is important to carry out the bimanual examination with the vaginal fingers in the posterior fornix. Examination of the posterior fornix is also important in the detection of 'nodules' in the pouch of Douglas. This may indicate endometriosis or rarely ovarian malignancy (Bloomer's Shelf).

Generally, uterine masses will move with the cervix and pushing the mass upwards will make the cervix move upwards from the vaginal fingers. A pedunculated fibroid may be an exception to this rule. Likewise, ovarian masses will be felt to move separately. However, adhesions between the ovarian mass and the uterus may make it move *en masse*. This is especially seen with endometriomas.

Rectal Examination

Lower genital tract is anatomically and embryologically closely related to the rectum and the anal canal. Hence, per rectal examination forms an important ancillary examination for a gynecologist. Gynecological disorders like endometriosis and malignancies of the ovary and the lower genital tract may involve the rectal wall or mucosa. Conversely, bowel pathology may present with gynecological symptoms. In utero-vaginal prolapse, rectal examination may help to confirm the presence of a rectocele. Examination of the tone of the anal sphincter is vital in patients with fecal incontinence to identify the underlying pathology.

Rectovaginal Examination

It is a 'combined' examination in which the middle finger of the right hand is inserted in to the rectum whereas the index finger of the same hand is inserted into the vagina. This examination is often performed by gyne-oncologists and it is very useful in assessing pathologies in the recto-vaginal septum and the parametrium. If carcinoma of the cervix is suspected this examination will help us in the clinical staging of the disease. If the two fingers can't be approximated together, it may indicate that the tumor may have spread to uterosacral and cardinal ligaments. If this extends to the lateral pelvic wall, it suggests Stage III B. This implies that there is no 'tumor free space' between the cervix and the lateral pelvic wall and makes the patient unsuitable for surgery (radical hysterectomy). In ovarian malignancy, rectovaginal examination may give us a clue about the 'fixity' of the tumor and possible tumor deposits in the pouch of Douglas.

CONCLUSION

We have made an attempt to discuss the important principles of history and gynecological examination. It is important to remember that each patient is different and therefore flexibility and innovation is required. The very development of the Sims' speculum illustrates the importance of innovation. Sim was a village physician, who was called upon to manage a woman who was having vaginal bleeding following a horse riding accident. He took a spoon and bent the handle to retract the vaginal wall to identify the source of bleeding. This marked the development of the Sims' speculum. In our practice, although unconventional, sometimes we may have to perform a gentle digital examination prior to a speculum examination to identify the capacity of the vagina to choose the right size of the speculum or to identify the cervix. This is especially so in an elderly postmenopausal woman or in a woman with the large uterine mass, in whom the cervix may be impacted against the symphysis pubis. Such deviations in the examination may help avoid discomfort and pain, thereby enabling the clinician to obtain maximum information to help the patient.

Good history and a thorough examination should be considered as the pillars of good clinical practice. They form very important pieces of the clinical 'Jigsaw' puzzle. Hence, it is important to make every effort to identify useful pieces of information from both history and examination so as to enable us to get an idea about the broader picture. This will help us choose the right and appropriate investigations for the patient and make an optimum management plan. Such a systematic approach may help us solve the clinical 'puzzle' leading to improved patient care.

5.

Pratap Kumar
Arun Nagrath
Rupinder Kaur Ruprai

Pediatric Gynecology

INTRODUCTION

The pathologic processes in infants and young children differ significantly from that of the adolescent or adult female. The gynecologic problems encountered in the pediatric population are unique to this age group and involve physician skills differing from those utilized with an adult population. It is important to understand the normal anatomy and physiology of the reproductive tract and genitalia in the prepubertal female in order to understand, evaluate, and manage the common problems seen in this age group.

NORMAL ANATOMY AND PHYSIOLOGY

At 5 to 6 weeks' gestation, the undifferentiated gonad is bipotential and is capable of differentiating into either a testis or an ovary.[1] Gonadal sex establishes under the influence of the chromosomal sex. The embryonic differentiation of the normal female genital tract begins in the presence of two normal X chromosomes and in the absence of the masculinizing Y chromosome. The Müllerian ducts fuse at the midline and subsequently migrate caudally to the urogenital sinus. In the female, the Wolffian duct system degenerates in the absence of testosterone. By 12 weeks' gestation the ovarian cortex begins to develop, with primordial follicles appearing at around 13½ weeks. At birth, the female infant has 1 to 2 million germ cells remaining.[2,3]

The fetal hypothalamic-pituitary-ovarian (HPO) axis is functioning at 12 weeks of age with unrestrained pulsatile release of embryonic hypothalamic gonadotropin-releasing hormone (GnRH). There is maturation of the HPO axis toward term with the development of a negative feedback to estradiol (E2).

Estrogen synthesis by the fetal ovary is low at term, however, the maternal estrogen, which readily crosses the placenta, estrogenizes the neonate. From birth through the first 8 weeks of life, the female infant is under the influence of maternal estrogen. Placental separation at birth causes an elevation in follicle-stimulating hormone (FSH) and luteinizing hormone (LH) with a brief neonatal stimulation of the ovarian axis. Thus, the young female has 2 reasons for an estrogen effect on the genital mucosa:[3]

1. Effect of high maternal estrogen levels that crossed the placenta and
2. Stimulation of the child's ovaries by their own gonadotrophins.

For the first one and a half years or so gonadotropins (Gn) continue to cause some ovarian stimulation and endogenous estrogen production.[4] Perinatal ovarian cysts have been described following delivery but resolve spontaneously as gonado-trophin levels fall physiologically.[5] Beyond 18 months, until puberty, ovarian quiescence occurs due to the exquisite pituitary and hypothalamic sensitivity to even low levels of estrogen.[2]

Anatomical Findings in the Newborn

Until the first 8 weeks of life, the influence of maternal estrogen has a profound effect on the appearance of the female genitalia.

- Owing to the estrogenization, the labia minora are thick and sometimes longer than labia majora.
- The mucosa is pink and covered with physiologic leucorrhea.
- Clitoral hood is thick. The ***clitoris*** is often disproportionately enlarged.
- Hymen is thick, pouting, and fimbriated, sometimes making the orifice and the ***urethral meatus*** difficult to visualize.
- Vagina measures 4 cm in length. Vaginal mucosa is thick.
- In the first 10 days of life, vaginal bleeding may be seen in the neonate.[3]

Maternal estrogen exposure may stimulate a *mucoid discharge* or a *small amount of bloody vaginal discharge* but these effects begin to recede in about 2 weeks. Higher estrogen levels promote the metabolism of glycogen in the cells, making the lower genital tract much more susceptible to monilial infections, but as estrogen levels fall the likelihood of monilial infections decreases. Discharge and vaginal bleeding persisting after 10 to 14 days is therefore not normal and should be investigated further.[6] Estrogen levels continue to fall until about 1½ to 2 years of age, although gonado-trophins continue to cause some ovarian stimulation and endogenous production of estrogen during this time.

From the age of 3 until 8 or 9 years the estrogen levels are at their lowest and this influences the appearance of the female genitalia. With low levels of estrogen, the genital tissues become increasingly atrophic.

- The ***clitoral hood*** and the ***clitoris*** (the most prominent landmark in the prepubertal female's external genital area) age take on less prominence as the clitoris does not increase in size as do the other structures.
- The ***urethral meatus*** is often quite small in the prepubertal child. Occasionally the ***periurethral tissue*** becomes patulous and appears as an area of bright pink tissue.[3,4]
- The ***labia majora*** appear as normal skin circling around the more central genital structures. The ***labia minora*** are very thin, sometimes short, ridges of tissue that edge the vestibulum interiorly and course upward toward the midline, meeting just beneath the clitoris.[4] Below this, the urethra and vagina open. Unlike in the older female they do not provide coverage or protection for the vaginal opening.
- ***Smegma***—thick white substance noted in the anterior labia folds (should not be mistaken for leucorrhea).
- The ***vestibule,*** is the recessed mucosa that has as its landmarks the urethral meatus anteriorly and the vaginal orifice posteriorly. The ***vestibular sulcus*** is the base of the vaginal orifice and appears very erythematous due to the marked density of capillaries that surround this area and with minor trauma may lead to excessive bleeding.[3,4]
- A normal ***clitoral glans*** in prepubertal child is 5 mm in length and 3 mm in transverse diameter on an average; it shows little variation after puberty.[7,8]
- The ***hymen***, which edges the vaginal orifice, varies in size and shape. The once thick, redundant hymen becomes thin and translucent with varying configurations. It may be:[2,9]
  a. Annular (age 3—beginning of puberty)
  b. Crescent-shaped (no hymenal suburethral tissue; age 3 to beginning of puberty)
  c. Redundant (common in girls < 3 years) and irregular
  d. Teardrop-shaped

  The less common variations include:
  a. Imperforate hymen
  b. Micro perforate
  c. Septated hymen.

  Usually, correction of these variations is not necessary until the girl reaches puberty.[3]
- Until age 5, **vaginal orifice** measures 4-5 mm and from then until puberty, it measures = 10 mm. It is

important to note that the diameter of vagina can vary with the position of the child, degree of perineal relaxation, hymen shape and the level of estrogenization.[10,11]

- A child's **vagina** measure 5 cm in length.[8] Vaginal mucosa is red, thin (lack of esrtogenization), and folded; it is quite sensitive to instrumentation (speculum/ vaginoscope, etc).[8,12] The pH of the vagina is alkaline and consists primarily of columnar epithelium. Monilial infections, due to the low estrogen levels, vaginal discharge or bleeding is not a normal finding at this time.

- The uterus grows progressively during fetal life. After birth, the uterine thickness and volume is relatively more than the prepubertal uterus, with endometrial and myometrial characteristics similar to that of adult uterus.[13] With withdrawal of maternal hormone, the size regresses and the size then remains constant until the age of 7 years.[14] From 7 years, there is a slow rate of increase in the uterine volume until appearance of secondary sexual characteristics, after which there is a sharp acceleration during puberty.

- The **cervix** is small with a centered opening and is flushed with the vaginal vault (therefore, sometimes difficult to visualize). The prepubertal **ratio of cervix to uterus** is 2/3:1/3; alteration in this ratio generally presents as onset of precocious puberty.

- The **ovaries** are abdominal structures and gradual descent into the pelvis occurs with the onset of puberty.[2] The ovarian size increases throughout childhood in relation to the increase in size of antral follicles and stroma. Until the age of 6 years, these antral follicles measure < 5 mm in size and in the early pubertal ovaries, these measure < 9 mm (giving a PCOS like appearance). Any enlargement of the ovary can present as *an abdominal mass with associated abdominal symptoms.*

Examination of the Prepubertal and the Newborn

The Premenarchal Girls

Examination of the child: It begins with[15] plotting the *height* and *weight* on a growth chart, followed by checking the ears, neck, heart, and lungs. *Sexual developmental stage of the breasts* is noted. This is followed by abdominal and gynecological examination. Many of the problems encountered in the prepubertal patient are vulvar and lower vaginal in origin and not all will require visualization of the upper vagina and cervix.

Position and technique(s)[15]

1. Supine with frog-legged position (supine, with legs flexed, knees apart and feet touching) or legs in stirrups.
2. Knee chest position can be used to try to visualize the upper vagina and cervix.

The external genitalia, hymen, and distal vagina can be visualized by the "**Lateral spread technique**" where index fingers are placed on the posterior aspect of the labia and gentle *downward-lateral* traction is applied.

- *Hymenal tags* and *periurethral grooves* are normal findings.
- Common **lower tract abnormalities** include: *hymenal and vaginal cysts, urethral prolapse, labial agglutination, vaginitis, foreign objects, imperforate hymen,* and *lichen sclerosis.*[15]

Examination of the upper vagina and cervix is done for:

- Vaginal bleeding
- Persistent vaginal discharge
- Suspected foreign object
- Trauma
- Suspected vaginal tumor.

Bimanual examination is avoided as the estrogen status of the child in latency limits the examination. Insertion of the small finger for a rectal examination to evaluate the vagina and uterus is better tolerated.

Rectal examination is usually the last step, which helps in determining the existence and size of the cervix. It should measure about 5 mm in transverse diameter. Ovaries at this stage are too small to be felt. Any mass felt should be further investigated. Vagina can be palpated to look for foreign body or discharge.[8]

Examination under anesthesia and/or vaginoscopy may be required in only select cases such as tumor, foreign body and conditions where ultrasonography

(USG) does not provide adequate information on source of vaginal bleeding/discharge.[12]

Collection of Specimens

Specimens (if necessary) should be obtained at the end of the examination. As the premenarchal vaginal mucosa is atrophic, obtaining specimens with dry cotton tip swabs can cause pain and bleeding. Therefore, swabs moistened with saline should be used. Specimens for cultures are indicated when there is:

- Vaginal discharge in absence of foreign body.
- Suspicion of specific causes of vulvitis (infections by yeast, streptococcus, etc.).

AMBIGUOUS GENITALIA[16]

Ambiguous genitalia is a medical, surgical and psychological emergency.

1. *Examples of ambiguity*:
   - Genital tubercle with development half way between that of penis and clitoris.
   - Genital folds completely fused with bifid scrotum.
   - Penis abnormally bent and buried inward.
   - Posterior fusion of labia majora and single perineal orifice at the base of genital tubercle.
   - True clitoral hypertrophy and oblong mass in the inguinal position with female phenotype.
2. *Objectives*:
   - Thorough examination of general features and genitals
   - Investigations
   - Sex assignment-decision must only be made when sufficient information is available. This requires a multi disciplinary team of pediatric endocrinologists, obstetricians, radiologists, surgeons, geneticists, biologists, and pediatric psychiatrists.

Diagnosis

Step 1. Thorough physical examination, that begins by a methodical general inspection and careful genital inspection. Precise measurement of the penis is made; mean stretched penile length in the normal term new born is 3.5 cm (± 0.5 cm).

Step 2. Note degree of ambiguity-define the extent of ambiguity by presence, number, size, symmetry and position of gonads if possible.

Step 3. Careful palpation to locate gonads below the genital folds/inguinal region:
- *If gonads are absent*: female pseudohermaphroditism.
- *If gonad or gonads are palpable*: male pseudohermaphroditism.
- In a masculinized female newborn, congenital adrenal hyperplasia (CAH) and undervirilized male newborn should be ruled out.

Step 4. Careful background history:
- Information on other siblings/family members with similar problem.
- History of neonatal death.
- Consanguinity.
- Maternal ingestion of drugs/exposure to chemical environmental agents during pregnancy.
- Questions about salt losing.

Step 5. Formulate a **differential diagnosis**[16]

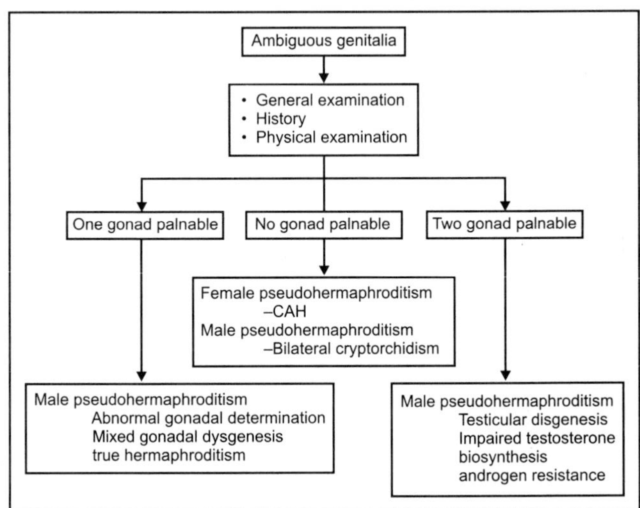

Step 6. Investigations:

a. Genetic:
- Buccal smears for Bar bodies (not reliable)
- Karyotyping
- PCR analysis of SRY gene on the Y chromosome (results available in one day)

b. Hormonal:
- Elevation of 17 hydroxylase (OH), progesterone (17 OHP) and plasma testosterone-CAH (due to 21 OH-lase deficiency).
- Basal plasma testosterone levels to evaluate Leydig's cell function
- Testicular stimulation with hCG determines (1000 U/day of hCG for 3 days or 1500 U every 2 days for 2 weeks):
  i. Functional value of testicular tissue (insufficient response of < 3 ng/ml suggests gonadal dysgenesis)
  ii. Inborn error of testosterone biosynthesis by showing augmentation in precursors: 17 OHP, dehydroepiandrosterone (DHEA), androstenedione.

c. Peripheral androgen receptivity—in all cases of undermasculinized external genitalia associated with elevated testosterone secretion:
- By clinical response of genital tubercle to exogenous testosterone (Augmentation of < 35 mm in phallic length in newborns with micropenis is insufficient); failure to respond → end organ resistance to androgens).
- By measurement of concentration of receptor sites in external genitalia (Concentration <300 fmol/mg of DNA → partial androgen insensitivity).

d. Imaging:
- USG: look for uterus and ovaries
- Genitography: for level of implantation of vaginal cavity on the urethra.

Etiology of Ambiguous Genitalia

The XX Newborn

Gonads are not palpable → female pseudohermaphroditism

- ***With SRY (–), causes of excessive androgen production include:***
  1. *Increased 17 OHP* (fetal cause): CAH is the most frequent cause of androgen excess in female newborn.
  2. *Normal 17 OHP*: Excessive maternal production or exposure to androgen/progestins causes virilization of female fetus:
     a. Exogenous steroids during pregnancy can cause posterior fusion of labia, clitoridal enlargement, and androgenization.
     b. Danazol because of its androgenic side effects.
     c. Ovarian tumors—luteoma of pregnancy, arrhenoblastoma, hilar-cell tumor, ovarian stromal cell tumor, Krukenberg tumor.
     d. Untreated maternal virilizing CAH.
  3. *Placental aromatase deficiency*: placental aromatase protects the fetus from excess androgenization and a defect in the same leads to virilization in female offspring
- ***SRY +***
  XX male
  XX true hermaphrodite—has both testicular and ovarian tissue. Two thirds of these are raised as males (for this potential for adequate penile length should be considered). For those raised as females 2/3 have clitoromegaly. In most cases, a small uterus is present, with potential for fertility.

XY Newborn

- Gonads are usually palpable → male pseudohermaphroditism.
- If testosterone rises normally after hCG stimulation → 5 α reductase deficiency/androgen insensitivity (complete/partial).

1. Complete androgen insensitivity:
- Female phenotype with blind vagina and no uterus.
- Under development of clitoris and labia minora.
- Presents as inguinal hernia in infancy and primary amenorrhea in puberty.
- Breast development is normal.
- Absent or scanty axillary and pubic hair.
- They develop female habitus.

Treatment: gonadectomy, ideally before puberty followed by estrogen therapy during puberty.

2. Partial androgen insensitivity syndrome has a spectrum of clinical phenotypes:
- Wolffian duct that is developed to a variable extent.
- Simple hypospadiasis
- Micropenis

- Undervirilization and gynecomastia in adolescent boys.

Management:

- Individualized depending on degree of genital ambiguity, growth response of penis to testosterone and type of androgen receptor mutation.
- Female rearing is preferred as they are azoospermic and would other wise require multiple reconstructive surgeries of external genitalia.

3. 5 α reductase deficiency

- At birth-undervirilized phenotype with hypospadic phallus resembling clitoris, bifid scrotum that is labia like and urogenital sinus opening on the perineum. Testes can be either in the inguinal canal, labia majora, or scrotum. Wolffian duct is differentiated normally in vas deferens, epididymis, and seminal vesicles.
- At puberty—virilization of external genitalia occurs along with acquisition of male genetic identity in these patients that are usually raised as females.

  Management: depends on the phenotype findings and gender at time of diagnosis.

- Gonadectomy should be performed early to prevent masculinization, along with vaginoplasty and clitoridal reduction.
- If diagnosed in puberty: one can consider raising child as male.

46 XY/XO Newborn

Diagnosis is mixed gonadal dysgenesis and characteristics include:

- A unilateral testis that is often intra-abdominal, a contralateral streak gonad, and persistent müllerian structures. There are varying degrees of inadequate masculinization and such males are infertile. Affected patients are at risk of gonadal tumors, therefore these should be removed, and patients should be reared as females.
- Distinction between mixed gonadal dysgenesis and Turner's syndrome with Y material is unclear.

Sex Assignment for Rearing

- The clinical examination provides an assessment of the degree of virilization and the presence of gonads.

- Biological assessments are mandatory for plasma 17 OHP and the SRY gene.
- Anatomic condition and functional abilities of genitalia; etiology of the genital malformation and family considerations should be kept in mind

In cases of female pseudohermaphroditism, the newborn should always be declared to be of female sex. With normal ovaries and uterus, they are potentially capable of bearing children.

In cases of male pseudohermaphroditism, great care should be taken as major considerations are: reconstructive surgery, probability of pubertal virilization, and response of external genitalia to exo- and endogenous testosterone. The presence of testicular tissue is not an essential factor in this decision.

GONADAL DYSGENESIS

- *Defect in 5 α reductase* → male sex rearing because pubertal virilization will lead to penile development (although it will be subnormal), normal pubic hair development, and the acquisition of male sexual identity.
- *Inborn errors of testosterone synthesis* → when a vagina and uterus are present, female sex rearing is preferred since vaginoplasty can be done and especially if male reconstructive surgery appears highly unlikely.
- *Androgen resistance* → female rearing.
- *True hermaphroditism* → female sex assignment since ovarian function is preserved
- *For male pseudohermaphroditism reared as girls→* castration.
- *For male pseudohermaphroditism reared as boys →* gonadal follow up through out life. Castration of XY intersex with testicular dysgenesis should be done, as there is a high chance of gonadal tumor.

VULVOVAGINAL DISORDERS

Labial Adhesions

Incidence: Labial adhesions occur in 1-38% of children aged from 13 months to 6 years.[17]

Labial adhesions result in partial to complete fusion of the labia minora.[18] The agglutination usually begins posteriorly and extends upward toward the clitoris, leaving a small opening anteriorly in most cases. The fused portion of the labia is usually identified by a thin line of demarcation or raphe.[19] Extreme cases of complete labial closure result in urinary retention, pruritus, and/or infection.

Etiology: It has been postulated that estrogen deficiency results in thinning of the superficial mucosal layers and any inflammation results in adhesions.

Treatment

- *Spontaneous resolution* can occur at puberty once estrogen is produced.
- *Application of estrogen cream* to the fine thin raphe twice a day for 2 weeks followed by once daily application for 2 weeks. As estrogen cream can be systemically absorbed. Parents may notice transient breast development, and it is not advised to continue therapy for longer than 4 weeks.
- **For recurrence**: A repeat course of treatment in 6 month to 1-year intervals is given.
- Once separation of the labia has occurred, a thin coating of *lubricant* once daily is suggested to keep the area moist and prevent recurrence.
- Surgical separation is done only if urinary problems result and estrogen therapy has failed.
- Forceful manual separation is *not advised* as this causes pain and trauma to the child. In addition, recurrence is much more common.

Vulvitis

Presentation: Vulvitis presents with vulvar discomfort or itching and urinary and/or anal signs. Symptoms can be persistent. Isolated erythematous areas can be seen. Lesions exclusively involve the vulva and there is no vaginal discharge, whereas, in vaginitis, there are both clinical vulvo-vaginal manifestations and a vaginal discharge due to an infection. Vulvitis is usually related to poor hygiene, irritants, and pinworms.

Management: A careful history with regard to use of any possible irritant should be taken. Questions should be directed to the level of hygiene, urinary incontinence, frequency of diaper changes, and bathing habits.

Conditions that Cause Vulvitis

- Diaper dermatitis
- Candidiasis
- Group A β-hemolytic *Streptococcus*
- Nocturnal pruritus-pinworm infestation
- Contact or allergic dermatitis
- Lichen sclerosis
- Nonspecific vulvovaginitis
- Infectious vulvovaginitis

1. *Diaper dermatitis* is associated with exposure to urine and stool in infants but also in girls, who are developmentally delayed and wearing diapers. Based on localization of lesion and their shape, they are described as Y-diaper dermatitis, W-diaper dermatitis, mixed diaper dermatitis, Jacquet erosive diaper dermatitis and Lucky-Luke diaper dermatitis.

Management:
- Keep the area dry.
- Regular change of diapers.
- Application of petroleum based ointment that serves as a moisture barrier.

Differential diagnosis:
- Seborrheic dermatitis
- Candidiasis
- Irritant contact dermatitis
- Atopic dermatitis
- Psoriasis

2. *Candida:* It is rarely seen in the non-estrogenized prepubertal girl but is common in infants under the age of 2.[20] It presents as erythematous rash with raised, well-demarcated borders and satellite lesions.

Predisposing factors:
- It may follow a course of antibiotics in the infant.
- Juvenile onset diabetes.
- Immunosuppression.

Investigation: KOH preparation helps identify hyphae.

Treatment: Antifungal creams such as clotrimazole, miconazole or butaconazole applied twice a day to the affected area for 10 to 14 days or until rash is cleared.

3. *Group A β-hemolytic Streptococcus:* It is treated with an antibiotic therapy for 2 weeks and occasionally for longer periods of time (up to 4 weeks). Additional therapy consists of sitz baths with baking soda or colloidal oatmeal added one to two times daily. Soap should be avoided and the area can be dried thoroughly with a hair dryer on low heat or cool air. Hygiene must be emphasized along with thorough hand washing before and after using the toilet.

4. *Nocturnal pruritus: Pinworms*, or *Enterobius vermicularis*, are 1 cm long, thin white worms that can migrate from the anus to the vagina and cause severe nocturnal pruritus.

Diagnosis: Inspection at night with a flashlight may show small threadlike worms exiting the anus. Alternatively, a morning inspection with "Scotch tape" to the anal region can identify the eggs.[3]

Treatment: Mebendazole 100 mg orally once and repeated in 1 week. It is advised to treat the entire family to prevent reinfection.

5. *Contact or allergic vulvitis*: This can lead to significant pruritis with scratching and excoriation.

Offending agents: Poison ivy, topical creams, ointments and lotions, perfumed or colored toilet paper, bubble baths and soaps, adult or baby wipes, as well as laundry detergents, fabric softeners and dryer sheets, and bleach used to wash undergarments.

Treatment:
- Removal of the irritant.
- If itching is severe:
  - Oral hydroxyzine hydrochloride, 2 mg/kg/day divided into four doses.
  - Application of topical hydrocortisone 2.5% twice a day for a week.

6. *Lichen sclerosus*: It presents as itching, irritation, soreness, bleeding, and dysuria.

On examination: The vulva is characteristically white, atrophic, with parchment like skin and occasionally evidence of sub epithelial hemorrhages, excoriations, fissures, and inflammation. It is usually symmetrically distributed (hourglass appearance) in the vulvar and perianal area.

Diagnosis: In the prepubertal age group the diagnosis is made clinically.

Treatment: Application of clobetasol cream 0.05% at nights to the affected area for 6 weeks. Follow-up should be scheduled at that time and if there is significant improvement, the dose is tapered progressively until it is being used only one time weekly at bedtime.[3]

7. *Nonspecific vulvovaginitis*: Vulvovaginal inflammation is the most common gynecological disorder of prepubertal girls and accounts for over 50% of visits to pediatric gynecological clinics.[21] Inflammation may involve the vulva, vagina, or both and can result from a variety of stimuli. Factors that contribute to nonspecific vulvovaginitis include:
1. Poor hygiene practices.
2. Inadequate front-to-back wiping.
3. Smaller labia minora, with a short ano-vaginal distance.
4. Thinner vulvovaginal epithelium that is not well estrogenized and thus more prone to irritation.
5. Foreign body such as toilet paper, small toys, or pieces of cloth, which may be inserted in the vagina by the child.
6. Chemical irritants such as bubble baths, shampoos, or bath oils, and deodorant soaps.
7. Dermatological conditions such as eczema and seborrhea.
8. Chronic disease and altered immune status.
9. Sexual abuse.

Pathogenesis: It is not well-defined. It may be associated with an alteration of the vaginal flora with an overgrowth of fecal aerobes or an over abundance of anerobes leading to symptoms of odor and discharge. *Escherichia coli* is often found on vaginal culture, suggesting poor hygiene; contamination with bowel flora may contribute to the problem.

Symptoms of nonspecific vulvovaginitis include itching, dysuria, and discharge.

Recommended vulvar hygiene measures *include*:
1. Use front-to-back wiping with warm water after a bowel movement.

2. Avoid deodorant soaps, bubble baths, or lotions.
3. Wear only white cotton underwear or if still in diapers, change soon after each urination or bowel movement.
4. Use unscented toilet paper.
5. Keep vulvar area clean and dry.
6. Wash hands before and after use of toilet.
7. Use mild bath soap.
8. Remove wet bathing suits soon after exiting pool area.

Occasionally, a child may be found to be in a "scratch and itch" cycle where the discharge and inflammation has led to pruritis and the subsequent scratching has led to bacterial infection.[3]

- Initially, sitz baths in lukewarm water with 2 tablespoons of baking soda, colloidal oatmeal, or Domeboro solution may soothe an acutely inflamed vulva.
- Antibiotics are commonly used if secondary bacterial infection is suspected and include amoxicillin, amoxicillin/clavulinic acid, or cephalosporin for 7-10 day courses.
- Topical estrogen cream once or twice a day for 7 to 14 days may promote healing if vulvovaginal denudation is suspected due to disturbed bacterial homeostasis.
- Occasionally a low-dose topical steroid (hydrocortisone 1% or 2.5%) will help relieve itching and inflammation.

8. *Infectious vulvovaginitis:* Specific vulvovaginal infections that occur in the prepubertal female are often from respiratory and enteric systems and, less frequently, sexually transmitted.

Respiratory pathogens found in the vagina of young girls include:

- *Hemophilus influenzae,*
- *Staphylococcus aureus,*
- *Group A β-hemolytic streptococci,*
- *Streptococcus pneumoniae* causing a yellowish to greenish purulent vaginal discharge.
- *Shigella flexneri,* an enteric pathogen, can cause a mucopurulent, sometimes bloody discharge following an episode of diarrhea in some young girls.

Treatment: It is based on individual's microscopic report specific for the organism.

PHYSIOLOGIC DISCHARGE

The newborn may experience some transient vaginal secretions resulting from maternal estrogen exposure *in utero.* This appears as clear mucous, whitish in color, or clear. On occasion, a bloody discharge is noted due to transient endometrial shedding. It often resolves within a few hours to days. Mucous secretions may appear again around the time of puberty as estrogen levels rise in the adolescent.

Premenarchal Vaginal Discharge

The hypoestrogenic hormonal milieu in a preadolescent child is a major factor contributing to the susceptibility of the vaginal mucosa to infection. The thin mucosa lacks cornification, has an alkaline pH, and is therefore more susceptible to invasion from pathogens. The premenarchal (with or without vulvovaginitis) vaginal flora contains both aerobic and anaerobic organisms.[22]

Vaginal discharge in children is a common gynecologic complaint and may be resistant to symptomatic and/or antibiotic treatment. Very copious discharge is a marker of unusual pathology.[23] In recurrent or unresponsive patients, an evaluation to rule out a foreign body is traditionally recommended.[24]

Common Sources for Vaginal Irritation or Discharge

- Fecal contamination from poor perineal hygiene.
- Spread of respiratory bacteria from hand to perineal contact.
- Local irritants such as bubble bath or nylon underwear.

Sexual Abuse as a Cause for Vaginal Discharge [3]

Evaluation is certainly warranted when organisms are found on cultures that are associated with sexual transmission.

- Genital infection with *Neisseria gonorrheae* is associated with a purulent thick yellow discharge along with vulvar erythema and edema.

- *Chlamydia trachomatis* may present with vulvo-vaginitis, pruritis, and discharge. Infants born to mothers with chlamydia may carry the organism for up to 18 months.[25]
- After 18 years, findings of chlamydia warrant a search for sexual abuse.
- *Trichomonas* observed on saline wet mount is uncommon in an unestrogenized vagina and therefore is rarely a cause of vaginitis in the prepubertal child.[21]

VIRAL INFECTIONS

1. *Condyloma acuminata*: **There anogenital warts are caused by the human papillomavirus (HPV).**

   Presentation: Condyloma appears as white or fleshy, papilloma like tumors in the unestrogenized vulvar mucosa but have more verrucous characteristics of adult lesions on the perineum and perianal areas. As in the adult, certain subtypes of the HPV warts are potentially oncogenic.

   Condyloma usually present as asymptomatic lesions and are noted by the parent or caregiver. Large lesions may present with a child complaining of pain on urination or defecation.

   Mode of transmission:
   - ***In children < 2 years of age***, mode of transmission generally, is vertical from mother to child during childbirth.
   - ***After age 2***, sexual abuse is a primary concern in children presenting with condylomatous lesions, as seen in one third of cases. It is postulated that the incubation period may be markedly prolonged in cases where sexual abuse is not suspected or found.[26]

   Treatment: Spontaneous resolution occurs often and so intervention is usually not required.[17] In the past, treatment was with trichloroacetic acid, podophyllin, cryotherapy or CO_2 laser vaporization therapy under anesthesia. However, more recently the imiquimod cream, an immune response modifier supplied in a cream base, has revolutionized therapy for external genital warts.[25] A thin layer of cream is applied to the wart(s) at bedtime and left on for 6 to 10 hours,

after which it is washed off. Therapy is for 3 alternate days a week and continued until the warts are completely gone, or up to 16 weeks.

2. *Molluscum Contagiosum*: It is caused by pox virus localized in the genital area. Presents as 1-10 mm dome-shaped papule, flesh, or pearly colored with umbilicated center. It is a self-limiting disease. As treatment is often painful (curettage or cryotherapy), non-intervention is preferred.

3. *Herpes and Zoster virus infection*: Genital HSV infections are rare in children.

URETHRAL PROLAPSE

Presentation: Urethral prolapse usually presents with **unexplained bleeding**, often thought to be vaginal. There is no recent history of vulvar trauma or pain.

On physical examination: Bright red, friable annular mass is seen just above the hymen surrounding the urethral opening.

Treatment: Estrogen cream to the area nightly for 1 to 2 weeks. If the prolapse does not resolve, a referral to an urologist is indicated.

FOREIGN BODIES

Incidence: It is 4-10% in the pediatric age group.[23]

Presentation: Unexplained bleeding, vaginal discharge, or genito-urinary complaints may indicate the possibility of the presence of a foreign body. The vaginal discharge is often dark brownish in color and occurs daily, requiring the use of a panty liner by the child. The discharge is often malodorous.

Methods to Rule out a Foreign Body

- Careful genital examination in the clinic
- Vaginal saline lavage or
- Examination under anesthesia with vaginoscopy (also useful in identifying other etiologies of vaginal discharge and its ability to execute an extensive vaginal irrigation). Vaginoscopy in the operating room is the traditional method of assessment of foreign bodies in children unresponsive to improved perineal hygiene and medical therapy, such as

antibiotics. The exam under anesthesia allows for a more thorough examination and for obtaining vaginal cultures and biopsies, if indicated.

- Pelvic ultrasound examination,
- Plain abdominal X-ray
- MRI in rare circumstances

Treatment: Vaginal irrigation may wash out any loose pieces of toilet paper, but objects such as safety pins or parts of toys may require that the child be anesthetized to remove the foreign body. Following removal, sitz bath is recommended until the residual symptoms subside.

IMPERFORATE HYMEN

Issues related to imperforate hymen are discussed in Chapter 2 that deals with disorders of the development of the Müllerian system.

PRECOCIOUS PUBERTY

The development of progressive isosexual secondary sexual characteristics before the age of 8 years in girls and before the age of 9 years in boys is termed "precocious puberty.[27] Increased growth is often the first change in precocious puberty. This is usually followed by breast development and growth of pubic hair. The rapid linear growth that characterizes precocious puberty is associated with premature and rapid skeletal maturation and fusion of the epiphyses. In many cases, this results in short adult stature compared with genetic height potential.

Precocity occurs in girls 5 times more frequently than boys and almost three quarters of precocity in girls is idiopathic.[28] Nevertheless, in the face of any precocious development, one should rule out a serious disease process in central or peripheral sites. The factors that regulate the HPO axis and modulate the timing of puberty remain elusive, but it is evident that some regulation is under genetic control. Identification of specific chromosomal abnormalities and gene mutations allows for diagnostic testing and enables the physician to offer accurate counseling of the recurrence risk for relatives.

Classification[29,30]

There are 2 major classes of precocious puberty: disorders that result from early reactivation of the HPO axis (referred to as Gn-dependent or central precocious puberty, CPP) and those that do not (referred to as Gn-independent precocious puberty). Most girls who present with precocious puberty have CPP, which results from the secretion of GnRH from the hypothalamus. Majority of girls have no discernible structural CNS lesion and are thus said to have an "idiopathic" form of the disorder.

GnRH-Dependent (True Precocity)
- *Idiopathic*   74%
- *CNS tumors*   7%
  - Craniopharyngioma
  - Hypothalamic hamartoma
  - Optic glioma, astrocytoma, and others
- *Other CNS disorders*
  - Static encephalopathy (secondary to infection, hypoxia, trauma, etc.)
  - Low-dose cranial radiation
  - Hydrocephalus
  - Arachnoid cyst
  - Septo-optic dysplasia
- *Secondary central precocious puberty (CPP)*
  - After late treatment of congenital adrenal hyperplasia (CAH)
  - Hypothyroidism with elevated follicle stimulating hormone (FSH)

GnRH-Independent (Precocious Pseudopuberty)
- Ovarian (Cyst or tumor)   11%
  - Granulosa or theca-cell tumors
  - Simple follicular cyst
  - Estrogen-secreting tumors (teratomas, dysgerminomas)
- McCune-Albright syndrome   5%
- Adrenal feminizing   1%
- Adrenal masculinizing   1%
- Ectopic gonadotrophin (Gn) production   0.5%

Other Disorders of Premature Sexual Maturation (Gn-independent)
- Premature thelarche.

- Premature thelarche variant (slowly progressive precocious puberty/ exaggerated thelarche)
- Isolated menarche.

Particular attention should be given to the following possibilities:

- Drug ingestion.
- Cerebral problems such as cranial trauma or encephalitis.
- Retarded growth with symptoms of hypothyroidism.
- Pelvic or abdominal mass.

GnRH-Dependent Precocious Puberty

- There is a premature maturation of the HPO axis, resulting in production of Gn's and sex steroids. It runs in families and usually occurs very close to borderline age of 8 years. On the other hand, idiopathic precocious puberty does not run in families and occur much earlier in childhood. These diagnosis should be made only by exclusion and deserve long-term follow up as cerebral abnormalities may not become apparent until adulthood.
- ***Clinical presentation*** of true precocity may not follow the usual progression of puberty. Adrenarche or menarche may be the first sign. There is normal reproductive life and it is not associated with premature menopause. Intellectual and psychosocial developments are also commensurate with chronological age rather than stage of puberty. The most serious effect is the resultant adult short stature.

GnRH Independent Precocious Puberty

Gn-independent precocious puberty is characterized by increased production of gonadal steroids, causing the typical physical changes of puberty, in the absence of reactivation of the HPO axis.[27] This form includes conditions that mimic the effect of pituitary Gn on gonadal function, such as those in which there is secretion of Gn from nonpituitary sources:

- Eleven percent of girls with precocious puberty have an *ovarian tumor*. The tumor is usually an estrogen producing neoplasm or cyst. Bleeding is irregular and menorrhagic—clearly anovulatory. A pelvic mass is readily palpable in 80% of cases.

- ***McCune-Albright Syndrome*** (MAS) is characterized classically by the clinical triad of cutaneous hyperpigmentation (café-au-lait spots), polyostotic fibrous dysplasia, and isosexual precocious puberty.[31] In addition, this syndrome can be associated with ovarian cysts, growth hormone, and prolactin secreting adenomas, hyperthyroidism, adrenal hypercortisolism, and osteomalacia. Premature menarche may be the first sign of the syndrome. However, these endocrine disturbances are not accompanied by increased plasma concentrations of the relevant trophic or stimulatory hormones. Thus, girls with precocious puberty caused by MAS have ovarian enlargement and follicular hyperplasia but have low serum levels of LH and FSH and a prepubertal response of LH to administration of GnRH.[32] Eventual fertility is unimpaired and adult height is usually normal.
- ***Autonomous benign ovarian follicular or luteal cysts***. The cysts may enlarge, involute, and then recur so that signs of sexual precocity and vaginal bleeding remit and exacerbate.

Diagnosis of Precocious Puberty

Aims of Diagnosis

- Rule out life-threatening disease (includes neoplasms of the CNS, ovary, and adrenal).
- Define the progression of the process.
- Rule out nonendocrine causes of vaginal bleeding (Trauma, foreign body, vaginitis, genital neoplasm).

Differential Diagnostic Steps

Diagnostic confirmation is based on demonstration of pubertal levels of Gn and sex steroid secretion. Diagnosis of CPP is classically made when magnetic resonance imaging (MRI) is negative and a significant LH response occurs following GnRH stimulation that is 2 to 3 times higher than the prepubertal response. Typically, stimulated LH levels rise to > 10 mIU/mL in CPP.[30] Physical examination should focus on determining whether the development reflects androgen action, estrogen action, or both.

Physical Diagnosis

- Record of growth, Tanner stages, height and weight percentiles.
- External genitalia changes.
- Abdominal, pelvic and neurological examination.
- Signs of androgenization.
- Special findings—McCune Albright syndrome, hypothyroidism.
- *If the all signs of sexual precocity are present and basal or GnRH stimulated Gn's are in the pubertal range*: suspect apituitary source of Gn.
- *When signs of sexual precocity are associated with accelerated growth and skeletal maturation in the absence of virilization*: suspect ovarian tumor or cysts.
- *If signs of sexual precocity are accompanied by virilization*: suspect an adrenal hyperplasia or a virilizing adrenal / ovarian tumor.
- *If breast and genital development, pubic hair growth, and vaginal bleeding are seen in a short child with a delayed bone age*: suspect primary hypothyroidism.

Laboratory Diagnosis:

- Diagnostic evaluation should **begin with an X-ray** to assess **bone age** as a marker for sex steroid hormone action. When skeletal age is concordant with chronological age continued close observation could be done.
- **When secondary sexual characteristics are associated with an advanced bone age**, measurements of: E2, DHEAS, testosterone, progesterone, 17-hydroxy progesterone, Gn's and thyroid hormones should be obtained, and a GnRH stimulation test is indicated to differentiate between CPP and peripheral precocious puberty.
- In most cases, the diagnosis of Gn-dependent precocious puberty warrants an USG of abdomen and pelvis and MRI or CT scan of the head.

Treatment of Precocious Development

The objective of management and treatment of precocious puberty include:

1. Diagnose and treat intracranial disease.
2. Arrest maturation until normal pubertal age.
3. Attenuate and diminish established precocious characteristics.
4. Maximize eventual adult height.
5. Avoidance of abuse, reduction of emotional problem. Contraception if necessary.

Long-term complications of true idiopathic precocious puberty include compromised adult height and psychosocial and behavioral issues. Adult height can be improved with treatment if treatment is instituted prior to epiphyseal closure.[33]

A number of therapies have been used to achieve these goals. These have included:

- **Medroxyprogesterone** and **cyproterone acetate** are not fully effective in inhibiting pubertal or skeletal maturation or improving adult height.
- **Danazol**
- **GnRH agonists** Continuous, nonpulsatile presentation of GnRH to the pituitary Gn's induces a state of secondary hypogonadism. Treatment is maintained until the epiphyses are fused or until appropriate pubertal and chronological ages are matched.
  - Substantial regression of pubertal characteristic, amenorrhea, and reduction in growth velocity are rapidly achieved and maintained within the 1st year of treatment.
  - The greatest improvement is obtained in children whose bone ages are relatively young at the onset of treatment. It does not substantially affect adult height in girls who enter puberty between 6 and 8.[34]
  - Majority experience no increase in breast development, and a third show regression to an earlier Tanner stage. Some experience transient vaginal bleeding ~2 to 4 weeks after initiation of therapy due to estrogen withdrawal.
  - Growth can get suppressed to a subnormal velocity due to the decreased estrogen (suppressed by the analogue). Supplementation with **mini-dose estrogen replacement** is safe and effective (for at least 2 years) in maintaining normal prepubertal growth without acceleration of bone maturation or pubertal development.[35]

- GnRH agonist treatment is not effective for **Gn-independent precocious puberty** such as Mc-Gune Albright syndrome, GnRH-independent sexual precocity or CAH. Treatment for MAS involves inhibiting the synthesis or action of sex steroids by inhibiting the synthesis of estrogen (aromatase inhibitors) and using a combination of drugs like cyperoterone acetate, MPA, spironolactone, ketoconazole and testolactone.
- **Neurosurgical excision** of hypothalamic, pituitary, cerebral or pineal tumors must be individualized in each patient.
- For **ovarian or adrenal tumor:** surgical excision is the treatment of choice.
- For primary hypothyroidism: give **thyroid replacement**
- For adrenal hyperplasia: **glucocorticoids** (and **mineralocorticoids** if salt wasting is present) is the treatment of choice.

Forms of Precocious Puberty

1. **Precocious pubarche** is most often a benign condition secondary to **early adrenarche**. In some patients, premature pubarche may predict the future development of chronic anovulation and androgen excess associated with polycystic ovarian syndrome.
2. **Premature thelarche** usually occurs in the first 2 years of life (classical type), is self-limiting, and regresses before puberty. There is asymmetrical breast development with no other signs of sexual maturation; growth is normal. Approximately 10 to 15% of these girls develop CPP, but in the majority of patients, the breast bud is a transient event that warrants only close follow-up for the appearance of other pubertal signs.[36] It is typically associated with:
   - Some degree of FSH secretion.
   - Antral follicular development.
   - Ovarian function that is greater than normal.
3. **Thelarche variant** represents a spectrum of conditions, which lie between premature thelarche and CPP. There is usually pubic hair development; growth prognosis is normal; and breast development arrests without advancing to full sexual maturation.
4. **Isolated menarche** young girls have 6 weekly cyclical uterine bleeding without any other form of sexual maturation and have normal growth. Resolution can occur after 1 or 2 years.[29]

OVARIAN CYSTS

Ovarian cysts can occur in early childhood (3-8 years of age), but are more common in neonatal and adolescent periods. The incidence is < 5 % between birth and age 8. Small cysts are more frequent than large cysts.[37]

Types

- Functional cysts-due to ovarian gonadotrophin stimulation and failure of follicular apoptosis.
- Ovarian neoplasia.
- Hormone secreting cysts can cause rapid pubertal development/precocious pseudopuberty (McCune Albright syndrome).
- The onset of pubertal signs can be transient with breast development increasing during ovarian cyst formation and decreasing with spontaneous resolution.
- Unilocular cysts < 5 cm should be followed up conservatively with USG until they regress. Beyond 5 cm size, there is risk of torsion with rapid progression.

Clinical Presentation

- Asymptomatic cyst
- Painful abdomino-pelvic syndrome (acute/ sub acute): associated with non-specific signs (nausea, vomiting, urinary disorders)
- Endocrine signs: marked by precocious development of sexual characteristics, associated with increased growth velocity and advanced bone maturation. Rapid breast development followed by metrorrhagia suggests pseudo precocious puberty due to ovarian cysts. Café-au-lait spots and polyostotic dysplasia characterizes McCune Albright syndrome.

Diagnosis

- ***Pelvic ultrasonogram***: Note the size, shape and volume of cyst; thickness and regularity of wall; nature of cyst contents. Functional cysts are anechoic with thin, regular wall. Condition of contra lateral ovary is also noted.

- **Color Doppler** for vascularization of mass (e.g. hemorrhagic cyst can be echogenic but avascular).
- **CT/ MRI**
- **Hormonal** E2, testosterone, and other androgens, LH and FSH. Hyper secretion of E2 with negligible LH and FSH that do not respond to stimulation with LHRH confirm autonomous independent Gn secretion and suggest secretory tumor.
- **Tumor markers** α fetoprotein $\rightarrow$ embryonic carcinoma and immature teratoma.
- **β hCG** $\rightarrow$ choriocarcinoma and dysgerminoma
- **Ca 125** $\rightarrow$ can be high even in functional cysts.

Other Condition Associated with Cysts

- *Acquired infantile hypothyroidism*
- *Adrenal disorder*
- *Benign teratoma*
- *Juvenile granulose cell tumors*
- *Sex cord-stromal and mixed germ cell tumors.*

Management

- *Anechoic cyst:* monitor for 4 weeks to 6 months. An increase in size beyond this period or persistence warrants excision.
- *In cases of adnexal torsion or if the cyst is heterogeneous:* emergency surgery should be performed.
- *Recurrence of secretory cyst* is suggestive of McCune Albright syndrome. Granulosa cell tumors are rare and associated with precocious pseudopuberty, therefore these are treated surgically.

SUMMARY

- An orderly approach to the history and physical examination aids in making a correct diagnosis.
- One should remember that it is important to gain the confidence of the child and make the process as pain-free as possible.
- Providing clear explanations of the problem assists in lowering the parents' anxiety and reassuring them that there are rarely any long-term consequences of these common problems.

REFERENCES

1. Emans SJ, Grace E, Hoffer FA, Gundberg C, Ravnikar V, Woods ER. Estrogen deficiency in adolescents and young adults: impact on bone mineral content and effects of estrogen replacement therapy. Obstet Gynecol 1990; 76:585-92.
2. Bradshaw K, George N, Moore A, Trump D. Mutations of the XLRS1 gene cause abnormalities of photoreceptor as well as inner retinal responses of the ERG. Doc Ophthalmol 1999;98:153-73.
3. Kass-Wolff JH and Wilson EE. Pediatric Gynecology: Assessment Strategies and Common Problems. Semin Reprod Med 2003;21(4):329-38.
4. Pokorny S. Pediatric & adolescent gynecology. Compr Ther 1997;23:337-44.
5. Speroff L, Glass R, Kase N. Clinical Gynecologic Endocrinology and Infertility. 6th edn. Baltimore: Williams & Wilkins; 1999.
6. Baldwin DD, Landa HM. Common problems in pediatric gynecology. Urol Clin North Am 1995;22:161-76.
7. Sane K, Pescovitz OH: The clitoral index: A determination of clitoral size in normal girls and in girls with abnormal sexual development. J Pediatr 1992; 120:264-66.
8. Elisabeth Thibaud. Gynecologic clinical examination of the child and adolescent. Sultan C (Ed): Pediatric and Adolescent Gynecology: Evidence-based Clinical Practice. Endocr Dev Basel, Karger, 2004;7:1-8.
9. Pokorny SF, Kozinetz CA. Configuration and other anatomic details of the prepubertal hymen. Adolesc Pediatr Gynecol 1998;1:97-103.
10. Gardner JJ. Descriptive study of genitalia variation in healthy, non-abused premenarchal girls. J Pediatr. 1992;120:251-57.
11. McCann J, Voris J, Simon M, Wells R. Comparison of genital examination techniques in prepubertal girls. Pediatrics. 1990;85:182-87.
12. Emans J. Office evaluation of the chilled and adolescent; Emans J, Laufer MM, Goldstein DF (Eds): Pediatric and Adolescent Gynecology. Philadelphia, Lippincott, 1998.
13. Eleonora Porcu. Imaging in Pediatric and Adolescent Gynecology. Sultan C (Ed): Pediatric and Adolescent Gynecology. Evidence-based Clinical Practice. Endocr Dev. Baasel, Karger, 2004;7:9-22.
14. Orsini LR, Salardi S, Pilu G, Bovicelli L, Cacciari E: Pelvic organs in premenarchal girls: Real time ultrasonography. Radiology, 1984;153:113.
15. Hewitt G. In-Training Section. Examining Pediatric and Adolescent Gynecology Patients. Strickland J (Ed). J Pediatr Adolesc Gynecol 2003;16:257-58.
16. Sultan C, Paris F, Jeandel C, Lumbroso S, Galifer RB, Picaud JC. Ambiguous Genitalia in the Newborn: Diagnosis, Etiology, and Sex Assignment. Sultan C (ed): Pediatric and Adolescent Gynecology. Evidence-Based Clinical Practice. Endocr Dev. Basel, Karger, 2004;7:23-38.
17. Dominique Hamel-Teillac. Vulvo-Vaginal Disorders. Sultan C (Ed): Pediatric and Adolescent Gynecology. Evidence-

Based Clinical Practice. Endocr Dev Basel, Karger, 2004; 7:39-56.

18. Christensen EH, Oster J. Adhesions of labia minora (synechia vulvae) in childhood: A review and report of fourteen cases. Acta Paediatr Scand 1971;60:709-15.

19. Pokorny SF. Prepubertal vulvovaginopathies. Obstet Gynecol Clin North Am 1992;19:39-58.

20. Sanfilippo JS, Muram D, Lee PA, Dewhurst J. Pediatric and Adolescent Gynecology. Philadelphia: WB Saunders; 1994.

21. Emans S, Laufer M, Goldstein D. Pediatric and Adolescent Gynecology. 4th edn. Philadelphia: Lippincott Williams & Wilkins; 1998.

22. Gerstner GJ, Grunberger W, Boschitsch E, Rotter M. Vaginal organisms in prepubertal children with and without vulvovaginitis. Arch Gynecol 1982; 231:47.

23. Smith YR, Berman DR, Quint EH. Premenarchal Vaginal Discharge: Findings of Procedures to Rule Out Foreign Bodies. J Pediatr Adolesc Gynecol 2002;13:227-30.

24. Widholm O: Genital bleeding during childhood. Pediatr Ann 1981;1016.

25. Tyring S, Arany I, Stanley M, et al. A randomized, controlled, molecular study of condylomata acuminata clearance during treatment with imiquimod. J Infect Dis 1998;178: 551-55.

26. McCune KK, Horbach N, Dattel BJ. Incidence and clinical correlates of human papillomavirus disease in a pediatric population referred for evaluation of sexual abuse. J Pediatr Adolesc Gynecol 1993;6:20-24.

27. Plant TM. Puberty in primates. In Knobil E, Neill JD (Eds). The Physiology of Reproduction. 2nd ed. New York: Raven Press; 1994:453-85.

28. Herman-Giddens ME, Slora EJ, Wasserman RC, et al. Secondary sexual characteristics in young girls seen in office practice: A study from the paediatric research in office settings network. Pediatrics 1997; 99:505-12.

29. Stanhope R, Traggiai C. Precocious puberty (Complete, Parial). Sultan C (Ed): Pediatric and Adolescent Gynecology, Evidence-Based Clinical Practice. Endocr Dev. Basel, Karger, 2004;7:57-65.

30. Kakarla N, Bradshaw KD. Disorders of Pubertal Development: Precocious Puberty. Semin Reprod Med. 2003;21(4):339-51.

31. De Sanctis C, Lala R, Matarazzo P, Balsamo A, Bergamaschi R, Cappa M. McCune-Albright syndrome: A longitudinal clinical study of 32 patients. J Pediatr Endocrinol Metab 1999;12 (6): 817-26.

32. Holland FJ, Fishman L, Bailey JD, Fazekas AT. Ketoconazole in the management of precocious puberty not responsive to LHRH analogue therapy. N Engl J Med 1985;312:1023-28.

33. Klein KO. Precocious puberty: Who has it? Who should be treated? J Clin Endocrinol Metab 1999;84:411-14.

34. Hillard PJA. Menstruation in young girls: A clinical perspective. Obstet Gynecol 2002;99:655-62.

35. Lampit M, Golander A, Guttmann H, Hochberg Z. Estrogen mini-dose replacement during GnRH agonist therapy in central precocious puberty: A pilot study. J Clin Endocrinol Metab 2002;87:687-90.

36. Bradshaw KD, Quigley CA. Disorders of pubertal development. In: Jameson JL (Ed): Principles of Molecular Medicine. Totowa, NJ: Humana Press; 1998:569-80.

37. Millar DM, Blake JM, Stringer DA, Hara H, Babiak C. Prepubertal ovarian cyst formation: 5 years' experience. Obstet Gynecol 1993;81:434-38.

6.
Adolescent Gynecology

Arun Nagrath
Pratap Kumar
Rupinder Kaur Ruprai

INTRODUCTION

Adolescence, the period between childhood and adulthood, is usually defined by the rapid onset of biological and psychological growth and development before or at the 2nd decade of life, ending before age 20. Major social and environmental factors influence the onset, duration, and completion of adolescence. In this phase of transition, psychological problems in a process of re-understanding oneself are rampant and are often associated with minor disorders which may prove to be of concern to their parents.

The gynecological problems encountered in adolescents (who are no longer children and not adults either) are often both medically and psychologically complex and thus require a highly skilled and coherent approach. The way to interact and manage them is not the same as dealing with adults. Certain conditions are specific to adolescents that require special skills in counseling and management and providing them special care to meet their medical and psychosocial needs. There is need for clinicians to extend a careful understanding of the biological and psychosocial changes of adolescence, the associated environmental changes, and the legal and ethical issues that affect the provision of health care services.

Adolescent health care services focus on the use of health guidance to promote the use of screening to identify conditions that occur relatively frequently and cause significant suffering either during adolescence or later in life.

Various problems can present in this age group[1] such as:

- Dysfunctional uterine bleeding (39%)
- Amenorrhea (25.7%)
- Vulvovaginitis (10%)
- Ovarian tumor (2.4%)
- Dysmenorrhea (5.7%)
- Oligomenorrhea (3.3%)
- Sexual abuse (2.4%)
- Others (11.5%).

PHYSIOLOGY OF PUBERTY

Puberty is defined as the period of development culminating in sexual maturity. The physical changes accompanying pubertal development (appearance of secondary sexual characteristics, acceleration of growth, onset of menarche, the capacity for fertility and psychological changes), result directly or indirectly from maturation of the hypothalamic-pituitary-ovarian (HPO) axis, stimulation of the sex organs and the secretion of sex steroids. Hormonally, puberty is characterized by the resetting of the classic negative gonadal steroid feedback loop, alterations in gonadotropin (Gn) rhythm and the acquisition in the women of a positive estrogen feedback loop, controlling the monthly rhythm as an interdependent expression of Gn's and ovarian steroids. The cascade of events initiated by the release of pulsatile GnRH from prepubertal feedback and central negative inhibition results in increased levels of Gn's and steroids with appearance of secondary sexual characteristics and eventual adult function (menarche and later ovulation). Normal and abnormal events related to puberty are discussed in Chapter 23.

EXAMINATION OF THE ADOLESCENT GIRL

Objectives:
- Clinical assessment
- Diagnosis and therapy
- Establishment of interpersonal relationship to support those especially with concerns of puberty, sexuality, and fertility.

Preparation for Examination

Adolescents should be given an opportunity to speak privately with their physician without parental involvement. While parental involvement should be respected and encouraged, it must be balanced with the patient's right to privacy and confidentiality.

Prior to the gynecological examination, it is important to note and assure:
- A thorough explanation of the pelvic examination with the use of diagrams.
- A full medical assessment.
- Consent.
- The least invasive examination that is will suffice in fulfilling the objective should be sought.
- Examinations should not be omitted solely because of age of the patient.
- Cultural issues should be respected.

Breast Examination

- The breast bud can be palpated before it actually appears. At this stage, examination can be tender. It appears as a small firm mound beneath an enlarged areola.
- The onset of development between the two breasts can be unequal with a time lag of 3 to 12 month difference. With in 2-4 years from then, it reaches its fully developed size. During the developmental phase, the breast is firm.[2]

For the sexually active adolescents: vaginal examination, speculum examination, PAP smear, and samples to look for genital infections should be done.

Bimanual examination is indicated in adolescents with *gynecologic complaints* or *unexplained abdominal or pelvic pain*.

Vaginal examination with the use of a speculum is indicated with:
- Irregular bleeding
- Menorrhagia
- Vaginal discharge
- Suspected sexually transmitted diseases (STD).

In this age group, the genital tissues are estrogenized and vaginal introitus is more elastic which can allow speculum insertion. However, the size of the hymenal opening should be considered when choosing the speculum.[3]

Radiological tests may be performed when in suspicion of an abdominal mass, abdominal pain, or precocious puberty. Pelvic ultrasonography (USG), computed tomography (CT), or a magnetic resonance imaging (MRI) scan can be scheduled if imaging is indicated.

Counseling and confidentiality plays an important role in this delicate age group. Potential therapy with the use of anatomical charts is helpful. A relationship of trust should be ascertained between the physician and the patient.

DELAYED PUBERTY

This is an important area for clinicians dealing with adolescent. This is discussed in the chapter dealing with puberty.

ABSENT OR PARTIAL VAGINA

Absent or partial vagina may be associated with some of the conditions that cause delayed puberty.

Frank technique or perineal dilation: The only non-surgical option, this technique is successful only in patients with a long rudimentary vagina. Patients apply progressive pressure to the perineum using a bicycle-seat stool to hold a dilator in place. Patient compliance is often poor due to discomfort.

Surgical care: The ideal repair provides the patient with an unscarred vagina that allows sexual functioning.[4] The surgical techniques are discussed in Chapter 2 that deals with disorders of the development of the Müllerian system.

SECONDARY AMENORRHEA/ OLIGOMENORRHEA

Abnormal uterine bleeding is a clinical problem that is encountered frequently during the adolescent years due to the lack of maturity of hypothalamus pituitary ovarian axis. This is discussed in Chapter 9 that deals with abnormal menstruation.

ABNORMAL UTERINE BLEEDING

Abnormal vaginal bleeding accounts for a significant portion of adolescent gynecological complaints. In adolescents, mean duration of menses is 4.7 days, cycle 21-40 days and average blood loss is 35 ml.

Menstruation

There is significant variability in post-menarchal menstrual cycles. Early menstrual cycles can range from 18 to 80 days in the 1st year following menarche, and usually over the next 5 years, they become more frequent, with normal variability from 20-40 days.[5]

During the first 2 years after menarche, most cycles are anovulatory. The transition from anovulatory to ovulatory cycles results from "maturation of HPO axis" characterized by positive feed back mechanisms in which rising estrogen level triggers a surge of LH hormones and ovulation.

* However, heavy, prolonged and recurrent menstrual periods are not normal adolescent patterns of bleeding and may represent an underlying **coagulation defect** in about 20% of patients.[6]
* Heavy bleeding can also be due to **acquired disorder of platelet dysfunction** including Immune thrombocytoplastic purpura, aplastic anemia, and leukemia. Incidence of 13% of thrombocytopenia was found among girls who presented with menorrhagia.[7] Detail discussion of abnormal uterine bleeding is given in Chapter 8.

Premenstrual Syndrome

Definition: The cyclic appearance of one or more of a large constellation of symptoms just prior to menses, occurring to such a degree that lifestyle or work is affected followed by a period of time entirely free of symptoms.

The most frequently encountered symptoms (usually occurring in last 7-10 days of the cycle) include:
* Abdominal bloating
* Anxiety
* Breast tenderness
* Crying spells
* Depression
* Fatigue
* Irritability
* Thirst and appetite changes
* Variable degrees of edema of the extremities.

Prevalence: Approximately 40% women report significant problems related to their cycles and about 2-10% report a degree of impact on work or lifestyle.

Diagnosis: There are guidelines for the diagnosis of PMS as described by American Psychiatric Association that called PMS as *luteal phase dysphoric disorder*. It gave the following criteria:

A. Symptoms are temporally related to the menstrual cycle, beginning in the last week of the luteal phase and remitting after the onset of menses.

B. The diagnosis requires at least five of the following and one of the symptoms must be either one of the first four:

1. Affective liability, e.g. sudden onset of being sad, tearful, irritable or angry.
2. Persistent and marked anger or irritability.

3. Marked anxiety or tension.
4. Markedly depressed mood, feelings of hopelessness.
5. Decreased interest in usual activities.
6. Easy fatigability or marked lack of energy.
7. Subjective sense of difficulty in concentrating.
8. Marked change in appetite, overeating or food craving.
9. Hypersomnia or insomnia.
10. Physical symptoms such as breast tenderness, headache, edema, joint or muscle pain, and weight gain.
C. The symptoms interfere with work, usual activities, or relationships.
D. The symptoms are not an exacerbation of a psychiatric disorder.

Treatment: Most women who seek care for PMS have symptoms not related to the timings of menstruation. Before the diagnosis is established, women must record symptom ratings daily for at least two full cycles. At the same time patient must be screened for other psychiatric disorders.

Women should be advised number of life style changes:
1. Elimination of caffeine from the diet
2. Smoking cessation
3. Regular exercise
4. Regular meals and a nutritious diet
5. Adequate sleep
6. Stress reduction by reducing responsibilities and by relaxation exercises like *yoga*.

Various Drugs Used in Management

1. **Alprazolam:** It has antidepressant, anxiolytic and smooth muscle relaxant properties. A dose of 0.25 mg BD or TDS during the luteal phase in very effective.
2. **Fluoxetine:** It is a selective serotonin reuptake inhibitor. It is effective for luteal phase dysphoric disorder. It is used in daily dosage of 20-60 mg for 1-2 weeks preceding menstruation.
3. **Other drugs**: OCPs, vitamin B_6, bromocriptine, monoamine oxidase inhibitors, and synthetic progestational agents. Women with PMS with deficiency of fatty acid metabolism were advocated evening of primrose oil. It provides linoleic and gamma linoleic acid (precursor PGE). Many have used spironolactone for women with a major complain of bloating.

4. **Medical and surgical oophorectomy:** Described to have dramatic success. A lasting response to surgical hysterectomy and oophorectomy was reported in women unresponsive to medical therapy, but in adolescent women, surgical management is not considered.
5. **GnRH agonist:** Treatment can produce hypogonadotropic hypoganadism, i.e. medical oophorectomy. GnRH agonist treatment has been effective. Estrogen and progestin is added to avoid the side effects of GnRH agonist, but this may diminish the improvement in PMS symptoms.

PELVIC PAIN AND RECURRENT ABDOMINAL PAIN

The pelvic pain can be:

Acute Pain

It is intense and characterized by sudden onset, sharp rise, and short course.

Causes:
  I. *Gynecological disease or dysfunction*:
    1. Acute Infection:
        a. Endometritis
        b. Pelvic Inflammatory disease (Acute salphingo oophoritis)
        c. Tubo ovarian abscess:
           i. Rupture
          ii. Torsion
    2. Adenexal Disorders:
        a. Hemorrhagic functional ovarian cysts
        b. Torsion of Adnexa
        c. Twisted Para ovarian cyst
        d. Rupture of functional ovarian cyst/ovarian neoplasm
  II. *Gastrointestinal:*
    1. Gastroenteritis
    2. Appendicitis
    3. Bowel obstruction
    4. Diverticulitis

III. *Genitourinary:*
1. Cystitis
2. Pyelonephritis
IV. *Musculoskeletal:*
1. Abdominal wall hematoma
V. *Others:*
1. Acute porphyria
2. Aneurysm.

Assessing the **character of pain** is very useful in analyzing the etiology.
- Rapid onset of pain is more consistent with perforation of hollow viscus or ischemia.
- Colic or severely cramping pain is commonly associated with contraction or obstruction of a hollow viscus such as an intestine or a uterus
- Pain perceived over the entire abdomen suggests a generalized peritonitis.

Chronic Pelvic Pain

It is defined as pain of greater than 6 months duration.

Causes:
I. *Gynecological:*
1. Adhesions/endometriosis
2. Salpingo-oophoritis:
   a. Sub-acute
   b. Chronic
3. Ovarian neoplasm's like teratomas
II. *Gastrointestinal:*
1. Recurrent appendiceal colic
2. Infectious diarrhea
3. Recurrent partial small bowel obstruction
III. *Genitourinary:*
1. Recurrent or relapsing cystourethritis
2. Pelvic Kidney
IV. *Musculoskeletal causes.*

Cyclic Pain

It is defined as pain that occurs at a definite time with a definite association to the menstrual cycle. Dysmenorrhea is the most common cyclic pain phenomenon.

Causes:
1. *Dysmenorrhea*
   a. Primary

b. Secondary:
- Imperforate hymen
- Transverse vaginal septum
- Cervical stenosis
- Uterine anomalies (bicornuate uterus, blind uterine horn)
- Endometeriosis[8]

2. *Mittelschmerz syndrome*

Dysmenorrhea

Dysmenorrhea is pain with menstruation usually cramping in nature and centered in the lower abdomen. This subject is discussed in detail in Chapter 7 that deals with dysmenorrhea.

PELVIC INFLAMMATORY DISEASE

It is a polymicrobial disease, which can cause endometritis, parametritis, oophoritis, and tubo-ovarian abscess. This presents in girls who are sexually active. Treatment involves broad-spectrum antibiotics. Failure to respond warrants diagnostic laparoscopy to rule out other causes and if needed to drain tubo ovarian abscess.

Vulvovaginal Complaints

Pruritis Vlvae

It is an itching sensation with a desire to scratch vulva. The various **causes associated with vaginal discharge** are:
- Trichomonas vaginalis
- Candida albicans: accounts for 80% of cases of pruritis vulva.

Causes not Associated with Vaginal Discharge

a. *General disease:* Diabetes, jaundice, uremia, cirrhosis, hemochromatosis
b. *Nutritional:* Iron deficiency anemia, vitamin A and B_{12} deficiency, achlorhydria
c. *Allergies:* Drugs, soap, detergents, antiseptics, deodorants, dusting powder, wearing tight synthetic undergarments, condoms, spermicidal agents
d. *Parasitic infections:* Pediculosis, scabies
e. *Vulval diseases:* Condyloma acuminate, granulomas Bchiet's syndrome, Paget's disease, vulvar cancer.

f. *Cervical causes:* Cervicitis, erosion causing excessive mucoid discharge

g. *Anal disease:* Thread worm infestation

h. *Urinary diseases:* Bacilluria, acidic urine, incontinence, glycosurea

i. *Psychological:* Psychoneurosis due to stress

j. Generalized/localized dermatitis, psoriasis, eczema.

Vaginal Discharge

May be physiological or pathological

Physiological Discharge

1. Normal increased amount of vaginal discharge as seen at time of ovulation (ovulation cascade from cervix):
   - Premenstrual phase
   - During pregnancy
   - During sexual excitement (outpouring of Bartholin's secretions).

2. Leucorrhea: Increased amount of normal vaginal discharge. The causes are:
   - At birth, due to stimulation of uterus and vagina by placental estrogens
   - At puberty
   - Active or passive congestion of pelvic organs especially cervix as seen in:
     i. Prolonged ill health
     ii. Anxiety states and neurosis
     iii. Sedentary occupation
     iv. Standing for long periods in hot atmosphere
   - Increase in glandular elements in the cervix as in case of cervical erosion or ectopy
   - Vaginal adenosis
   - Estrogen-progesterone OCPs use.
   - Regular douching of vagina, which washes away natural secretions and protective lactobacilli.

Pathological Discharge

1. Inflammatory discharge:
   - Vulvovaginitis: gonococcus, *Trichomonas vaginalis, Candida albicans,* bacterial vaginosis, nonspecific organisms in childhood and old age.
   - Cervicitis: gonorrhea, Chlamydia, anaerobic organisms, puerperal infection.
   - Endometritis: puerperal or senile
   - Secondary infection of wounds, abrasions, burns, chemical injuries.

2. Neoplasms

3. Urinary and feculent discharge due to presence of fistula.

4. Rarely, intermittent emptying of hydrosalpinx, discharge of ascitic fluid through fallopian tubes and uterus.

OVARIAN ENLARGEMENTS IN ADOLESCENT GIRL

The ovarian tumor represents the major diagnostic and therapeutic challenge to the gynecologist today. Ovarian masses, cystic and solid, may occur at any age. They can be non-neoplastic or neoplastic.

Non-neoplastic Enlargements of the Ovary

Follicular Cyst

This is the most frequent type, but from the neoplastic standpoint, the least important variety of ovarian cyst. It arises from the ovarian follicles through the process called atresia folliculi where every month a number of follicles undergo atresia with death of the ovum. They appear as tiny, often microscopic cysts lined by one or more layers of granulosa cells and found in considerable numbers even in normal ovaries. They may attain the size of 8 to 10 cm and they can then become of clinical importance producing discomfort in the pelvis.

Nevertheless these cysts spontaneously regress in most instances, as do the evidences of precocity, it must be assumed that a surge of pituitary gonadotropic hormone has occurred that is transient and thus self-limiting. When symptoms like amenorrhea are prolonged, stimulation of postovulatory change by administering oral medroxy progesterone acetate 10 mg three times a day over a period of 5 to 7 days will generally bring on menstruation. Clomiphene citrate 50 mg given orally for 5 consecutive days helps to induce ovulation and brings about menstruation or pregnancy.

Neoplastic Enlargement of Ovary

An ovarian tumor in adolescents is more often malignant than benign. Most of the germ cell tumors (60%) occur in young girls.

Dysgerminoma

Before the age of 20 its occurrence is 40–45%. It presents with abdominal pain. In 90% of cases, menstrual history is normal. In younger age group, its recurrence is most likely.

Endodermal Sinus (yolk sac) Tumor

It is a rare tumor but the 2nd most common of yolk sac origin, thought to originate from multipotential embryonal tissue as a result of selective differentiation of yolk sac structures. The tumor characteristically presents with papillary projections composed of a central core of blood vessels enveloped by immature epithelium, Most of the patients are children or young women presenting with abdominal pain and pelvic mass. It responds to chemotherapy with good survival rate.

Choriocarcinoma

Rarely seen in a pure form. Generally, it is a part of a mixed germ cell tumor. It secretes large quantities of human chorionic gonadotrophin (hCG), which forms an ideal tumor marker in the diagnosis, and management of the tumor. The tumor is highly malignant and metastasizes by blood stream to the lungs, brain, bones, and other body viscera.

Embryonal Cell Carcinoma

It is a rare, highly malignant tumor accounting for about 5% of all germ cell tumors that occurs in prepubertal girls. It elaborates both a fetoproteins and hCG. It is associated with symptoms of precocious puberty and menstrual irregularities.

Granulosa Cell Tumor

It is a sex cord stromal tumor with feminizing functioning mesenchymoma. These tumors are interesting growths of the ovary composed of cells closely resembling the granulosa cells of the graffian follicles. The main clinical features depend on the estrogenic activity of the tumor and only larger ones cause pain and abdominal swelling. It can result in precocious puberty with development of secondary sexual characteristics, hypertrophy of the breast and external genetalia, pubic hair and myohyperplasia of the uterus. The endometrium shows an estrogenic anovulatory pattern. Removal of the tumor causes regression of all these manifestations.

Concern with use of oral contraceptive pills in adolescents with ovarian tumor[9]

In adolescents with malignancy and a central venous line, the added risk for VTE in the presence of prothrombotic states (e.g. OCs) is unknown, but may be increased.[10,11]

- Female adolescents with malignancy often are treated with OCPs. An association between hormonal therapy and venous thromboembolism (VTE) is well established. Presence of a central venous line (CVL) is also a major risk factor for development of VTE.[12,13]

- The mature hemostatic system may be the cause of adolescents having an increased incidence of VTE compared to other younger children.[14]

The mechanism of OC-associated VTE: It is not known but is probably due to its estrogen component. However, recent studies have found that the progestin component also has an effect on VTE risk as third-generation OCs confer a two to three-fold greater risk of VTE than second generation OCs, which contain a different progestin component.[15]

POLYCYSTIC OVARIAN SYNDROME (PCOS)

It was earlier known as **Stein Leventhal syndrome**. It is estimated to occur in 5% of the population. The patients are mostly 15 – 25 years of age. PCOS includes chronic non-ovulation and hyperandrogenemia associated with normal or raised estrogen, raised LH, and low FSH/LH ratio. The girl complains of oligo-menorrhea and often amenorrhea of a few months. Infertility occurs in 30%. Obesity and hirsutism are the additional features. Ultrasonogram (USG) shows several subcapsular cysts of varying size diagnostic of PCOS.

In order to prevent its long-term consequences, it is best diagnosed early. Unfortunately, it is difficult to make the diagnosis in early puberty as most girls after menarche have anovulation, multiple small cysts on their ovaries, elevated LH and testosterone levels, and decreased SHBG.[16]

The actual risk of an adolescent with a PCOS-like condition of developing adult PCOS is unknown.

- In adolescents with anovulatory cycles and increased levels of testosterone and androstenedione, 70% get normal menstrual cycles after 5 years.[17]
- However, with very high levels of testosterone and androstenedione as well as hirsuitism, the anovulatory cycles are likely to persist into adulthood. In adolescents with anovulatory cycles and high LH levels 4 years after menarche, 57% of patients continue to have anovulation and increased LH levels.[18]
- Adolescents who develop adult PCOS have irregular menstrual cycles and increased androgens and LH, but they rarely have increased insulin levels, unlike in adults, as girls in puberty have an increased sensitivity to insulin that later normalizes as they become adults.[19]

Menstruation

Many PCOS patients have irregular menstrual cycles or are amenorrheic. Physicians must ensure that these patients are having menstrual cycles at least 4 times per year. If the patient is not able to regulate her cycles with diet and exercise, she must be given periodic progestins to allow her endometrium to shed. Endometrial cancer can occur in PCOS patients in their 20s who have had years of unopposed endogenous estrogen. Another way to regulate these patients is to place them on the OCPs, but they must be warned that their irregular cycles will return when they discontinue the medication.[20]

Pregnancy

Women with PCOS have a higher early miscarriage rate compared to the general population.[21] They are at increased risk of developing gestational diabetes and pregnancy-induced hypertension. These effects are independent of the patients' BMI.[22]

Treatment

- **Weight loss** is important as it helps in restoring the hormonal milieu to some extent.

- **Cigarette smoking** raises DHEA and androstenedione levels and should be avoided.
- **Estrogen** suppresses androgen and adrenal production. It is best given with progestogens with no androgenic properties, especially as in oral contraceptives.
- **Dexamethasone** 0.5 mg or prednisone 5 mg at bedtime also reduces androgen production.
- Hirsutism is treated with **cyproterone acetate** or **spironolactone**
- Infertility is treated with **clomiphene citrate** 80% ovulate and 40% conceive.

EATING DISORDERS

The incidence peaks in the 13 to 18 years old age group in women. These girls present with amenorrhea or infertility. Oligomenorrhea can also be caused by eating disorders including over eating. Eating disorders can also exacerbate an underlying menstrual problem as seen in PCOS.[23]

The prognosis for patients with eating disorders follows the rule of thirds: 1/3 recover completely, 1/3 have persistent lifelong concerns about their weight, and 1/3 have a chronic relapsing illness where death occurs in 2%–5%.[24]

- **Sexuality:** OCPs do not work well in this population. Induced vomiting does not allow consistent hormonal levels to prevent ovulation. Thus, there is a high rate of therapeutic abortions in the bulimic population.[25]
- **Menstruation:** Oligomenorrhea and amenorrhea can be the result of weight gain or loss, caloric restriction, excessive exercise, or psychogenic stress. A weight 10% below the normal for the patient's height can delay menarche from the expected time by causing hypothalamic dysfunction.[25] Likewise, a gain or drop in weight from the patient's baseline can cause menstrual changes and are usually anovulatory.

ATHLETIC ADOLESCENTS

The female athlete triad consists of amenorrhea, an eating disorder, and osteopenia. A caloric deficit leads to a disruption in the pulsatile release of GnRH, resulting in low levels of gonadotrophins and secondarily reduced levels of estrogen and progesterone, leading to amenorrhea and osteopenia.[24]

- **Amenorrhea:** There is a higher incidence of delayed menarche and menstrual dysfunction in girls who start intensive athletic training and dieting before menarche or early post-menarchal period.[26] Amenorrhea varies from 6%–43% depending on the intensity of the exercise (intensity is a more important factor than total time). A shortening of cycle length is frequently observed in exercising females.[27]

- **Osteopenia:** The vast majority of bone mass is acquired by the end of the 2nd decade of life. Adolescent athletes who are amenorrheic are osteopenic in their early adult years.[28] A bone mass density should be measured after 6 months of amenorrhea and if osteopenia is found, hormonal treatment should be started, such as oral contraceptive pill with calcium supplementation. Adequate calcium intake is important in achieving peak bone mass (current recommendation for adolescent females is 1500 mg/day).

TURNER'S SYNDROME

Turner's syndrome is the most common form of gonadal dysgenesis in females that leads to premature ovarian failure. Incidence is 1 in 2500 female live births. Most Turner's patients require HRT to undergo pubertal development and protect their bones and heart. These patients also have an increased incidence of other associated anomalies and concerns with their cardiovascular systems.[20]

Most patients are sterile with streak ovaries. However, 5%–10% of Turner's mosaic patients undergo spontaneous pubertal development, and 2% of these are fertile.[29] It is very important to discuss contraception with spontaneously menstruating Turner's patients as their pregnancies are at risk for chromosomal problems and malformations.[30]

CONGENITAL ADRENAL HYPERPLASIA (CAH)

Ninety-five percent of childhood CAH cases are of classic 21-hydroxylase deficiency. Approximately 75%

of these are salt wasters. Girls are usually virilized *in utero* and born with abnormal external genitalia. The internal genitalia are normal.[20]

Puberty and Menstruation

- Pubertal development occurs normally if adequately treated from an early age. However, most CAH girls have delayed menarche.[31]

- If the disease is left untreated/under-treated with glucocorticoids, the child will enter puberty early with an advanced bone age. Likewise, if the disease is over-treated, puberty is often delayed and menarche can be absent.

- They have oligomenorrhea and anovulation, as the LH surge is inhibited by steroid substrates. Some never ovulate normally, even on adequate replacement medication. Polycystic ovaries in them are also common, which produce more androgens and prevents ovulation.

Sexuality

- They are more likely to have delayed heterosexual milestones as lesbians or to have bisexual imagery.[32] Negative body image, less sexual activity, and decreased sex drive[33] is seen in them due to high levels of progesterone in the follicular phase (acts like a biological minipill, preventing regular ovulation and decreasing libido).[34]

CYSTIC FIBROSIS

Cystic fibrosis (CF) is the most common serious autosomal recessive genetic disease with a mean age of survival of 28 years. Cystic fibrosis girls have normal secondary sexual development; however, their puberty and menstruation may be delayed in severe disease. These women have normal reproductive tracts with slightly decreased fertility.[20] The reasons for the subfertility includes thick cervical mucus, poor nutritional status, severe respiratory disease, and increased incidence of anovulation.

- An increased incidence of stress incontinence (due to frequent coughing) is also seen.

- Oral contraceptive pills (OCPs) can exacerbate their respiratory tract, diabetes, malabsorption, and hepatic dysfunction. The progestins increase the production and viscosity of respiratory tract mucus, impair glucose tolerance, and promote hyperplasia of goblet cells, causing increased intrahepatic cholestasis and cholelithiasis. Despite the concern with OCP use, the overall experience has been favorable and without significant adverse events.

EPILEPSY

Epilepsy is the most common neurological disorder seen in the reproductive years with a prevalence of 1%. Seizure disorders that continue into adolescence often remain into adulthood.[20]

Menstruation

A seizure disorder may be exacerbated with menarche in 37% of patients. Up to 50% of epileptic women, have seizures that occur at predictable times in the menstrual cycle, with 70% in the premenstrual time when estrogen and progesterone are high.[35]

Oral contraceptive pills (OCPs) are often used in epileptic patients to regulate their menstrual cycle, but on anti-epileptic drugs, seizure medications decrease the effectiveness of low-dose OCPs.

CHILDHOOD CANCER SURVIVORS

Cytotoxic cell damage is progressive and irreversible in the ovary, where the number of germ cells is fixed and cannot be regenerated. Gonadal function is more likely to be preserved if treatment occurs prepubertal. Strategies to decrease ovarian damage from cancer treatments include substitution of alkylating agents, cyclical rather than continuous regimens, surgically tacking the ovaries out of the radiation field, ovarian suppression during treatment (with OCPs, GnRH agonists, GnRH antagonists), and cryopreservation of ovarian tissue before treatment.[36]

Radiation

Permanent ovarian failure occurs if the ovary receives > 1000 rads of radiation.[37] Premature menopause is more common if the teenager received radiation therapy in addition to chemotherapy.[38] Ovary decreases in size with loss of follicles, and FSH levels are found in the menopausal range. Prepubertal abdominal or pelvic radiation exposure can cause delayed menarche.

Chemotherapy

Chemotoxic agents act on primordial follicles by inducing apoptotic changes in the pregranulosa cells and causing follicle loss. The alkylating agents (such as cyclophosphamide, melphalan, and chlorambucil) are the most harmful to undeveloped oocytes (4.5-fold risk), whereas antimetabolites and plant alkaloids are safer for the ovary.[36]

ADOLESCENT PREGNANCY

Adolescent pregnancy is always an accident associated with high-risk behavior. More than 40% of women in the United States become pregnant before they reach 20 years of age. In UK, 9 in 1000 girls aged 13-15 and 63 in 1000 girls aged 16-19 become pregnant. Other than abortion as an outcome of this, other problems of concern include aggression during course of pregnancy, addictive behavior, and congenital malformations. Teenagers that are pregnant consistently have less prenatal care, they are more likely to smoke, and they deliver infants with lower birth weights. Besides the numerous pregnancy related complications, early parenthood tends to curtail opportunities for education and employment, hampering social and cultural development. Efforts to teach sexuality and contraception have resulted in decrease in sexual activity in adolescents.[39]

TERMINATION OF PREGNANCY

Twenty percent of the therapeutic abortions done in the United States are performed on women who are less than 19 years of age.[39] Termination of pregnancy in an adolescent girl is a serious problem from medical, legal, and social angles. Legally no girl can be pregnant before 15 years of age. If a girl below 18 years becomes pregnant, she cannot give a valid consent for medical termination of pregnancy (MTP). Consent of parent/ legal guardian is required for termination on a girl below 18 years of age. Any abortion that is not performed in accordance of MTP Act amounts to illegal abortions and the doctors performing such an operation is liable for punishment. These laws vary from country to country.

SEXUALLY TRANSMITTED DISEASE (STD)

Sexually transmitted disease (STD) rates have always been higher in adolescents compared to adults. About 60% of these infections occur in young people <25 years of age, and 30% of this age group is <20 years. Between ages of 14 and 19, STDs occur more frequently in girls than boys by a ratio of 2:1 (due to deficiency in progesterone as a result of HPO instability, which results in increased vulnerability of female genital tract to infection). These diseases are caused by bacterial, viral, fungal or protozoal infection. Besides HIV and hepatitis B, most common infections include Chlamydia, *N. gonorrheae,* human papilloma virus (HPV), herpes simplex virus (HSV), and syphilis.

- ***Future Fertility:*** Future tubal damage from common STDs can be severe despite minimal or no clinical signs. The severity of the infection influences future outcome. Those with severe infections have a five-fold higher rate of infertility compared to mild cases.[40] Although the prognosis for future fertility is improved with appropriate use of antibiotics, the real need is to prevent episodes of PID.

SEXUAL ABUSE

Clinicians are frequently asked to determine whether a child has been sexually abused. In such cases, one should be familiar with the locally mandated reporting laws. Young children who have been sexually abused do not always present with physical signs of injury as the abuse may have occurred some time ago, or there may not have been actual attempt to penetrate the vagina. Behavioral symptoms vary for each individual. Sleep disturbances with nightmares may be seen. Children who perform sexual acts on others are often found to have a history of abuse. Physical symptoms may include enuresis, encopresis, dysuria, vaginal bleeding, and pelvic or abdominal pain.[41] Collection of forensic evidence should be handled by an experienced practitioner with recognition of the emotional needs of the child as well as the legal requirements.

SUMMARY

Failure to address both the physical concerns and their reproductive implications can have profound lifelong consequences, especially if the reproductive desires cannot be fulfilled. Not *every* condition encountered can be rectified, but with sensitive physiological management, appropriate treatment, and the use of new reproductive technologies, most of these patients with early gynecological concerns can live normal sexual and reproductive lives.

REFERENCES

1. Paula J, Adams Hillard. Gynecological Needs of Children and Adolescents: One-Year Experience of a Pediatric and Adolescent Gynecology Clinic. Cincinnati Children's Hospital Medical Center, Cincinnati, OH. NASPAG 18th Annual Clinical Meeting.
2. Elisabeth Thibaud. Gynecologic clinical examination of the child and adolescent. Sultan C (Ed): Pediatric and Adolescent Gynecology. Evidence Based Clinical Practice. Endocr Dev Basel, Karger, 2004;7:1-8.
3. Hewitt G. In-Training Section. Examining Pediatric and Adolescent Gynecology Patients. Strickland J (Ed). J Pediatr Adolesc Gynecol 2003;16:257–58.
4. Edmonds DK. Congenital malformations of the genital tract and their management. Best Pract Res Clin Obstet Gynaecol 2003; 17(1):19-40.
5. Treloar A, Boynton R, Behn B, et al. Variation of the human menstrual cycle through reproductive life. Int J Fertil 1967; 12(1):77.
6. Claessens EA, Cowell CA. Acute adolescent Menorrhagia. Am J Obstet Gynecol 1981;139(3):277-80.
7. Beven JA, Maloney KW, Hillery CA et al. Bleeding disorders: A common cause of Menorrhagia in adolescents. J Pediatr 2001; 138(6): 856-61.
8. Gidwani G. Endometriosis is more common than you think. Contemp Ob/Gyn 1989; 33:75.
9. Douketis J, Chan AKC, and Massicotte P. Opinions in Pediatric and Adolescent Gynecology. Does Oral Contraceptive Therapy Do More Harm than Good in Adolescents Who Are Receiving Chemotherapy? Jamieson MA (Ed). J Pediatr Adolesc Gynecol 2003;16:377–79.
10. Revel-Vilk S, Chan AK, Bauman M, et al. Prothrombotic conditions in an unselected cohort of children with venous thromboembolic events. J Thromb Haemostas 2003; 1:915.
11. Nowak-Gottl U, Junker R, KreuzW, et al. Risk of recurrent venous thrombosis in children with combined prothrombotic risk factors. Blood 2001; 97:858.
12. Massicotte MP, Dix D, Monagle P, et al. Central venous catheter related thrombosis in children: Analysis of the Canadian Registry of Venous Thromboembolic Complications. J Pediatr 1998; 133:770.

13. Monreal M, Alastrue A, Rull M, et al. Upper extremity deep venous thrombosis in cancer patients with venous access devices–prophylaxis with a low molecular weight heparin (Fragmin). Thromb Haemost 1996; 75:251.

14. Andrew M, Vegh P, Johnston M, et al. Maturation of the hemostatic system during childhood. Blood 1992; 80:1998.

15. Vandenbroucke JP, Rosing J, Bloemenkamp KW, et al. Oral contraceptives and the risk of venous thrombosis. N Engl J Med 2001; 344:1527.

16. Rosenfield RL, Ghai K, Ehrmann DA, et al. Diagnosis of polycystic ovary syndrome in adolescence: Comparison of 76 Elford and Spence: The Forgotten Female adolescent and adult hyperandrogenism. J Pediatr Endocrinol Metab 2000; 13(5):1285.

17. Apter D, Vihko R. Endocrine determinants of fertility: Serum androgen concentrations during follow-up of adolescents in the third decade of life. J Clin Endocrinol Metab. 1990; 71:970.

18. Venturoli S, Porcu E, Flamigni C. Polycystic ovary syndrome. Curr Opin Pediatr 1994; 6:388.

19. Van Hoof M, Voorhorst F, et al. Polycystic ovaries in adolescents and the relationship with menstrual cycle patterns, luteinizing hormone, androgens, and insulin. Fertil Steril 2000; 74(1):49.

20. Elford KJ, Spence JEH. Mini-Review-The Forgotten Female: Pediatric and Adolescent Gynecological Concerns and Their Reproductive Consequences. J Pediatr Adolesc Gynecol 2002;15:65–77.

21. Tulppala M, Stenman U, Cacciatore B, et al. Polycystic ovaries and levels of Gn's and androgens in recurrent miscarriage: Prospective study in 50 women. Br J Obstet Gynaecol 1993;100:348.

22. Urman R, Sarac E, Dogan L, et al. Pregnancy in infertile PCOD patients. Complication and outcome. J Reprod Med 1997; 42(8):501.

23. Morgan J. Eating disorders and reproduction. Aust N Z J Obstet Gynaecol 1999; 39(2):167.

24. Gidwani G, Rome E. Eating disorders. Clin Obstet Gynecol 1997;40(3):601.

25. Katz M, Vollenhoven B. The reproductive endocrine consequences of anorexia nervosa. Br J Obstet Gynaecol 2000;107:707.

26. Hergenroeder A. Bone mineralization, hypothalamic amenorrhea, and sex steroid therapy in female adolescents and young adults. J Pediatr 1995; 126(5):683.

27. Allen D. Effects of fitness training on endocrine systems in children and adolescents. In: Advances in Pediatrics. New York, Mosby Inc., 1999;41-66.

28. Warren M, Steihl A. Exercise and female adolescents: Effects on the reproductive and skeletal systems. JAMWA 1999; 54(3):115.

29. Hovatta O. Pregnancies in women with Turner's syndrome. Ann Med 1999; 31:106.

30. Tarani L, Lamperiello S, et al. Pregnancy in patients with Turner's syndrome: Six new cases and review of literature. Gynecol Endocrinol 1998; 12:83.

31. Brook CG. The management of classical congenital adrenal hyperplasia due to 21-hydroxylase deficiency. Clin Endocrinol 1999; 33:559.

32. Money J, Schwartz M. Dating, romantic and nonromantic friendships and sexuality in 17 early treated adrenogenital females aged 16–25. In PA Lee, LP Plotnick, AA Kowarski (Eds): Congenital Adrenal Hyperplasia. Baltimore: University Park Press, pp 419–31.

33. Kuhnle U, Bollinger M, et al. Partnership and sexuality in adult female patients with congenital adrenal hyperplasia. J Steroid Biochem Mol Biol 1993; 45:123.

34. Helleday J, Siwers B, Ritzen E, et al. Subnormal androgens and elevated progesterone levels in women treated for congenital virilizing 21-hydroxylase deficiency. J Clin Endocrinol Metab 1993; 76:933.

35. Penovich P. The effects of epilepsy and its treatment on sexual and reproductive function. Epilepsia. 2000; 41(2):553.

36. Blumenfeld Z, Avivi I, et al. Preservation of fertility and ovarian function and minimizing chemotherapy induced gonadotoxicity in young women. J Soc Gynecol Invest. 1999; 6(5): 229.

37. Schover L. Psychosocial aspects of infertility and decisions about reproduction in young cancer survivors: A review. Med Pediatr Oncol 1999; 33:53.

38. Chatterjee R, Goldstone A. Gonadal damage and effects on fertility in adult patients with haematological malignancy undergoing stem cell transplantation. Bone Marrow Transplant 1996; 17:5.

39. Adolescent Pregnancy Facts 2000 pamphlet. American College of Obstetricians and Gynecologists.

40. Westrom L, Mardh P, et al. Acute pelvic inflammatory disease. In: Sexually Transmitted Diseases (2nd edn). New York, McGraw-Hill Co., 1987.

41. Kass-Wolff JH, Wilson EE. Pediatric Gynecology: Assessment Strategies and Common Problems. Semin Reprod Med 2003; 21(4):329-338.

7. *Dysmenorrhea*

PK Shah
Sheetal Dholakia

INTRODUCTION

This chapter deals with dysmenorrhea which is one of the commonest gynecological disorders affecting women in the reproductive age group. Dysmenorrhea is defined as pain associated with menstruation.

It describes the various types of dysmenorrhea with their risk factors and etiology. The management protocol has been schematically represented using flowcharts, describing the various medical and surgical methods. Dysmenorrhea is preventable to some extent and the preventive measures have also been listed. A brief mention has been made of the recent advances made in the management of this disorder and the various differential diagnosis of this condition. The aim of this chapter is to enable the student to have a concise and complete overview of this menstrual disorder.

The term dysmenorrhea is derived from a Greek word: *Dys*—difficulty, *Menorrhea*—monthly flow.

Thus meaning difficulty in monthly flow and practically implying difficult or painful menstruation.

DEFINITION

It is defined as pain associated with menstruation.

It is a major cause of absenteeism from work amongst women thus decreasing efficiency and quality of life among affected women.[1,9]

INCIDENCE

Dysmenorrhea is one of the commonest gynecological complaints among women, but the exact incidence is difficult to estimate. Pain is a subjective symptom and cannot be accurately estimated by an outside observer, since different women may perceive pain with different severity and tolerance. It is now estimated that almost 50% of all women experience some degree of dysmenorrhea while 10% are incapacitated by it.

RISK FACTORS FOR DYSMENORRHEA

The following are some of the proposed risk factors for dysmenorrhea:

Menstrual Factors[7]

1. Early Menarche—A study conducted on adolescent girls revealed that early age of menarche was associated with a higher incidence of dysmenorrhea.
2. Long and heavy menstrual flow—It was also seen that women with long and heavy cycles had more severe dysmenorrhea.

Parity

The incidence of dysmenorrhea is lower in multiparous women. It was seen that the incidence of primary dysmenorrhea decreased after the first delivery. It was also found to be decreased in terms of severity.[8]

Diet

Lower consumption of fish, eggs and fruits are believed to increase the incidence of dysmenorrhea but the association is not clearly established.[8]

Exercise

Various types of exercises were advocated to reduce dysmenorrhea. It was also seen that among athletes the incidence of dysmenorrhea was lower, probably due to anovulatory cycles. But good evidence for that explanation same is lacking.[10-12]

Cigarette Smoking

Heavy smoking was found to be associated with decreased duration of bleeding but increased duration of dysmenorrhea. Thus duration of dysmenorrhea was increased in heavy smokers with no effect on cycle length.[13]

Psychological

Emotionally dependent and overprotected girls are more likely to develop dysmenorrhea. It is also more commonly seen in girls whose mothers suffered from dysmenorrhea, since the mother becomes overzealous and apprehensive around the time of menarche of her daughter which thereby makes the young girl more conscious, aware and paranoid of her forthcoming menses. Rather than being the cause of the pain, it is more likely that the psychological factors modify the pain causing depression and anxiety.[14]

CLASSIFICATION OR TYPES

A. *Primary or spasmodic dysmenorrhea:*
Synonyms—Essential/Intrinsic/Functional. It is defined as painful menstruation in the absence of pelvic pathology.

B. *Membranous dysmenorrhea:*
It is actually a type of spasmodic dysmenorrhea characterized by the passage of an endometrial or decidual cast.

C. *Secondary dysmenorrhea:*
Painful menses secondary to underlying organic disease of the pelvic organs.

Primary Dysmenorrhea

Etiology: There are various theories for the etiology of primary dysmenorrhea and are as follows:[1,4,6]

The prostaglandin theory: This is the most widely accepted theory suggested by Pickles as early as the 1960s. He extracted the smooth muscle stimulant from menstrual fluid which was identified as a mixture of prostaglandins.

Prostaglandins are derived from arachidonic acid. The three main prostaglandins concerned with menstruation are:

$PGF_{2\alpha}$

PGE_2

PGI_2

The main effects of the prostaglandins on dysmenorrhea are as follows:

$PGF_{2\alpha}$ is a potent vasoconstrictor and causes increased myometrial contractility.

PGE_2 increases the sensitivity of the nerve endings.

PGI_2 causes vasodilatation, decreases prior to menstruation leading to ischemia.

Thus there is enough evidence to suggest that prostaglandins play an important role in the etiology of dysmenorrhea:

- Both PGE_2 and $PGF_{2\alpha}$ are present in high quantities in menstrual fluid.
- The established actions of both PGE_2 and $PGF_{2\alpha}$ have been mentioned earlier.

- Prostaglandin synthetase inhibitors are found to relieve dysmenorrhea, decrease menstrual fluid prostaglandin concentration and decrease uterine contractility.

Hormonal or endocrine theory: Dysmenorrhea is characteristically seen in ovulatory cycles where progesterone plays a key role.

The evidence to support this theory is seen in the following facts:

- Anovulatory cycles are usually painless and that is why primary dysmenorrhea starts 1 to 2 years after menarche.
- Oral contraceptive pills which abolish ovulation improve dysmenorrhea dramatically.
- Prostaglandin concentrations are higher in the secretory phase.

Progesterone plays an important role. It is believed that prostaglandin synthesis by the endometrium requires priming by progesterone but the mechanism is not clear.

It is also seen that high doses of oestrogen relieve dysmenorrhea and decrease uterine contractility. Thus it is established that steroid hormones play a role in causing dysmenorrhea but the exact mechanism is not clearly understood.

Vasopressin, which is found in menstrual fluid is also a potent vasoconstrictor.

Myometrial contractility: It is well known that the myometrium contracts in order to shed the endometrium during menstruation.There is no evidence to show presence of uterine hyperactivity at the time of menses but it is believed that irregular dysrhythmic contractions of the uterus or simply increased uterine tone causes dysmenorrhea. The myometrial contraction thus puts a stretch on the uterine nerve fibres thus causing pain.

Myometrial ischemia: In a normal menstrual cycle there is vasodilatation during the secretory phase which increases the tortuosity of the spiral artery. The spiral arteries are the main sources of blood supply to the endometrium.

Just prior to the menses the spiral arteries undergo vasoconstriction. The decrease in uterine blood flow causes ischemia. Ischemia is a known cause of pain and thus this theory compares dysmenorrhea to the pain of angina.

Cervical obstruction: In the earlier years cervical stenosis was believed to be the single most important cause of dysmenorrhea.

Abnormal uteri like septate or bicornuate may be associated with narrow cervices but normal uteri in patients with dysmenorrhea revealed no hysterosalpingographic evidence of cervical narrowing. Thus this theory is less likely to be the cause of dysmenorrhea in anatomically normal uteri.

Psychological: Psychological cause for dysmenorrhea was earlier believed to be the single etiological factor for dysmenorrhea. Later psychological and physiological dysmenorrhea were believed to be mutually exclusive causes. In modern day practice we understand that though dysmenorrhea is proven to be a physiological disorder, psychological factor do play an important role. It is now believed that psychological factors modify pain or its intensity rather than causing it. Thus a *severe* recurring pain can easily cause depression in any woman especially when it alters efficiency.

Thus girls with lower threshold for pain can be completely incapacitated in comparison to women with a higher threshold for pain.

A combination of the above: This is the actual theory of dysmenorrhea wherein pain is a result of the concerted occurrence of two or more factors for, e.g. hormones are precursors of prostaglandins which alter myometrial contractility and thus pain is caused. The psychological factors may play a part in all of the above.

Pathogenesis

The pain pathway for dysmenorrhea is as follows:

Sympathetic fibres pass from the uterus through the posterior roots of T10, T11, T12 and L1 and from the cervix through S2, S3 and S4.[6]

Thus uterine pain is referred to the cutaneous distribution of lower abdominal wall in front, groins, upper and medial aspects of the thighs nearly to the knees and posteriorly to the sacral area and buttocks while that from the cervix to the lower sacral area and buttocks.

Clinical Features[3]

History

Age: usually seen among younger women upto 25-30 years.

Time of onset: 2-3 years after menarche thus corresponding to the beginning of ovulation.

Duration of pain: It starts just prior to the menses lasting for 2 days.

Type of pain: Cramping pain in the above described areas.

Examination

General and abdominal examination: usually normal

Local examination: essentially normal pelvic organs

Management of dysmenorrhea[1]

It can broadly be classified as general and specific measures and is given in Figure 7.1. The management options can be selected based on the severity of dysmenorrhea and is given in Table 7.1.

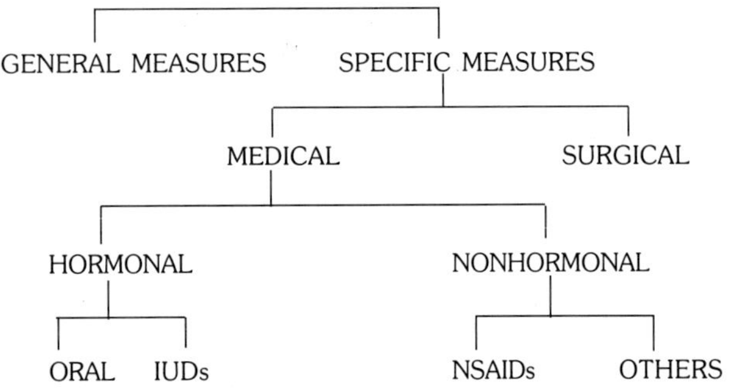

IUD—Intrauterine device
NSAID—Nonsteroidal anti-inflammatory drugs

Figure 7.1: Management of dysmenorrhea

General Measures

These include:

- *Improvement in nutritional state and dietary changes*—A healthy and nutritious diet is a prime factor in the betterment of general health. Thus the inclusion of fruits, eggs and fish in the diet of the

Table 7.1: Severity of dysmenorrhea

Mild	*Moderate*	*Severe or incapacitating*
* Psychotherapy	* NSAIDs	*OC pills
* Counseling to allay anxiety	* OC pills	*Conjugated estrogens
* Occasionally NSAIDs		* Surgery
* Laxatives.		

OC—Oral contraceptives
NSAID—Nonsteroidal anti-inflammatory drugs

patient may help to alleviate the pain of dysmenorrhea to some extent. Recent literature advocates the use of phytoestrogens, i.e. estrogens derived from plant and vegetable sources like soyabeans, chick peas, etc. to reduce dysmenorrhea.

- *Regular exercise*—Various remedial exercises were advocated for dysmenorrhea like floor polishing movements, bending, twisting, swaying, rowing movements and other similar routines. These must be done for at least 15 minutes daily between and during the periods. These can be done in addition to or instead of various game.

- *Explanation regarding the condition and reassurance*—This plays an extremely important role in the management of dysmenorrhea and should be included as an essential component in the treatment plan. The patient must be reassured that dysmenorrhea is not a sign of abnormal reproductive organs or future infertility. One should explain the normal menstrual cycle, its physiology and the cause of dysmenorrhea. She must be told that it is a physiological symptom (except in cases of secondary dysmenorrhea) that could be relieved.

- *Palliative measures like laxatives and hot baths*—These are believed to cause pain relief by increasing the blood supply and thus taking away the ischemic element as the cause of dysmenorrhea.

- *Psychotherapy*—is a vital part and must be offered to all patients of dysmenorrhea—As explained earlier an in depth analysis of the family history of the patient, her personality, her home atmosphere, beliefs in the family towards menstruation and dysmenorrhea and her attitude towards dysmenorrhea must be made and then the patient should be appropriately counseled.

Specific Measures

Medical management

i. **Hormonal**—The use of hormones to reduce dysmenorrhea is on the rise. The pharmacological basis for the use of hormones is simply that anovulatory cycles are not associated with dysmenorrhea. Thus conversion of an ovulatory cycle into an anovulatory one is the principle of treatment using hormones.

a. *Oral hormonal therapy:* Oral contraceptive pills of the combined variety are the best agents in order to convert ovulatory cycles into anovulatory ones. It serves a dual purpose for women with dysmenorrhea and also requiring contraception. They are usually started on the 3rd day of the cycle and continued for 21 days. Recently conjugated estrogens are also being promoted, especially in women suffering from progestogenic side effects like acne, bloating etc. with the combined pill.

b. *Intrauterine device (IUD):*[5] Progestasert, which is a progesterone containing IUD, is being advocated for the treatment of dysmenorrhea. The principle of action of this IUD is that the progesterone is maintained in low concentrations and the prostaglandin concentration will be reduced. It may cause anovulation. The disadvantage of this method is the increased incidence of ectopic pregnancy and its high cost.

ii. **Nonhormonal**

a. *NSAIDs:*[2] Nonsteroidal anti-inflammatory drugs or Prostaglandin synthetase inhibitors (PSI'S) form the mainstay of treatment of primary dysmenorrhea. Amongst the NSAIDs the following are important.

- Fenamates
  Mefanamic acid 250-500 mg 3-4 times a day
  Flufenamic acid 10-200 mg 3 times a day
  Tolfenamic acid 133 mg 3 times a day
- Indomethacin 25 mg 3-6 times a day
- Ibuprofen 200-400 mg 4 times a day
- Naproxen sodium 275 mg 4 times a day

NSAIDs can be started just prior to menses and continued for 5 days.

The doses are as mentioned above but may be altered as required.

b. *Others*

i. *Calcium antagonists:*[5] Calcium antagonists—relax the uterine muscle and reduce pain but they cause bradycardia and hypotension. The common ones used are Nifedepine, Verapamil and Diltiazem.

ii. *Beta adrenergics:*[5] These increase the endometrial flow and thus decrease ischemic pain. They are not commonly used.

Surgical management

The surgical management could be conservative or radical, but are not commonly advocated except in severe cases.

Conservative surgeries[6]

1. Dilatation of the cervix is especially helpful in cases of cervical stenosis.
2. Injection of alcohol into the pelvic plexus is rarely practiced.

Radical surgeries

Cotte's operation or prelumbar sympathectomy

Resection of the hypogastric nerve where it lies in front of the fourth and fifth lumbar vertebrae. The management depends on the severity of dysmenorrhea.

There are various alternative modalities which are currently available:

- *Heat fermentation*—Application of heat over the painful areas especially the back, lower abdomen and thighs often produces relief.
- *Microwave diathermy*[15]—It has been tried in women suffering from severe dysmenorrhea not responding to other medical line of management and has proved to be successful in relieving the same.
- *Acupuncture and Acupressure*—They often prove to be helpful especially in women who have a strong psychological factor and those who have a strong faith in alternative remedies.
- *Yoga*—This provides some form of exercise and at the same time allays anxiety by relaxation thus helping to relieve dysmenorrhea.
- *Ayurveda and Homeopathy*—This century is seeing a lot of alternative types of medicines in practice on the rise. Thus these two major sciences have also proved successful in treating dysmenorrhea.

Membranous Dysmenorrhea

It is a type of spasmodic dysmenorrhea with passage of endometrial cast.

Etiology: Unknown, but is proposed to be due to a hypersecretory endometrium thus leading to thick endometrium which is eventually shed as large fragments or casts.

Histologically the cast is decidua with blood clot.

Patient profile: Usually a young patient and the periods are heavy associated with colicky pain.

Treatment: Is the same as that for primary dysmenorrhea.

Secondary Dysmenorrhea

Synonyms—Extrinsic, congestive or organic.

Etiology

Painful menses secondary to the following underlying organic diseases of the genital tract.

I. Uterine abnormalities
   Congenital:
   1. Redundant uterine horn
   2. Imperforate hymen
   3. Cryptomenorrhea
   Acquired:
   1. Uterine fibroids
   2. Endometrial polyps
   3. Adenomyosis
II. Infections
   Pelvic inflammatory disease of any etiology.
III. Endometriosis
   It is one of the commonest causes of secondary dysmenorrhea.
IV. Foreign bodies
   Intrauterine device.
V. Iatrogenic
   Cervical stenosis following surgery like cone biopsy.

Clinical Features

Age: usually seen among older women in the 3rd–4th decade.

Time of onset: usually follows initial years of normal painless cycles.

Duration of pain: onset few days prior to menses and continues throughout the cycle and even after cessation of menses.

Type of pain: continuous dull aching or dragging type of pain.

On Examination

General: look for anemia.

Abdomen: presence of a mass or doughy abdomen in cases of tuberculosis.

Per vaginum: enlarged uterus or uterine mass altered mobility of the uterus, fornicial tenderness due to adhesions or fornicial mass, e.g. chocolate cysts.

Management

Investigations: Routine investigations like complete blood count to look for anemia or any evidence of infection seen as leucocytosis or raised erythrocyte sedimentation rate.

Urine microscopy to rule out any urinary tract infection.

Stool examination for worm infestation or amoebiasis causing colitis.

Specific investigations
- Ultrasonography to look for any pelvic mass, ectopic pregnancy (positive urine pregnancy test), uterine anomaly or chocolate cysts.
- Hysteroscopy for small polyps which maybe missed on routine pelvic examination.
- Dilatation and curettage for endometrial pathology like carcinoma endometrium, Tuberculosis of the endometrium, cervical stenosis or uterine polyp.
- Laparoscopy for pelvic adhesions, uterine anomalies, infections or ovarian mass.

Treatment

Treatment of the cause and symptoms:
I. Medical—NSAIDs and OC pills.
II. Surgical
   1. Laparoscopic adhesiolysis for pelvic adhesions.
   2. Cystectomy in cases of ovarian cysts including chocolate cysts.

3. Hysteroscopic septum resection in case of septate uterus.
4. Myomectomy for fibroids.
5. Hysteroscopic polypectomy in case of uterine polyps.

Summary of management

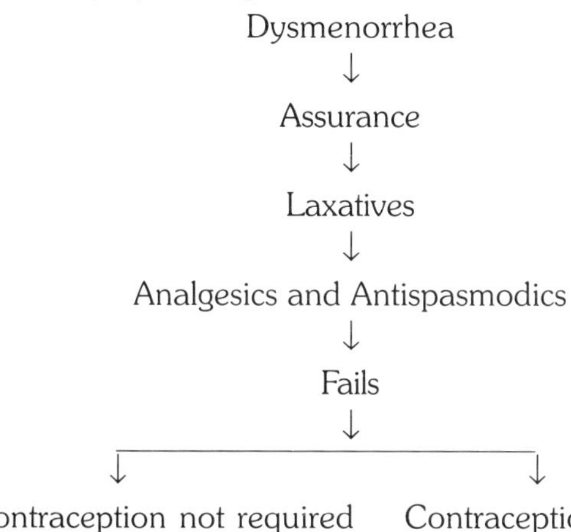

Differential Diagnosis

1. Chronic pelvic pain due to gastrointestinal tract disease.
2. Ectopic pregnancy.
3. Premenstrual tension.
4. Mittelschmerz pain or ovulation dysmenorrhea.
5. Arthritic pain.

Recent Advances in Management

- Laser or laparoscopic presacral neurectomy.
- Progesterone containing IUCD
- Lysine clonixinate for treatment of primary dysmenorrhea—This is a newer NSAID given in a dose of 125 mg tablets 4 times a day. It acts like an analgesic and antispasmodic.[16-18]
- Sublingual piroxicam in a fast dissolving form tablet has been used with minimum side effects and good efficacy.[19]
- Transdermal glyceryl trinitrate acts by relieving myometrial contractions and thus acts as a uterine relaxant.[20]
- Rofecoxib a specific cycloxygenase—2 inhibitor in a dose of 25-50 mg every 24 hours inhibits prostaglandin synthesis.[17]

CONCLUSION

Thus the management of dysmenorrhea starts from correct diagnosis of the condition, differentiation between primary and secondary dysmenorrhea and whether there is need for contraception. Once the correct diagnosis has been made the patient must be reassured and appropriate therapy started. Laparoscopy should be advocated in patients not responding to medical treatment for more than six months to one year. Thus dysmenorrhea is no longer believed to be a psychological problem but often physiological and at times due to pathology which deserves treatment due to its ability to alter efficiency and quality of life for a woman.

REFERENCES

1. Parsons. Primary Dysmenorrhea. Text Book of Gynecology 2nd edn, 325-29.
2. Novak. Pelvic Pain and Dysmenorrhea. Berek J (Eds) General Gynecology 6th edn, Williams and Willians; 408-14.
3. Kistner. The Menstrual Cycle. Kistner's Gynecology 6th edn, USA; Harcourt Brace and Co., 1995;44-46.
4. Shaw R. Disorders of Menstruation. Shaw's textbook of Gynecology 12th edn, New Delhi; Churchill Livingstone, 1999;227-29.
5. Dutta. Dysmenorrhea and other disorders of menstrual cycle, Text Book of Gynecology 4th edn, Kolkatta; Central; 1997;168-71.
6. Dawood YM. Dysmenorrhea. Clinical Obstet and Gynecol 1983;26(3): 719-27.
7. Lumsden MA. Dysmenorrhea. Progress in Obstetrics and Gynecology 5:276-89.

8. McLure Browne. Dysmenorrhea. Post graduate Obstetrics and Gynecology, 3rd edn 89-99.

9. Balbi C, Musone R, Menditto A, Di Prisco L, Cassese E, D'Ajello M, Ambrosio D, Cardonel A. Influence of menstrual factors and dietary habits on menstrual pain in adolescence age. Eur J Obstet Gynecol Reprod Biol 2000;91:143-48.

10. Di Cinto E, Parazzini F, Tozzi L, Luchini L, Mezzopane R, Marchini M, Fedele L. Dietary habits, reproductive and menstrual factors and risk of dysmenorrhea. Eur J Epidemiol 1997; 13(8):925-30.

11. Coco AS. Primary dysmenorrhea. Am Fam Physician 1999; 60(2): 489-96.

12. Golomb LM, Solidum AA, Warren MP. Primary Dysmenorrhea and physical activity. Med Sci Sports Exerc 1998;30(6):906-09.

13. Hornsby PP, Wilcox AJ, Weinberg CR. Cigarette smoking and disturbance of menstrual function. Epidemiology 1998; 9(2):193-96.

14. Lawlor CL, Davis AM. Primary dysmenorrhea. Relationship to personality and attitudes in adolescent females. J Adolesc Health Care 1981;1(3):208-12.

15. Vance AR, Hayes SH, Spielholz NI. Microwave diathermy treatment for primary dysmenorrhea. Phys Ther 1996; 76(9):1003-008.

16. Di Girolamo G, Zmijanovich R, et al. Lysine clonixinate in the treatment of primary dysmenorrhea. Acta Physiol Pharmacol Ther Latinoam 1996;46(4): 223-32.

17. Morrison BW, Daniels SE, et al. Rofecoxib, a specific cyclooxygenase—2 inhibitor, in primary dysmenorrhea: randomized controlled trial. Obstet Gynecol 1999; 94 (4) : 504-08.

18. Hernandez Bueno JA, de la Jara Diaz J et al. Analgesic-antispasmodic effect and safety of lysine clonixinate and L-hyoscinbutylbromideo in the treatment of dysmenorrhea. Ginecol Obstet Mex 1998; 66:35-39.

19. Ragni N, Ciccarelli A. Primary Dysmenorrhea treated with sublingual piroxicam. Minerva Ginecol 1993; 45(7-8): 365-75.

20. Moya RA, Moisa CF, et al. Transdermal glyceryl trinitrate in the management of primary dysmenorrhea. Int J Gynecol Obstet 2000;69(2): 113-18.

8.

PK Sekharan

Abnormal Uterine Bleeding

INTRODUCTION

Abnormal uterine bleeding is a common gynecological problem accounting for nearly 15% of the outpatient attendance and almost 20% of the gynecological operations. Abnormalities of cycle length, duration of flow and amount of blood loss are causes for concern for the patient and her relatives. It may be due to organic causes or as a result of the dysfunction of the hypothalamus-pituitary-ovary-endometrial axis—designated as dysfunctional uterine bleeding (DUB). Abnormal uterine bleeding is clinically grouped as bleeding abnormalities in childhood and adolescence, in the reproductive age group and in perimenopause—as the etiology and approach to management is entirely different in these groups of patients. Majority of cases of dysfunctional uterine bleeding may be treated medically, surgical options being considered for those resistant to medical intervention.

This chapter deals mainly with the diagnosis and management of DUB although other causes of abnormal uterine bleeding are mentioned, to stress the point that DUB is a diagnosis of exclusion and that all the organic causes of abnormal uterine bleeding are to be considered in the clinical approach to DUB.

DEFINITION OF DUB

Dysfunctional uterine bleeding (DUB) is a symptom complex that includes any condition of abnormal uterine bleeding in the absence of pregnancy, neoplasm, infection and other pathology of the female genital tract as well as other systemic causes of abnormal bleeding. Such bleeding is most often the result of endocrinologic dysfunction.

PATHOPHYSIOLOGY

Normal Menstruation

Cyclical menstruation is the culmination of programmed hormonal stimulation on the endometrium involving the hypothalamic gonadotropin releasing hormone (GnRH), the two pituitary gonadotropins—follicle stimulating hormone (FSH) and luteinizing hormone, (LH) and the two ovarian steroid hormones—estradiol-17β and progesterone. Between menarche and menopause, 400 to 500 menstrual cycles occur in the average female. Menstruation has three clinical characteristics: the interval or cycle length, the duration of flow and the amount of blood loss. One-fifth of women have the problem of heavy menstrual blood loss at some period during their reproductive life. The average menstrual cycle is of twenty-eight days with an average flow of four days and a mean blood loss of 40 ml. A blood loss of 80 ml or more is considered as menorrhagia.

Table 8.1: Characteristics of normal menstrual cycle

	Average	Range	Abnormal
Cycle	28 days	21-35 days	<21 or >35 days
Duration	4 days	1-7 days	>7 days
Blood loss	40 ml	20-80 ml	>80 ml

Abnormalities in Menstrual Cycle

Abnormal Uterine Bleeding (AUB) is characterized by either:

- Bleeding at abnormal or unexpected times or
- Excessive flow at the time of an expected period.

Table 8.2: Types of abnormal bleeding

Menorrhagia	Excessive bleeding at regular intervals, more than 80 ml.
Menometrorrhagia	Prolonged, irregular, excessive bleeding.
Polymenorrhea	Frequent periods at less than 21-day intervals.
Polymenorrhagia	Excessive bleeding at less than 21-day intervals.
Oligomenorrhea	Infrequent periods at more than 35-day intervals.
Intermenstrual bleeding	Bleeding that occurs between normal cycles.
Postmenopausal bleeding	Bleeding occurring after menopause.

Pathogenesis of Dysfunctional Uterine Bleeding

1. The most common cause for dysfunctional uterine bleeding is anovulation. This is seen in:
   - Perimenarchial and perimenopausal age
   - Polycystic ovary syndrome
   - Obesity-associated anovulation

   Anovulation results in a lack of progesterone and the resultant excessive proliferative response to unopposed estrogen causes stromal cell growth that exceeds the structural integrity of its supporting matrix, and the endometrium breaks down with irregular, heavy bleeding. In the absence of normal mechanisms to limit menstrual blood loss, bleeding can be prolonged and heavy. The amount of blood loss correlates directly with the level of estrogen stimulation.

   Unopposed estrogen stimulation can, over a period of time, induce hyperplasia and lead to cytological changes of atypical adenomatous hyperplasia or even low-grade adenocarcinoma. Such cellular transformation may take 10-20 years and therefore, endometrial sampling should be an integral part of investigations in all elderly patients with abnormal uterine bleeding.

2. Ovulatory cycles may also cause abnormal uterine bleeding in upto 20% of cases as proven by histological studies. Causes are:
   - Persistent corpus luteum, which does not regress in 12-14 days.
   - Luteal phase defect (LPD), an inadequate corpus luteal function.

   Ovulatory patients with abnormal uterine bleeding are more likely to have an underlying organic condition.

CLINICAL PRESENTATIONS OF ABNORMAL UTERINE BLEEDING

Vaginal Bleeding in Prepubertal Girls

- Scanty vaginal bleeding can occur in newborn due to stimulation of the endometrium by placental estrogen, which will resolve spontaneously.
- Vulvitis with excoriation, urethral prolapse, foreign body in the vagina and trauma (sexual abuse) are causes for vaginal bleeding in young girls.
- Vaginal bleeding with the appearance of secondary sexual characteristics before the age of 8 years is called precocious puberty.
- A serious but rare cause of vaginal bleeding in prepubertal age group is rhabdomyosarcoma ("sarcoma botryoides"), which presents with bleeding and a "bunch of grapes" like clustered mass in the vagina.

Points in Diagnosis

- In young girls brought with complaints of vaginal bleeding, especially before the age of 10, one must focus on examining the genitalia, looking for foreign bodies, vaginitis, or genital injury.
- A foul smelling discharge points to the possibility of foreign body or even malignancy.

- Examination maybe aided by general anesthesia and the use of endoscope.
- Abdominal ultrasound will help to identify ovarian tumors.

The management of bleeding in the prepubertal age group is directed to the cause of the bleeding. Sarcoma botryoides is managed by pre-operative chemotherapy followed by conservative surgery or radiation.

Abnormal Uterine Bleeding in Adolescent Girls

- Menorrhagia in the pubertal age is commonly due to anovulation and estrogen excess secondary to a lack of maturation of the negative feedback in the hypothalamo-pituitary axis and may settle by itself within 2 to 3 years of menarche.
- Polycystic ovary syndrome is an important etiological factor for anovulatory bleeding in pubertal age group.
- It is important to remember that coagulation defects is the cause in up to 20%. These include idiopathic thrombocytopenic purpura (ITP), von Willebrand's disease and Glanzmann's thrombasthenia. Menorrhagia may be the only symptom of an inherited bleeding disorder.
- Organic conditions like bicornuate uterus, functioning ovarian tumor and genital tuberculosis can also cause puberty menorrhagia.
- The possibility of pregnancy must be considered when an adolescent presents with abnormal vaginal bleeding.
- Abnormal bleeding can be associated with thyroid dysfunction.

Points in Diagnosis

- History suggestive of coagulation disorders should be elicited, like excessive flow at menarche, petechiae, epistaxis and excessive bleeding at trivial injury or tooth extraction.
- On examination, general appearance suggestive of endocrine disorders, obesity, hirsutism and the presence of any pelvic or abdominal mass should be noted.
- Investigations of abnormal bleeding in the perimenarchial age includes complete blood count, hemoglobin level, platelet count, coagulation studies, and bleeding time to exclude bleeding and clotting disorders.
- A pregnancy test is not out of place in adolescent girls with irregular bleeding.
- An abdominal ultrasound examination is helpful in diagnosis of functioning ovarian tumors, PCOS, bicornuate uterus and pregnancy.

The management of abnormal uterine bleeding in the adolescent girls depends on the severity.

Mild excess bleeding as decided by adequate hemoglobin levels, are best treated with iron supplementation, close follow-up and reassurance.

Patients with *moderate bleeding* may be treated by a combination low-dose oral contraceptive or cyclical progesterone which prevents excessive endometrial build up and excessive bleeding.

In *acute heavy bleeding* not due to coagulation disorders, high dose estrogen followed by long-term hormonal suppression is used.

Surgical intervention like D&C and endometrial sampling are best avoided, but may be necessary to remove thick endometrial debris and to diagnose endometrial tuberculosis.

Abnormal Uterine Bleeding in the Reproductive Age Group

The diagnosis of dysfunctional uterine bleeding in patients of reproductive age is made by exclusion.

- Pregnancy-related conditions like ectopic pregnancy, abortion, and gestational trophoblastic disease are common causes of abnormal uterine bleeding in the reproductive age group.
- Fibroid uterus, endometrial polyp, endometriosis and pelvic inflammatory disease are important organic conditions leading to abnormal uterine bleeding in the reproductive age.
- Polycystic ovary syndrome and obesity will cause hyper-estrogenic anovulatory menorrhagia and may require specific interventions.
- Neoplastic conditions like carcinoma cervix, endometrial hyperplasia and endometrial carcinoma as causes of abnormal bleeding are to be ruled out by proper examination and investigations if suspected.

- Both hypothyroidism and hyperthyroidism may cause abnormal uterine bleeding, as does hepatic and renal failure.
- Irregular bleeding associated with contraceptive use.

Points in Diagnosis

- Medical and gynecological history and exclusion of pregnancy
- History of exogenous hormone intake.
- Hematological studies including coagulation profile
- Pregnancy test
- Trans-abdominal and trans-vaginal ultrasound to aid the diagnosis of organic conditions like fibroid, endometrial polyps and neoplasia.
- Endometrial sampling to diagnose endometrial hyperplasia and carcinoma.
- Hysteroscopy and biopsy has replaced D&C in the diagnosis of intrauterine pathology.

Once organic conditions are ruled out, DUB in patients of reproductive age group is managed by medical therapy. Ablative therapy or hysterectomy may be considered in patients with intractable and recurrent menorrhagia not responding to medical management, if they are not concerned about further child bearing.

Abnormal Bleeding in Perimenopausal Women

The normal perimenopausal menstrual bleeding pattern is that of less frequent and less heavy menses. Irregular and heavy bleeding at perimenopause is usually associated with organic conditions like endometrial polyps and sub-mucous fibroids (18-20%), endometrial cancer (3-5%) and endometrial hyperplasia (1-7%) (Figures 8.1 and 8.2).

The management should always include endometrial sampling, trans-vaginal ultrasonography and hysteroscopic evaluation of intra-uterine pathology. Patients with endometrial hyperplasia are best treated by hysterectomy and attempts at controlling symptoms with hormonal therapy are to be avoided in patients with atypical endometrial hyperplasia. Patients without endometrial hyperplasia or organic conditions are treated with cyclical estrogen—progesterone therapy.

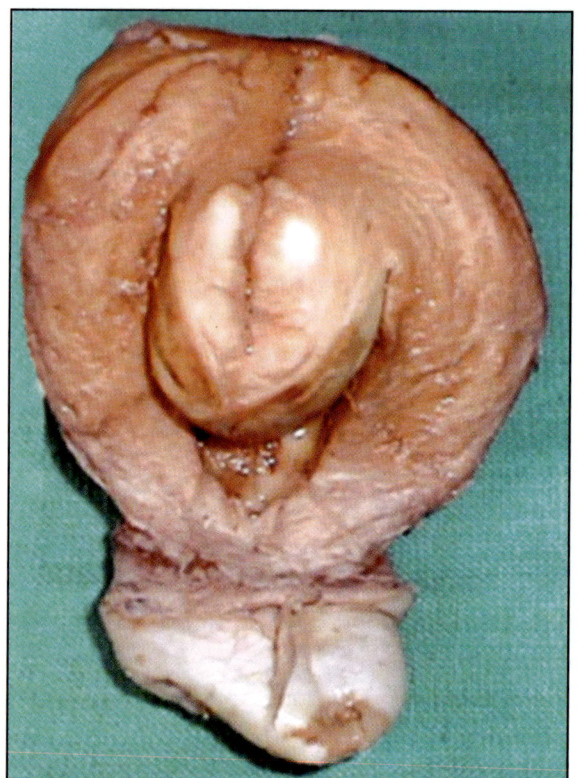

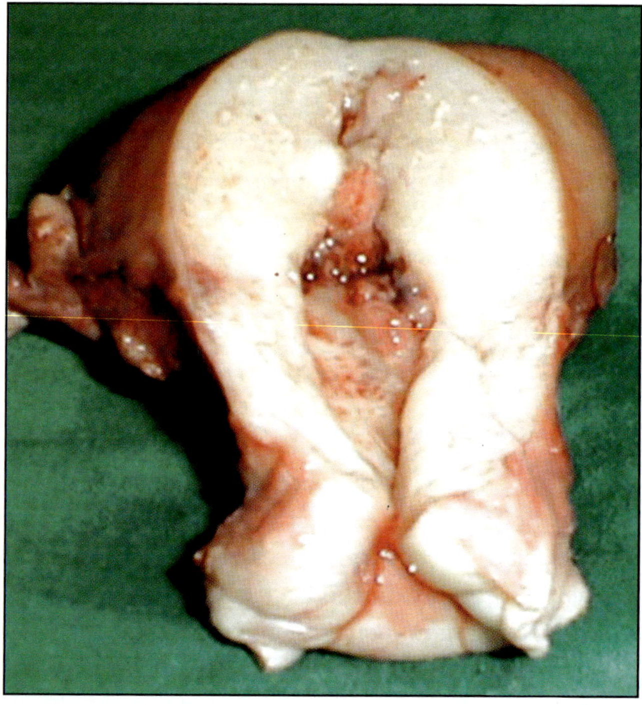

Figures 8.1 and 8.2: Common organic causes of abnormal uterine bleeding in the reproductive age group

Post-menopausal Bleeding

Any bleeding in post-menopausal women should be considered abnormal. The significance of post-menopausal bleeding is its frequent association with gynecologic malignancy, especially endometrial carcinoma. The incidence of post-menopausal bleeding in the age group 50 to 55 years is reported to be 1.3% and at 70-75 years nearly 0.2%. The risk of endometrial cancer is around 11%.

Table 8.3: Causes of post-menopausal bleeding

Benign conditions	Malignant conditions
Endometrial polyps	Endometrial carcinoma
Cervical polyps	Carcinoma cervix
Senile vaginitis	Carcinoma vagina
Vulval dystrophies	Carcinoma vulva
Trauma	Carcinoma of the fallopian tube
Hormone replacement therapy	Secondary tumors

Points in Diagnosis

- Organic conditions and malignancies are always to be kept in mind in this age group.
- A thorough history of the nature of the bleeding and the associated risk factors like diabetes, nulliparity and use of hormones help in diagnosing endometrial carcinoma.
- A thorough physical examination including examination per speculum helps the diagnosis of carcinoma vagina, carcinoma cervix and cervical polyps.
- PAP smear helps in detection of carcinoma cervix in 90% and endometrial carcinoma in 30%.
- Fractional curettage under anesthesia was the standard method of assessing women with post-menopausal bleeding in the past. Recent evaluation of the procedure has shown that adequate tissue is obtained in only 50 to 60% of the cases and being a blind procedure, areas of neoplasia may be missed.
- Vaginal Ultrasonography and hysteroscopy will complement the diagnostic accuracy of endometrial biopsy in post-menopausal bleeding.

Management of post-menopausal bleeding is directed towards the organic conditions detected. In the absence of abnormal hyperplasia and other organic conditions, perimenopausal and post-menopausal women are started on Hormone Replacement Therapy (HRT). Cyclical estrogen for 21 days (conjugated equine estrogen-Premarin 0.625 mg or estradiol valerate-Progynova 1 mg) with medroxy progesterone acetate 10 mg for 12 days in the second half-will be beneficial without the risk of endometrial hyperplasia.

TREATMENT MODALITIES IN DUB

The main concern in DUB is heavy menstrual blood loss and this is the most distressing symptom as far as the patient is concerned. Therefore, the following passage deals with the various medical and surgical modalities in the treatment of menorrhagia. Other aspects of treatment like regularization of cycles and management of anovulatory cycles maybe dealt with elsewhere.

Table 8.4: DUB management

I   *Medical management*
   1. Non-steroidal Anti-inflammatory Drugs (NSAIDs)
      Mefenamic acid, Naproxen, Ibuprofen, Meclofenamate.
   2. Anti-fibrinolytic agents
      Tranexamic acid
   3. Hormones
      - Synthetic Progetogens: Norethisterone, Medroxy progesterone acetate
      - Progesterone impregnated Intra Uterine Devices: Levonorgestrol (Mirena®)
      - Combined Oral Contraceptive Pills
      - Estrogens: conjugated equine estrogen (Premarin®) estradiol valerate (Progynova®)
      - Synthetic Androgen: Danazol
      - Gonadotropin-Releasing Hormone agonists (GnRHa)
      - Anti-estrogen: Gestrinone
   4. Miscellaneous agents: Desmopressin
II   *Surgical management*
   1. Endometrial resection
      - Trans Cervical Resection of Endometrium (TCRE)
   2. Endometrial ablation
      - Microwave endometrial ablation
      - Thermal Balloon ablation
      - LASER ablation
      - Cryo-ablation
   3. Hysterectomy
      - Vaginal hysterectomy
      - Laparoscopic Assisted Vaginal Hysterectomy (LAVH)
      - Total abdominal hysterectomy
      - Laparoscopic supracervical hysterectomy

Non-steroidal Anti-inflammatory Drugs for Heavy Menstrual Bleeding

There is evidence to suggest that the endometrium of women with excessive menstrual bleeding has higher levels of prostaglandins with a change in ratio. There is an increase of PGE_2 and prostacyclin (PGI_2), which are vasodilatory in their effect compared to PGF2-α and thromboxane A_2, which are vasoconstrictor PGs and this results in abnormal hemostasis. Non-steroidal anti-inflammatory drugs or prostaglandin synthetase inhibitors reduce vasodilatory prostaglandin levels in women with excessive menstrual bleeding by inhibiting the enzyme cyclo-oxygenase and so, may have an additional beneficial effect on dysmenorrhea.[2]

NSAIDs used in the management of menorrhagia include mefenamic acid, naproxen, ibuprofen, flurbiprofen, meclofenamic acid, diclofenac, indomethacin, and acetylsalicylic acid. The clinical efficacy of individual NSAIDs is comparable though some may respond well to one agent than to another. Side effects of treatment, especially gastro-intestinal effects like gastritis are variable in frequency but are not usually severe. Gastro-intestinal side effects are less with mefenamic acid than with naproxen.

Dosage

- Mefenamic acid 500 mg TID × 5 days or until bleeding stops.
  (It may be started a few days prior to the anticipated onset of flow with benefit).
- Naproxen 500 mg BD × 5 days.
- Ibuprofen 600 mg to 1200 mg OD × 5 days.
  Mefenamic acid and related compounds will help to reduce the menstrual loss by 25% and thus form an effective first-line medical treatment.

Antifibrinolytic Agents

Fibrinolytic activity is in excess in the endometrium of women with menorrhagia and will adversely affect the local hemostasis. Antifibrinolytic agents like tranexamic acid has been found to reduce menstrual blood loss up to 50%.

Dosage

- Tranexamic acid 1 g QID × 5 days, starting from day 1 of the cycle. Epsilon aminocaproic acid (EACA), another antifibrinolytic agent, is found to be less effective in the management of menorrhagia.

Cyclical Progestogens for Heavy Menstrual Bleeding

Anovulatory cycles are more common at extremes of reproductive life and in women having polycystic ovary syndrome, which will manifest as infrequent menstruation with bouts of heavy bleeding. Prolonged estrogen stimulation of the endometrium without progesterone withdrawal bleeding may cause a build up of the endometrium with erratic heavy bleeding. Supplementing exogenous progesterone, therefore breaks the continuity of proliferative change under estrogen and this forms the rationale for using cyclical progestogens in anovulatory menorrhagia. Progestogen therapy will be sufficient to control heavy bleeding once uterine pathology is ruled out. Progestogens act as anti-estrogens accelerating the conversion of estradiol to estrone which is quickly eliminated from the target cells, inhibiting the augmentation of estrogen receptors, and act as antimitotic anti-growth factors on the endometrium. [3]

Dosage

In anovulatory cycles:
- Norethisterone (Primalut N®) 5 mg TID in the luteal phase for 10-15 days
- Medroxy progesterone acetate (Provera®) 5-10 mg OD in the luteal phase for 10-15 days
- Dydrogesterone (Duphastone®) 10 mg OD in the luteal phase for 10-15 days

There after progestogens are given for 10 days every cycle for 3-6 cycles to have therapeutic effect.

In Ovulatory Cycles

Given cyclically for 21 days starting from 5th day of the cycle for 6 cycles.

This regimen of progestogens may have a role in the short-term management of menorrhagia.[4]

These agents cause withdrawal bleeding—the so called "medical curettage." The different agents have different levels of efficacy, the overall effect ranging from 15-50% reduction of menorrhagia.

Combined Oral Contraceptive Pills for Heavy Menstrual Bleeding

Combined low-dose oral contraceptive pills are effective in heavy menstrual bleeding and reduce blood loss by 60% in DUB.[5]

Dosage

- Ethenyl estradiol 30 µg + Levo norgestrel 150 µg (Ovral L®) BD × 7 days to stop the bleeding and allow withdrawal bleeding to occur, which may be slightly heavy.

  From 5th day of the withdrawal bleed, start the OC pill once a day for 21 days cyclically to allow withdrawal bleed, which becomes progressively lighter.

  For those desiring contraception, this regimen may be continued till desired. In others, 3-6 cycles of therapy may be sufficient. On stopping the pills, some may go in for anovulatory cycles with a short period of amenorrhea followed by menorrhagia as before. To prevent this relapse into menorrhagia, oral progestogens maybe given for 10 days in the second-half.

Progesterone/Progestogen Releasing Intrauterine Devices for Heavy Menstrual Bleeding

It was observed that intrauterine devices, with the addition of progesterone developed as contraceptives and as a uterine relaxing agent to reduce expulsion rate, resulted in a large reduction in menstrual blood loss. This "side effect" is now used in the treatment of menorrhagia.

Agents Used

- Progestasert® (the first hormone impregnated device releasing 65 µgm of progesterone per day) Effective for 18 months.
- Mirena® (a device releasing 20 µgm of levonorgestrel per day) Effective for 5 years.

  These intrauterine devices have been reported to reduce heavy menstrual bleeding by up to 90% with relief of dysmenorrhea.[6] The incidence of pelvic inflammatory disease is also reported to be less due to thickening of cervical mucus. The incidence of amenorrhea at the end of one year is around 20% and during the first year of use the major disadvantage is intermenstrual bleeding and spotting. The levonorgestrel—releasing device (Mirena®), though costly, is a useful treatment for heavy menstrual bleeding with the additional advantage of being a contraceptive, which is effective for five years with return of fertility after removal. The Levonorgestrel intrauterine device is more effective than cyclical oral norethisterone given for 21 days but not as effective as transcervical resection of the endometrium (TCRE) (vide infra).

Estrogen for the Control of Acute Heavy Bleeding

Continuous heavy bleeding can occur in anovulatory DUB in pubertal girls due to prolonged hemorrhagic desquamation of the endometrium. Progestogens in this situation are not going to be effective as there is insufficient tissue for progesterone action. Short-term exposure of the endometrium to estrogen at high-dose will exert a healing effect on the desquamated endometrium and will promote clotting at capillary level.

Dosage

- In acute severe bleeding:
  conjugated equine estrogen (Premarin®) 25 mg IV 4th hourly for 24 hours or until bleeding stops + Progestogen or a combined oral contraceptive (COC) pill, started simultaneously for a week, then stopped to allow withdrawal bleeding. Cyclical progestogen/COC pill is given for 3-6 cycles.
- In less severe bleeding:
  conjugated equine estrogen (Premarin®) 1.25 mg oral for 7 days or estradiol valerate (Progynova®) 2 mg oral for 7 days along with a progestogen/COC pill as above.

Danazol

Danazol is a synthetic androgen introduced initially for the treatment of endometriosis which can result in significant reduction in menstrual blood flow and leads to amenorrhea. It can cause androgenic side effects and is not a first-line treatment for menorrhagia. It is usually used as a short-term pre-operative endometrial-thinning agent prior to endometrial resection.

Dosage:
- Danazol (Ladogal®) 400 mg OD × 3-6 months.

GnRH Analogues

GnRH analogues causes pituitary down regulation and can be used for control of heavy menstrual bleeding but will lead to hypo-estrogenic state if used for more than 6 months unless estrogen/progestogen "add back" therapy is given. GnRH analogues can be given for endometrial suppression before ablation. In patients with renal failure, blood dyscrasias or after organ transplantation, GnRH analogues can be given for short-term relief. Agents used are Buserelin(subcutaneous), Goserelin(nasal spray), leuprolide etc.

Desmopressin

Desmopressin, a synthetic analogue of vasopressin, is of special use in managing heavy menstrual bleeding associated with von Willebrand's disease. It can be administered as a nasal spray or by intravenous route. This is a last resort in selected cases.

Endometrial Resection and Ablation for Heavy Menstrual Bleeding

Surgical treatment of heavy menstrual bleeding often follows failed or ineffective medical therapy although this may be used as a first line therapy.
- Hysterectomy has been regarded as the definitive surgical treatment for intractable heavy menstrual bleeding, but is a major surgical procedure with significant physical and emotional complications. Many women prefer less invasive surgical procedures.
- Endometrial resection is an alternative to hysterectomy that should be offered to women with heavy menstrual bleeding. There are high satisfaction rates, shorter operation time and hospital stay, earlier recovery and reduced post-operative complications, but is less effective than hysterectomy.

In one study, 38% of those who had endometrial ablation required further surgical treatment in the form of repeat endometrial ablation or hysterectomy at the end of four years.[7]

The endometrium has great ability of regeneration and to suppress menstruation successfully it is essential to remove the full thickness of the endometrium with the superficial myometrium, including the deep basal glands, which are believed to be the primary foci for endometrial re-growth.

Trans-cervical resection of the endometrium (TCRE) is performed using an operative hysteroscope with a diathermy loop (resectoscope) usually in combination with roller ball diathermy ablation.

Endometrial destruction up to 4-6 mm can be achieved using neodymium:yttrium-aluminum-garnet (Nd:YAG) laser which is reported to be safer than TCRE. It is advisable to prepare the endometrium with prior administration of danazol, progesterone or GnRH analogue to make it thinner.

The newer techniques of endometrial ablation are uterine thermal balloon ablation, cryo-ablation, photo-dynamic therapy and microwave endometrial ablation. Microwave and endometrial balloon ablation has the potential to allow acceptable and effective treatment in the outpatient setting. A significant reduction in the hysterectomy rate for abnormal uterine bleeding would be achieved if ablation techniques are used as first line surgical treatment.

Dilatation and Curettage

Dilatation and curettage is both diagnostic and therapeutic in cases of abnormal uterine bleeding. Removal of the structurally fragile bleeding endometrium allows restoration of normal hemostatic events with regeneration of the endometrium and restoration of the normal proliferative response.

Hysterectomy

It has been estimated that 2 million women in the United States are seen annually with complaints of heavy menstrual bleeding and that about 150,000 undergo hysterectomy, which accounts for 20% to 30% of all hysterectomies performed.[8] Ovulatory type of bleeding has less success with medical management and requires surgery.

Principles

- Hysterectomy is a method of treating refractory and recurrent type of dysfunctional uterine bleeding in older women.
- In parous women it is always better to do a vaginal hysterectomy with correction of vaginal relaxation.
- In difficult situations, a laparoscopic assisted vaginal hysterectomy (LAVH) or an abdominal hysterectomy may have to be performed.
- In premenopausal women healthy ovaries are to be retained.
- Laparoscopic supra-cervical hysterectomy with removal of the uterus using a mechanical morsellator can also be performed where the cervix is healthy.
- Hysterectomy is the option in treating women with atypical adenomatous hyperplasia, if they are not concerned about future child bearing.
- Hysterectomy is resorted to in patients with recurrence of symptoms following endometrial ablations.

Endometrial Hyperplasia

In anovulatory type of DUB, unopposed estrogenic stimulation can lead to the development of endometrial hyperplasia. The histologic changes described as cystic glandular hyperplasia, simple hyperplasia and adenomatous hyperplasia without atypia are usually not precursors of carcinoma and will regress spontaneously or with progesterone therapy. Lesions with cytological atypia, described as atypical adenomatous hyperplasia, are best treated by hysterectomy.

CONCLUSION

The systematic approach to abnormal uterine bleeding is given in Figure 8.3.

REFERENCES

1. Chimbira TH, Anderson ABM, Turnbull AC: Relation between menstrual blood loss and patients subjective assessment of loss, duration of bleeding, number of sanitary towels used; Br J Obstet Gynecol 1980;87:603-609.
2. Lethaby A, Augood C, Duckitt K: Nonsteroidal anti-inflammatory drugs for heavy menstrual bleeding (Cochrane Review). In Cochrane Library, Issue1, 2001. Oxford: Update Software.
3. Krikland JL, Murthy L, Stancel GM: Progesterone inhibits the estrogen induced expression of cfos messenger ribonucleic acid in the uterus, Endocrinology 1992; 130: 322.
4. Lethaby A, Irvine G,Cameron I: Cyclical progestogens for heavy menstrual bleeding (Cochrane Review). In The Cochrane Library, Issue 1, 2001, Oxford: Update Software.
5. Nelson L, Rybo G: Treatment of menorrhagia, Am J Obstet Gynecol 1971;110:713.
6. Lethaby AE, Cook I, Rees M: Progesterone/progestogen releasing intrauterine systems verses either placebo or any other medication for heavy menstrual bleeding (Cochrane Review). In The Cochrane Library, Issue 1,2001. Oxford: Update Software.
7. Lethaby A, Sheppered S, Cook I, et al: Endometrial resection and ablation versus hysterectomy for heavy menstrual bleeding (Cochrane review). In The Cochrane Library , Issue 1,2001,Oxford: Update Software.
8. William J Butler: Normal and abnormal uterine bleeding, Te Linde's operative gynecology, 8th edn, J.B. Lippincott Company.

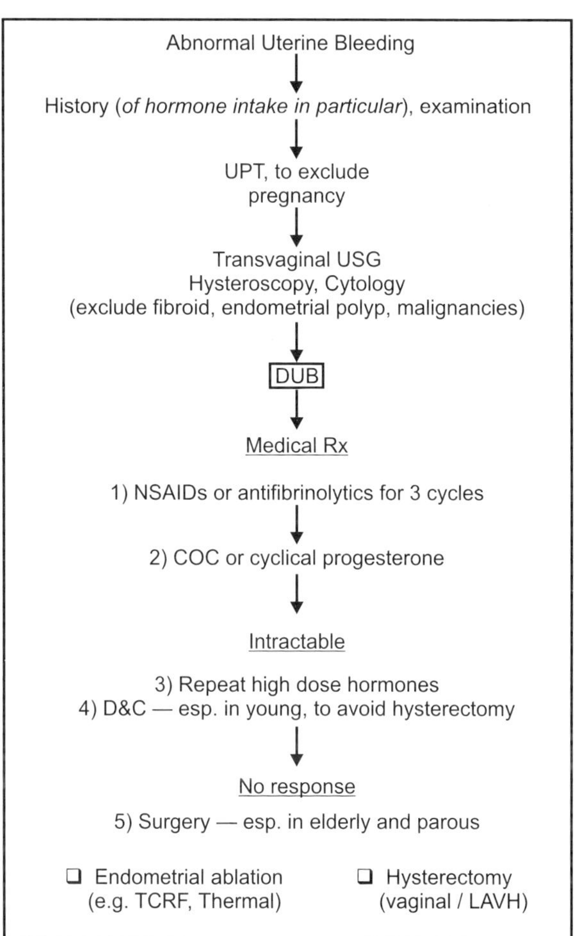

Figure 8.3: Approach to DUB

9.

N Pandiyan

Amenorrhea and Oligomenorrhea

INTRODUCTION

Amenorrhea and oligomenorrhea are common gynecological problems. Thirty percent of women attending the gynecology outpatient department at a large teaching hospital had these menstrual disturbances. Amenorrhea and oligomennorhea, though not disabling conditions, could be disturbing to the woman who is used to regular menstrual cyclicity. They may also be indicators of other sinister disabling conditions. Proper evaluation of the cause of amenorrhea is essential for its rational management. We will now briefly outline the physiology of menstruation. A clear understanding of the physiology is essential for the proper planning and treatment of amenorrhea and oligomenorrhea.

PHYSIOLOGY OF MENSTRUATION

Menstruation is the periodic physiologic shedding of the endometrium. During the follicular phase of the ovulatory cycle, the growing follicle secretes estrogens, which act on the endometrium inducing proliferative changes. With ovulation the follicle is transformed into a Corpus Luteum and the progesterone secreted induces secretory changes in the endometrium in preparation for nidation. When pregnancy fails to take place the endometrium lining is shed and is recognized as menstruation. Normal menstruation has a cyclicity of 28 days +/– 4 days. The blood loss is about 80 ml and mild crampy pains accompany the blood flow.

Menstrual abnormalities can occur because of endocrine disorders of ovulation, endometrial pathologies or due to systemic conditions.

The commonly encountered menstrual abnormalities are:
- Amenorrhea—absence of menstruation.
- Oligomenorrhea—infrequent menstruation.
- Hypomenorrhea—scanty menstruation.
- Polymenorrhea—frequent menstruation.
- Menorrhagia—excessive menstruation.
- Dymenorrhea—painful menstruation.
- Metrorrhagia—midcycle bleeding.

Endocrine Causes of Menstrual Abnormalities

The cyclical release of a fertilizable oocyte is the main function of the female reproductive system. This requires synchronized action of the higher cortical centers, hypothalamus, pituitary, ovary and endometrium. Asynchrony of this axis may lead to menstrual abnormalities and amenorrhea.

Endometrial Pathology Causing Menstrual Abnormalities

Infections of the endometrium—particularly endometrial tuberculosis, may cause menstrual abnormalities and amenorrhea.[1,2] Endometrial tuberculosis may cause menometrorrhagia in early stages and amenorrhea in advanced stages.

Systemic Diseases

Severe systemic illnesses by causing generalized ill health and severe weight loss may lead to menstrual abnormalities and particularly amenorrhea. A critical body mass is essential for normal hypothalamo-pituitary ovarian and menstrual function. Hemotological disorders like hemophilia and other bleeding disorders may cause menorrhagia.

AMENORRHEA

Definition: Absence of menstruation for 6 months or longer or for a period of 3 cycle lengths or longer is called as amenorrhea.

Amenorrhea is physiological under the following conditions:

1. Pre-pubertal/pre-menarchal.
2. Pregnancy.
3. Lactational.
4. Post-menopausal.

Physiology of Menarche

The age of onset of menarche has steadily declined over the last century and has now stabilized. The early onset of menarche is attributed to good nutrition and better living standards.

The higher cortical centers exhibit constant inhibitory control over the hypothalamo-pituitary ovarian axis. When a critical body mass is reached, the inhibitory control is lost and this permits the generation of GnRH pulse from the pulse generator in the hypothalamus. The release of GnRH leads to release of FSH/LH from the pituitary and further development of the ovarian and endometrial axis. In the early post-menarchal years this circuit is not mature and may lead to anovulatory cycles. There is enough data to indicate that endogeneous opioid have a crucial inhibitory role in the control of gonadotrophin secretion.[3]

Primary Amenorrhea

When a girl has not attained menarche by the age of 18 years she is said to have primary amenorrhea.

Causes

Primary amenorrhea can be caused by:

1. Endocrine causes.
2. Endometrial causes.
3. Systemic causes.

Endocrine causes: Lesions of the higher centers and those involving the hypothalamus may lead to defects in GnRH pulse generation, causing disruption in the hypothalamo hypophysial axis. This would lead to failure of gonadotrophin production and hence cause secondary ovarian failure leading to amenorrhea. The classical example of this condition is Kallmann's syndrome. Patients with Kallman's syndrome, besides amenorrhea also have defects in their olfactory neurons and hence have anosmia/hyposmia. Defects in the olfactory sulci in the brain have been demonstrated at MRI.[4] Hypothalamic dysfunction may also be a post encephalitic sequel.

   i. *Pituitary lesions* particularly those involving the non-gonadotroph cells may lead to pressure effect on the gonadotroph leading to decreased gonadotrophin production. Prolactinomas causing hyperprolactinemia may impair pituitary function both by pressure effect and by interfering with the GnRh pulse generator. Pituitary destruction as occurs with Sheehan's syndrome may lead to pituitary failure, non-production of gonadotrophins and hence, amenorrhea.

ii. *Primary ovarian failure* either due to chromosomal disorders like Turner's syndrome or due to premature ovarian failure may lead to non production of gonadal steroids and consequently amenorrhea.[5]

Endometrial pathologies: These may cause amenorrhea. Vigorous curettage of the uterine cavity may lead to adhesions between the uterine wall (synechiae) leading to amenorrhea.[6]

Genital tract tuberculosis, though primarily tubal extends to the endometrium, causing menorrhagia in early days and amenorrhea in the advanced stages due to destruction of the endometrium and sub-endometrial layers.

Endometrial receptor defects may lead to inadequate proliferation of the endometrium and poor or inadequate secretory changes causing menstrual abnormalities oligomenorrhea and amenorrhea.

In Mullerian agenesis, the uterus and upper vagina are absent and hence, the girls presents with primary amenorrhea. As she has normally functioning ovaries she has normal secondary sexual characters.

Systemic diseases: Many chronic illnesses like chronic liver failure and chronic renal failure lead to significant ill health, weight loss and to amenorrhea. Chronic renal failure also leads to elevation of prolactin levels and this may cause amenorrhea. Significant weight loss of any etiology, including eating disorders like anorexia nervosa may lead to amenorrhea.[7]

Clinical Approach to Primary Amenorrhea (Figure 9.1)

In a girl presenting with primary amenorrhea, a detailed personal history, sibling history, family history, clinical examination and a few relevant investigations will help in establishing a proper diagnosis and aid in appropriate management.

History of developmental delay in milestones may point to lesions in the higher centers. Consanguinous marriage among parents may suggest inherited disorders causing primary amenorrhea.

History of mother or sisters attaining menarche late may point to constitutional, familial 'delayed menarche'. Past history of trauma to the head or encephalitis may suggest a post-traumatic, post encephalitic sequel.

History of pulmonary tuberculosis may indicate genital tract tuberculosis as the cause of the amenorrhea.

Clinical examination is done to evaluate the state of nourishment, height and weight of the child and for evidence of other systemic diseases. Malnourished children have a greater risk of primary amenorrhea and delayed puberty. Evaluation of secondary sexual characteristics is done to estimate the degree of pubertal development. Normal secondary sexual development appropriate for age may indicate normal ovarian function and the cause for amenorrhea could be 'delayed menarche' or uterine pathology. Imperforate hymen should be considered. The clinical presentation and management has been discussed in the earlier chapter.

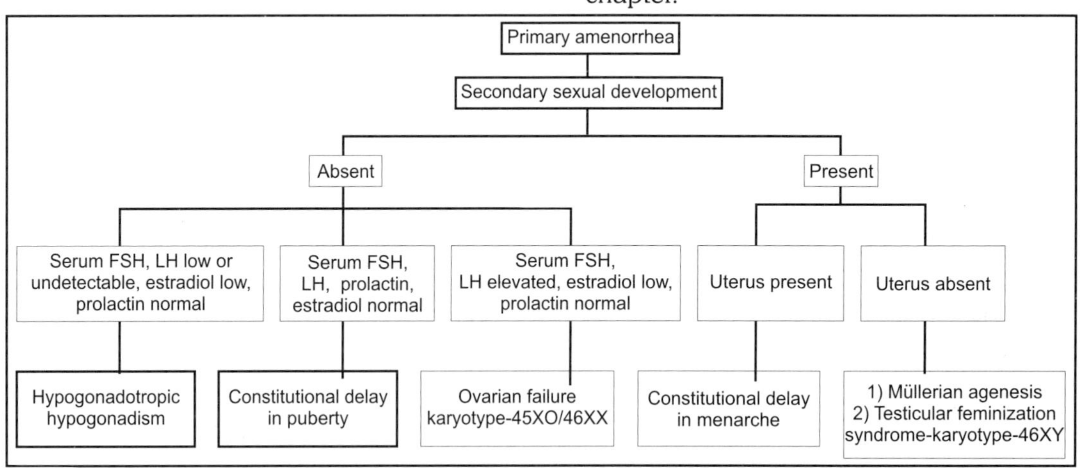

Figure 9.1: Clinical evaluation of primary amenorrhea

Estimates of serum, FSH, LH, prolactin and estradiol will help in identifying the site of lesion and in planning future management. All the hormone investigation may not be essential for all the patients.

Peripheral blood karyotypes may help in identifying Turner's syndrome, Turner mosaic and testicular feminization syndrome.

Galactosemia may be a rare cause of primary amenorrhea due to ovarian dysfunction.[9]

Clinical Features of Some Common Conditions Associated with Primary Amenorrhea

Turner's syndrome is the commonest cause of primary ovarian failure and primary amenorrhea. In the classical condition the ovaries are dysgenetic and present as streak gonads. The gonadotrophin levels are markedly raised.[8] Turner's syndrome occurs in around 1 in 2500 births and the usual karyotype picture is 45X. Mosaic forms are also common with karyotype picture presenting 45X/46XX, 45X/46XY, or with partial deletion of one arm of the X chromosome.

The presence of Y chromosome may be dangerous as they may have a testes and these children may require gonadectomy to prevent the risk of gonadoblastoma or dysgerminoma.

The classical features of Turner's syndrome include:

1. Short stature
2. Web neck
3. Lymphoedema
4. Shield chest with wide spread nipples
5. Scoliosis
6. Wide carrying angle
7. Sharp metacarpals
8. Soft, curling nails
9. Low set ears, low hairline, micrognathia and high arched palate.
10. Coarches of the ankle
11. Horse-shoe kidney
12. Strabismus
13. Ptosis
14. Multiple nevi.

All the features may not be present in all the patients. However, most patients present varying combinations of these elemental features.

A high index of suspicion is essential for prepubertal diagnosis of the condition and proper management of these children

Constitutional delay: The onset of puberty and the occurrence of menarche, even under normal physiological conditions, is influenced largely by nutritional, environmental and familial factors. In some girls despite the normal development of secondary sexual characters, the onset of menarche is delayed. This could be a case of 'delayed menarche'. A family history of similar condition in the mother and/or the siblings could clinch the diagnosis. However, in other girls, even the development or onset of puberty may be delayed— 'delayed puberty'—all these girls, after a few basic investigations, require only 'reassurance'. All these girls require FSH, LH estimation and ultrasound to confirm the presence of uterus and ovaries.

Hypothalmo-pituitary dysfunction: A heterogeneous group of conditions may present with the hypothalmo-pituitary dysfunction and cause secondary ovarian failure and primary amenorrhea.

Inflammatory lesions or tumors of the hypo-thalamus-pituitary region may lead to decreased secretions of FSH and LH and to ovarian failure. Lesions of the pituitary, like craniopharyngioma and hydro-cephalus, may cause such a condition.

The syndromes associated with hypogonadotrophic hypogonadism are:

- *Laurence-Moon-Biedl syndrome*: This is an autosomal recessive disorder characterized by obesity, retinitis pigmentosa, mental retardation, polydactyly and hypogonadism.
- *Prader–Willi syndrome*: It presents with hypotonia, mental retardation, characteristic facies, obesity and hypogonadism.
- *Kallmann's syndrome or olfactory genital dysplasia*: Patients present with primary amenorrhea due to defect in the hypothalamic pulse generator and consequently hypopituitarism and hypogonadism. Incomplete/complete agenesis of the olfactory bulbs may lead to anosmia/hyposmia. It is inherited as an autosomal dominant trait.
- *Testicular feminization syndrome*: Children with this condition though genetically male with a karyotype

of 46XY and are almost always raised as girls in view of the female phenotype. Often the girls present in their late teens with good secondary sexual development and primary amenorrhea. The condition is an X linked recessive disorder where the primary defect is in the 'insensitivity of the androgen receptor'. The gonads are testes, which are functional and produce normal amounts of testosterone and müllerian inhibiting substance. Therefore, these girls do not have uterus tubes and upper vagina. Due to androgen insensitivity, secondary sexual characteristics and the external genitalia have a female configuration. As there is adequate conversion of testosterone to estrogens and as the ovary is exposed to unopposed action of the estrogens, the breast development is normal. The gonads may be intra-abdominal or in the inguinal region and need removal after attainment of secondary sexual characteristics followed by hormone replacement therapy.

- *Müllerian agenesis*: These girls present with normal secondary sexual characteristics and primary amenorrhea. Karyotype reveals 46XX. These children have congenital absence of the müllerian tract leading to absence of uterus, tubes and upper vagina. These girls have normal functioning ovaries.

Management of Primary Amenorrhea

A detailed history, clinical examination and a few relevant investigations would help in identifying the cause and aid in the proper management of primary amenorrhea.

History of consanguinity amongst parents and/or history of similar problems among siblings may all point to a genetic origin. History of delayed milestones, past history of head trauma or encephalitis may suggest a central cause for the 'primary amenorrhea'.

Short stature, web neck and increased carrying angle with cardiac defects with no secondary sexual development may point to Turner's syndrome. Normal secondary sexual characteristics with a blind vagina may indicate 'Testicular Feminization Syndrome' or 'Mullerian agenesis'.

Normal secondary sexual characteristics with normal internal and external genitalia may indicate 'delayed menarche'.

Poor or absent secondary sexual development with normal genitalia by clinical and ultrasonography may indicate 'delayed puberty' or hypogonadism. Serum FSH estimation would help in diagnosing and differentiating hypogonadotrophic from hypergonadotrophic hypogonadism.

The treatment of primary amenorrhea depends upon the cause, what is desired at that point in time and what is possible under prevailing conditions. The treatment is summarized in Table 9.1.

Secondary Amenorrhea

If a lady who has previously menstruated spontaneously, does not menstruate for 6 months or longer or 3 cycle lengths or longer, she is considered to have 'secondary amenorrhea'. In practice many patients with primary amenorrhea are given inappropriate hormonal treatment and made to menstruate and are subsequently wrongly diagnosed as 'secondary amenorrhea'.

Causes

The commonest cause of secondary amenorrhea is pregnancy.

The other causes are:

1. Polycystic ovarian disease—though it often produces oligomenorrhea.
2. Hyperprolactinemia.
3. Tuberculosis of the genital tract.
4. Postpartum hemorrhage, postpartum collapse, pituitary necrosis and Sheehan's syndrome.
5. Post-pill amenorrhea.

The clinical evaluation of secondary amenorrhea is given in Figure 9.2.

Polycystic Ovarian Disease: Most patients with polycystic ovarian disease present with varying periods of amenorrhea/oligomenorrhea followed by menorrhagia. However some patients may have only anovulation with no irregularity in menstrual pattern.

The diagnosis is based on clinical findings, biochemical features and ultrasonographic findings.

Table 9.1: Management of primary amenorrhea

Condition	Clinical features	Investigations	Management
Delayed puberty/Menarche	Poor or absent or normal secondary sexual development	Normal serum FSH, LH and Prolactin.	Reassurance
Turner's syndrome	Poor or absent secondary sexual development. Uterus and tubes present.	Elevated Serum FSH, LH.Normal Prolactin. Karyotype—45XO or Mosaic-46XX/45XO.	Estrogen and progesterone for normal secondary sexual development and oocyte or embryo donation for conception. Rarely normal sexual development, menstruation and conception have been reported.
Mullerian agenesis	Normal secondary sexual development. Poorly developed or absent tubes, uterus and upper vagina.	Normal serum FSH, LH and Prolactin. Karyotype-46XX.	If fertility were desired, surrogacy would be the choice. In some women with rudimentary Mullerian structures uterine reconsruction have been done and pregnancies have been reported.
Testicular feminization syndrome	Normal secondary sexual development. Absent uterus, tubes and upper vagina. Inguinal swellings (hernia) may be present which may contain the testes.	Normal Serum FSH, LH and Prolactin. Karyotype-46XY.	Gonadectomy after normal pubertal development. Fertility cannot be restored. May function as women with normal sexual function. Some women may require vaginoplasty.
Genital tuberculosis	If post-pubertal—normal secondary sexual characters. If pre pubertal—before the development of secondary sexual characters and if ovaries are involved—poor or absent secondary sexual development.	Normal FSH, LH, Prolactin. Karyotype-46XX. Endometrium—Tuberculosis. Laporoscopy—Tuberculosis of the tubes.	Antituberculosis treatment may re-establish the cycle in many women. Pregnancies by IVF have been reported in cases where the tubes were damaged.
Hypothalamic amenorrhea as in Kallmann's syndrome or other hypothalamic lesions.	Poor or absent secondary sexual characters.	Low or undetectable serum FSH, LH. Normal Prolactin. karyotype-46XY.	Estrogen/Progestogen for restoration of secondary sexual characters. GnRH pulastile infusion for induction of Ovulation and restoration of fertility. Gonadotropins can also be used.

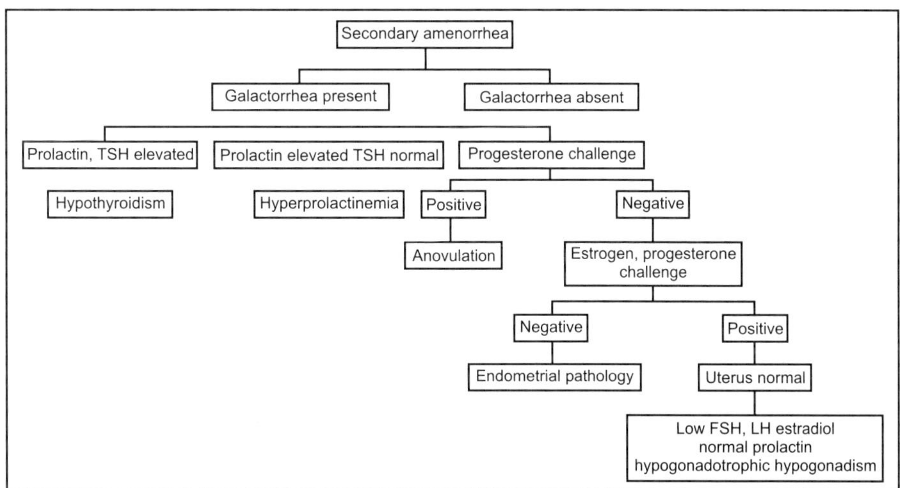

Figure 9.2: Clinical evaluation of secondary amenorrhea

(Vide separate chapter). The management is dependent on patient's presenting feature—infertility or irregular cycle. (Vide separate chapter).

Hyperprolactinemia: Hyperprolactinemia may lead to anovulation and amenorrhea.

Milder forms of hyperprolactinemia are often due to hypothyroidism.[10] Moderate elevation can be due to 'hyperplasia or neoplasia.'

Hyperprolactinaemia regardless of its etiology may produce varying degrees of ovulatory disturbances and amenorrhea.

Mild elevation may produce 'luteal phase defects' and moderate elevation may cause anovulation and amenorrhea.

Prolactinomas are almost always benign. They present clinically with galactorrhea, amenorrhea and if large with pressure symptoms. The diagnosis is based on history, clinical findings laboratory findings and CT/MRI parameters. The management depends on the cause of hyperprolactinaemia and the desire for childbearing.

When hypothyroidism is the cause of hyperprolactinemia correction of hypothyroidism leads to correction of hyperprolactinemia.

In moderate and severe hyperprolactinemia, medical management would be the first line of management. Bromoergocryptine is the drug of choice. In patients intolerant to Bromoergocryptine or not responding to Bromoergocryptine, Cabergoline can be used.

In some patients, particularly those with macroadenoma and pressure symptoms, transphenoidal microsurgery may have to be undertaken. Patients with hyperprolactinemia on medical management may have to take it for a long time, sometimes for several years.

Tuberculosis of the genital tract: Tuberculosis is a major killer disease in many developing countries including India. Genital tuberculosis is not uncommon. Tuberculosis of the genital tract primarily involves the tubes, but subsequently spreads to the endometrium. Women with genital tuberculosis develop tubal damage and block, which is usually not amenable to surgery. Destruction of the endometrium by tuberculosis leads to amenorrhea. Effective treatment of tuberculosis may help in regeneration of the endometrium in some women, but others may continue to be amenorrheic with poor prognosis for menstrual function and fertility.

Tubal tuberculosis often leads to irreparable tubal damage and even in women in whom menstrual function has been restored, IVF may be the only option left for restoration of fertility.

Postpartum pituitary necrosis—Sheehan's syndrome: In some women who suffer from postpartum hemorrhage and collapse, the pituitary may undergo necrosis leading to hypopituitarism. This often involves all the trophic hormones from the anterior pituitary, but it could also be gonadotrophin specific. This could lead to hypogonadotrophic hypogonadism and amenorrhea. These patients respond well to gonadotrophin therapy.

Table 9.2: Secondary amenorrhea

Condition	Clinical features	Investigations	Management
Polycystic ovarian disease	Anovulation, amenorrhea, oligomenorrhea, +/– hirsuitism, +/– obesity,	USG—bilateral enlarged ovaries; subcapsular cysts. Altered LH/FSH ratio>2:1	Induction of ovulation or Combined oral contraceptive pill.
Hyperprolactinemia	Luteal phase defects, galactorrhea, amenorrhea and hypopogonadism.	Serum prolactin is elevated. Serum TSH elevated when hyperprolactinemia is due to hypothyroidism. CT scan/MRI for evidence of prolactinoma.	Thyroxine if the hyperprolactinemia is due to hypothyroidism. Bromoergocryptine in patients with Hyperprolactinemia. Trans-sphenoidal micro surgery in selected cases.
Sheehan's syndrome or postpartum pituitary necrosis.	Failure of lactation. Other features of hypopituitarism. Amenorrhea	Low serum FSH, LH, prolactin, progesterone. May also have low TSH, ACTH.	Estrogen/progesterone therapy for restoration of menses. Gonadotrophins for induction of ovulation.

Menstrual function can be restored by oestrogen/progestogen therapy.

Oligomenorrhea is mostly due to anovulation. Spells of oligomenorrhea may precede amenorrhea. These patients require evaluation for hypothalamo pituitary dysfunction.

The treatment depends upon the cause and whether the patient requires re-establishing menstrual cyclicity or desires fertility.

Combined oral contraceptives pill given cyclically would re-establish menstrual cyclicity.

Induction of ovulation with clomiphene, cyclofenil, tamoxifen, or gonadotrophin would help in restoring fertility in many of these women.

In some women, during the spells of amenorrhea there may be a build up of endometrium leading to menorrhagia subsequently. This is called as 'oligo-menorrhagia'.

Prognosis

Amenorrhea and oligomenorrhea can be effectively treated in most women with these menstrual disorders. However, it is important to understand the basic pathophysiology of the condition and treat appropriately. The treatment depends also on the patients presenting complaint and her desire for childbearing.

REFERENCES

1. Tripathy SN (Mrs), Tripathy SN. Endometrial Tuberculosis. J Ind Med Assoc 1987;85:136-140.
2. Misra R, Sharma SP et al. Female genital tract tuberculosis with special reference to sterility in eastern UP. Jr O & G India 1996;46:104.
3. Ferin M, Vande Weile R. Endogenous opiod peptides and the control of menstrual cycle. Eur J Obstet Gynecol Reprod Biol 1984;18:365.
4. Knorr JR, Ragland RL,Brown RS,Gelber N. Kallman's syndrome. MRI findings, AJNR Am J Neuroradiol 1993; 14:845.
5. Blumenfeld Z, Halachmi S et al. Premature Ovarian Failure the prognostic application of auto immunity to conception after ovulation induction.Fertil Steril 1993;59:750, 1993.
6. Asherman JG. Traumatic intra uterine adhesions. J Obstet Gynecol Br Emp 1950;57:892-96.
7. Abraham S, Mitra M, Llewellyn-Jones D. Should ovulation be induced in women recovering from an eating disorder or who are compulsive exercisers? Fertil Steril 1990;53:566.
8. Rebar RW, Connolly HV. Clinical features of young women with Hypergonadotrophic Amenorrhea. Fertil Steril 1990;531:804.
9. Kaufman FR, Kogut MD, et al. Hypergonadotrophic Hypogonadism in female patients with galactosemia. New Engl J Med 1981;304:994-998.
10. Contreras P, Generini G, et al. Hyperprolactinaemia and galactorrhea; spontaneous versus iatrogenic hypothyroidism. J Clin Endocrinol metab 1981;53:1036.

10. Reproductive Health

Sambit Mukhopadhyay
Sabaratnam Arulkumaran

Globally, combination of social economic and cultural factors affects reproductive health of women. The extent of the problem varies in different countries. A large difference exists in the indices of reproductive health between developed and developing countries. Factors which influence reproductive health are discussed below.

ADOLESCENT HEALTH

The WHO defines adolescent as a person between 10-19 years of age. One in 5 people in the world is an adolescent and 85% of them live in developing countries. Adolescence is the period of transition from childhood to adulthood. Significant anatomical and physiological changes occur and the child matures to adulthood. Puberty occurs before adolescence. Series of physiological or biologic changes take place, which makes one capable of reproduction.

The maturation of hypothalamo-pituitary-ovarian axis takes place between 8-10 years. This is associated with series of events, which appear in a typical sequence. The sequences of events are growth spurt, thelarche, pubarche and finally menarche. Increased estrogen production brought about by increasing FSH production by the pituitary, is responsible for breast development, maturation of internal and external genitalia and finally menarche. Adrenal androgens contribute to pubic and axillary hairs. The whole process is usually completed in 3-4 years, however, both the order and the time of appearance can occasionally vary. Nutrition and general health influences the changes of puberty. Improved nutrition and better health lowers the age of menarche. Total amount of body fat also determines the onset of menarche. It is now believed that at least 17% of body should be fat for initiation of menarche.

Disorders of adolescent health and puberty are discussed in the chapter 'Pediatric and Adolescent Gynecology'. We discuss some important points that may have an effect on overall reproductive health of a woman.

Endocrine changes also trigger emotional and psychological development. A sense of identity develops and this is influenced to some extent by peer groups and family background. Sexual pairing may take place. Girls mature earlier than boys and may experience romantic interest. This may lead to sexual activity although it may depend on the social and cultural environment. Certain 'risk taking' behavior may be seen at this age. It can range from exploring sexual relationship to alcohol, smoking and substance abuse. Therefore, adequate access to family planning services, sex education and counseling services for young people is necessary to promote good sexual and mental health.

Sexuality and Fertility

Of all the changes in adolescence, sexuality draws more attention. The implications are different globally. Early age of sex and late marriage is mostly seen in the West. Nearly one third of the girls below sixteen are sexually active and many will have more than two sexual partners. Adolescents who engage in early sexual activity run the risk of acquiring sexually transmitted disease (STD), unwanted motherhood, relationship problem, loosing out in education, physical aggression, early use of tobacco and even addiction to drugs. Therefore, provision of contraceptive services and abortion services are important in such society. The situation is grave in certain parts of the world where adequate facilities of contraceptive and abortion services do not exist. In the absence of access to safe abortion services an adolescent girl may often resort to unsafe abortion with its attendent complications.

The other extreme is early marriage and child-bearing. Marriage usually happens close to menarche and early and frequent childbearing follows this. The girl usually loses out in education and does not have the choice to negotiate in safe sex and childbearing. This picture is common in the developing countries. Repeated childbirth leads to chronic ill health, anemia and in extreme situation death due to complications of pregnancy particularly in places where maternity services are not adequate.

Therefore, measures should be taken to reduce the effect of unwanted pregnancy and STD. This is possible and would require different interventions in different countries. Most important in developing country is to improve female literacy thereby making women aware of their choices and rights to decide their reproductive health at an early stage of their life.

Uncontrolled Fertility

More than 95% of population growth takes place in developing countries. If there was universal access to family planning and women could control the number of children they wanted, the total fertility rate in many countries would fall by one third.

India has only 2.4% of world's land area but contains 16% of world's population. The population has crossed the 1 billion mark and is increasing by 17 millions per year. Therefore, from demographic perspective its role in the world is crucial.

The rapid population growth not only has an effect on the environment, the resources of the country and its economy but it also has serious effects on women's health. Globally, 600,000 deaths occur during childbirth and 25% of these maternal deaths are from India alone. Therefore, prevention and spacing of pregnancy is important. Seventy percent of women in reproductive age use contraception whereas the similar figure for South Asia is only 33%. Thousands of deaths occur annually from illegal or unsafe abortions and certainly availability and accessibility of reliable contraception could make a huge difference. The UNFPA (United Nations Population Fund) estimates that approximately 120 million women will use contraception if they had access to it.

There are wide variety of contraceptive choices but there are barriers that lead to low use of contraception. Majority of women in India have little control over decision-making. It is often their husband or even family who decides about her contraception. Access to clinics may be difficult without the husband's permission.

Therefore, providing better information and improving access to contraceptive services are essential to reduce fertility and improve reproductive health. Family planning nurse or specially trained health workers can counsel women for contraceptive use. This could increase the uptake of contraception.

Unsafe Abortion

After malnutrition, lack of drinking water and sanitation, unsafe sex is the third most common cause of global ill health. Nearly 75,000 women die every year in the world of unsafe abortion. Most of deaths occur in developing countries where abortion services do not exist or competent person does not perform abortion. In India it is estimated that nearly 22,000 mothers die annually of illegal abortion. Although termination of pregnancy is legally approved (Abortion Act 1971) for more than three decades the services are not easily accessible to majority of women, particularly in rural areas. Facilities available across the country are also not uniform. Some states have very well-organized services whereas others with huge population have a very few centres for carrying out safe abortion. Consequently, women resort to unsafe abortions risking their lives. Ninety percent of the 6-8 million estimated abortions performed in India are conducted by untrained village practitioners using unsafe methods under poor hygienic condition.

Therefore, the primary aim of any services to reduce maternal mortality and improve reproductive health is to make provision of effective contraceptive and safe abortion services. Medical termination of pregnancy using RU-486 and Misoprostol is safer and can potentially avoid dangers of unsafe abortion.

Pelvic Inflammatory Disease (PID)/ Sexually Transmitted Disease (STD)

It is a clinical syndrome of polymicrobial infection, which usually occurs, in sexually active women characterized by inflammation and infection of the upper genital tract, typically involving the fallopian tubes, ovaries and surrounding structures.

The exact incidence of the disease is unknown because the disease cannot be diagnosed reliably from clinical signs and symptoms alone. Visualization of the fallopian tubes by laparoscopy is the best diagnostic test when there is doubt. This invasive test is not always necessary and possible to use routinely on all patients. PID accounts for one of the commonest causes of emergency gynecological admission. The exact prevalence of the disease is unknown as most PID is asymptomatic.

Factors associated with pelvic inflammatory disease are: young age, low socio-economic class, lower educational attainment, African ethnic origin and new sexual partner. Most of the infection is ascending in origin. The initial epithelial damage is done by *Chlamydia* or *Neisseria gonorrhoeae*. This is followed by opportunistic entry of other organisms. Isolation of organism from the upper genital tract is difficult and is usually polymicrobial in nature including organisms like *Mycoplasma* and anaerobes. The spread of infection to the upper genital tract may be influenced by instrumentation of the cervix and use of contraceptives (IUCD).

Pelvic inflammatory disease carries a high morbidity: about 20% of affected women become infertile, 20% develop chronic pelvic pain, and 10% who conceive develop ectopic pregnancy. Therefore, education and promoting good sexual health, especially for the younger age group is of paramount importance. Barrier method of contraception goes a long way to prevent sexually transmitted infection. Early diagnosis and prompt treatment with broad-spectrum antibiotics in proper dosage can prevent sequeale of pelvic inflammatory disease. The details of treatment of PID and STD is discussed in another chapter and therefore not repeated here.

Childbirth and Maternal Mortality

Of about half a million deaths occurring globally, only 0.4% are in the developed countries and 99.6% are in the developing countries. In South-east Asia a mother dies every 3 minutes and in India 1 mother dies every 4 minutes. This loss is mostly preventable. Mothers die at a young age at the prime of their life when they actually attempt to fulfil their social obligation of maintaining the continuity of human race.

For each maternal deaths, there are at least few near deaths due to severe morbidity.

Causes of maternal deaths
- Hemorrhage particularly postpartum hemorrhage (PPH)
- Sepsis
- Unsafe abortions
- Obstructed labor and/or ruptured uterus
- Over 80% of maternal deaths are due to direct causes and the rest are due to indirect causes like anemia, malaria, viral hepatitis, cardiac diseases, etc.

The average maternal mortality rate (MMR) is 380 per 100,000. However, the national average varies according to the socio-economic condition, gender, geographic location, ethnicity and other variables. The MMR in Uttar Pradesh is 707, whereas similar figure for Gujarat is only 29.

Neonatal death rates closely follow the figures of maternal mortality. Over 50% of infant deaths occur during the neonatal period, nearly two thirds of which occur during the first week of birth, mostly due to perinatal causes.

Globally, women from the poorest household with income less than $1 per day are 300 times more likely to die from maternal deaths than their better off counterparts. There exists safe and cost-effective technology to prevent maternal deaths but what is lacking in many countries is fully functioning health care system that can deliver good quality services during pregnancy and childbirth to all women irrespective of socio-economic status.

How can we make pregnancy safer?

Making pregnancy safer (MPS) is a health sector strategy to improve maternal health and reduce the combined problems of maternal and perinatal mortality. This initiative is launched by WHO to reduce the global burden of unnecessary death, illness and disability associated with pregnancy and childbirth.

Strategies needed to prevent maternal mortality and morbidity death are multiple. Some important ones are:

1. Better education, particularly health education for women.

   Education will raise awareness to seek health care.

2. Prevention of unwanted pregnancy

   Globally, 39% pregnancies are unplanned. Unsafe abortion is an important cause of maternal mortality in the developing world. Provision of good quality contraceptive services including emergency contraceptive services will prevent many unwanted pregnancy. Equally important is delivery of safe abortion services. This will go a long way to prevent perils of unsafe abortion.

3. All pregnant women and their infants should have access to skilled care.

   This includes both antenatal and intrapartum period. The number of intrapartum complications decreases with the presence of skilled attendants at delivery. Eighty percent of maternal deaths are due to direct causes and most of them are preventable by following certain guidelines.

4. Appropriate referral centres for treating complicated pregnancies

   Provision of referral centres with skilled personnel is important to deal with life-threatening complications. Accessibility of this service in many instances are due to lack of communication and transport facilities.

5. Audit of maternal deaths or near deaths is essential to evaluate the quality of care. It also provides an excellent mechanism of learning from mistakes. The UK confidential enquiry of maternal deaths provides an excellent example.

   'Making pregnancy safer' aims to achieve massive increases in proportion of women and infants having access to essential health care in 50 target countries by 2005. This may be achieved by collaboration with the government and other nongovernmental organisations.

CONCLUSION

Reproductive health of women should be a national priority. The priorities are different in developing and developed countries. It should start at the adolescent period when proper parental guidance and health education are important. With increasing literacy, better earnings and empowerment, it is likely women will be able to make reproductive choices in their life. This would mean negotiating safe sex, reduction in STD, avoiding early childbearing and reducing family size. Access to quality health service for all pregnant women and infants should be made available. Reduction in maternal mortality should be the topmost priority for any national health strategy. Making pregnancy safer (MPS) is an initiative launched by WHO to reduce maternal deaths. Collaboration with the government and nongovernmental organisations and key health professionals will be needed to achieve the unmet need of health for all pregnant women and their babies.

11. *Endometriosis and Adenomyosis*

Dev Kumar Menon

INTRODUCTION

Clinicians have been fascinated by endometriosis since Rokitansky first described it in 1860. It arouses interest because endometriosis is one of the commonest gynecological conditions and is responsible for considerable morbidity. Despite this, however, we are still unclear as to its etiology and treating the disease can often be extremely challenging.

This chapter aims to give the most up-to-date facts about endometriosis and adenomyosis. Special attention should be paid to the pathophysiology of endometriosis because understanding this enables the clinician to deduce the possible symptoms and complications of the disease. Emphasis has been placed upon the principles behind managing endometriosis. A flow chart of this is included to aid recall. The drugs used are described in detail, as clinicians use these regularly. A summary of key points is given at the end of the chapter.

ENDOMETRIOSIS

Definition

Endometriosis is the presence of endometrial tissue outside both the uterine cavity and myometrium. *Adenomyosis* is endometrial tissue found within the myometrium. These two conditions have different clinical features and should be viewed as distinctly different entities.

Sites

Endometriotic foci typically occur within the pelvic cavity and most commonly on the ovaries, broad ligament, pouch of Douglas and the uterosacral ligaments. They can rarely occur in distant parts of the body such as in the lungs, skin, kidneys and skeletal muscle.

Incidence

Endometriosis is estimated to be present in 10% to 25% of women presenting to the gynecologist.[1]

Prevalence

Endometriosis is prevalent during the reproductive years with a peak incidence between 30 and 45 years of age. It has also been reported in teenagers and post-menopausal women (where it perhaps has been reactivated by use of hormone replacement therapy).

Etiology

The exact cause of endometriosis is unknown. There are several theories proposed regarding its pathogenesis. But it is unlikely that any one single theory accounts for all forms of endometriosis. The theories suggest either that the endometrial cells get to their ectopic sites by being transported there (metastatic theories) or that non-endometrial cells in foreign sites change into endometrial cells (metaplasia theories).

Metastatic Theories

Sampson's theory suggests that endometriosis is a result of *retrograde menstruation*.[2] This means that during menstruation, blood containing endometrial cells may pass up the fallopian tubes, and enter the pelvic cavity where the cells may implant and grow. The finding of endometriotic foci in laparotomy scars and in episiotomy scars has also suggested that some endometriosis may be the result of *transplantation* of cells at surgery or delivery. Halban proposed that endometriosis might be spread by *hematogenous* or *lymphatic* dissemination. This may explain the finding of endometriosis in distant sites such as the lung and kidneys.

Metaplasia Theories

Meyer and Meigs both proposed that endometriosis might result from metaplastic change. Meyer described *coelomic metaplasia*.[3] This means that adult cells anywhere in the body may be induced to undergo de-differentiation back to their primitive origin, the embryonic coelom, before then transforming into endometrial cells. This is an attractive theory because it could explain the presence of endometriosis in nearly all its ectopic sites. Meigs described *müllerian metaplasia*. The uterus, fallopian tubes and upper vagina are derived from the müllerian ducts, and these cells may undergo metaplasia to form endometrial cells. What induces this transformation is uncertain, but it has been suggested that hormones, immunological factors, drugs or genetic factors may be responsible.

Pathophysiology

Endometriosis consists of viable endometrial tissue superficially implanted on another tissue. Just like normal endometrium, this tissue is dependent on cyclical ovarian hormone production and can proliferate and bleed in response to estrogen and progesterone fluctuations. The resultant bleeding within the pelvic cavity is not normal and is responsible for much of the patient's symptoms and complications.

The presence of blood may produce adhesions within the pelvis as the body tries to contain the bleeding and limit its spread. Peritoneal inflammation due to the bleeding may cause acute pelvic pain whilst adhesions may cause fixation of the pelvic organs and chronic pelvic pain. Adhesions may result in tubal blockage and thus cause infertility. Extensive endometriosis may cause marked scarring and distortion of the pelvic anatomy.

The presence of blood also increases the number of macrophages in the peritoneal fluid. Although these phagocytes help to remove the cellular debris, they may also attack sperms and embryos. This may explain why endometriosis patients may experience infertility even if their tubes are patent.[4]

The ectopic endometrial tissue produces prostaglandins, which act on the uterus to cause contractions and vasoconstriction.[5] Both the uterine contractions and the transient myometrial ischemia caused by vasoconstriction, may lead to the symptom of dysmenorrhea.

The body may wall off bleeding from the ectopic endometrium and give rise to a blood-filled cyst called an endometrioma. Endometriomas (sometimes called endometriotic cysts) may occur on the ovary, and they can undergo any complication that an ovarian cyst can have. Thus they may expand in size or rupture to cause acute abdominal pain. As these cysts are often adherent in the pelvis, torsion of the ovary seldom occurs.

Finally, patients with endometriosis may have irregular and abnormal uterine bleeding. This may be due to inflammation in the pelvis, which may inhibit normal ovarian function. Patients may experience anovulatory cycles or impaired ovarian hormone production, which can then result in abnormal bleeding.

Symptoms

Dysmenorrhea and pelvic pain are the most common symptoms.

The *dysmenorrhea* is usually secondary dysmenorrhea rather than primary. Typically, the pain begins prior to the onset of the menses, increases in intensity during the flow, and gradually improves as the bleeding settles. It may become progressively more severe over time.

The *pelvic pain* in endometriosis can be acute or chronic. It can vary in location from the lower abdomen, to the back or the perineum. Involvement of the rectovaginal septum can result in rectal tenesmus. Severe pelvic pain is likely to indicate the presence of deep infiltrating endometriosis.[6]

Deep *dyspareunia* is a common symptom but may not be volunteered by the patient unless the clinician specifically asks about this. The dyspareunia described is felt deep within the body rather than superficially over the vaginal introitus.

The clinician should enquire if the pelvic pain and dyspareunia worsen during each menses. Although other gynecological pathology can cause these symptoms, pain that is more prominent during the menses is very suggestive of endometriosis.

Infertility is more common in patients with endometriosis. Thus, in married couples who have not conceived, the clinician should ask if contraception is being used and whether the couple has been actively trying to conceive or not. A failure to conceive after 12 months of trying is sufficient to warrant further investigations for causes of infertility. Fertility related enquiry is essential because infertile patients with endometriosis are managed differently to those in whom conception is not an issue.

Abnormal bleeding may occur. The clinician should ask if the periods are irregular, heavy and if intermenstrual bleeding occurs.

Endometriosis in sites outside the pelvic cavity is rare, but when they occur they can cause cyclical pain and bleeding locally. Endometriosis in the *gastrointestinal tract* can cause *cyclical rectal bleeding.* Endometriosis in the *bladder* can cause *cyclical dysuria and hematuria. Lung endometriosis* may cause *cyclical* chest pain and *hemoptysis.* If any pain or bleeding described by the patient follows a cyclical pattern related to menstruation, the clinician should have a high index of suspicion of endometriosis.

The severity of the patient's symptoms does not necessarily correlate with the severity of her endometriosis. Thus, a patient may have minimal or no symptoms but still have severe endometriosis.

Signs

Abdominal examination may identify areas of *tenderness,* or a *palpable mass* arising out of the pelvis. The mass may be due to adhesions of the pelvic organs or an endometrioma. The finding of a rigid abdomen and marked rebound tenderness should alert the clinician to the presence of an acute abdomen. In this situation a laparotomy or laparoscopy is often needed urgently. Endometriosis may cause an acute abdomen if a large endometrioma ruptures, spilling blood into the peritoneal cavity.

Vaginal examination may also reveal areas of tenderness or a palpable mass due to adhesions or an endometrioma. However, the most characteristic sign of endometriosis is the presence of *tender nodular indurations along the uterosacral ligaments.* The clinician can feel for these uterosacral nodules by performing a rectovaginal examination. The clinician should also check the mobility and flexion of the uterus. A fixed retroverted uterus is a common finding in advanced endometriosis and results from pelvic adhesions.

Rarely, the clinician may be able to see endometriotic *deposits on the cervix, vagina or skin.* These may appear as clear, red or blue cysts or nodules. They may be seen to bleed at the time of menstruation. However, to confirm that these lesions are endometriotic, a biopsy and histological diagnosis is essential.

Diagnosis

There are no pathognomic symptoms or signs of endometriosis. The only way to make a definitive diagnosis is to visualize endometriotic deposits within the pelvis at laparoscopy or laparotomy.

Blood tests may show a mild leukocytosis, an elevated erythrocyte sedimentation rate and a raised CA-125 level. The level of CA-125 depends on the severity of the disease. Often, it is only mildly elevated. However other pathology can cause identical findings and blood tests can never be conclusive in establishing the diagnosis of endometriosis.

An ultrasound scan may be useful in identifying a possible endometrioma. The clinician would look for a cyst containing echogenic material (the inside of the cyst looks full of white shadows with 'layering' rather than being uniformly dark). This suggests the presence of blood rather than clear fluid within the cyst. Also, the walls of an endometrioma appear irregular unlike the smooth walls of a typical simple ovarian cyst. However, an ultrasound cannot conclusively distinguish between an endometrioma and an ovarian tumor with bleeding within it. At best the ultrasound scan can suggest the need for a laparoscopy or laparotomy to confirm the diagnosis.

The typical endometriotic appearance at laparoscopy is described as being a "powder burn". These are small brown/black puckered lesions that look like the remains of cigarette burn (as if someone has stubbed out a cigarette onto the peritoneal surface). An endometrioma is also easily distinguished at laparoscopy from a bleeding ovarian cyst because the content of an endometrioma does not look like fresh blood. It has a thick consistency and a dark brown appearance similar to chocolate. Because of this, endometriomas are also known as chocolate cysts. The visualization of an endometrioma or the typical powder burn lesions at laparoscopy is enough to make the diagnosis. A biopsy of the lesion is only necessary if more subtle appearances of endometriosis are present. These are much more difficult to identify and diagnose correctly. Such lesions include red flame like lesions, yellow-brown spots (called café-au-lait spots), pink glandular lesions (that look like the mucosa of the endometrium as seen at hysteroscopy), white areas of opacification of the peritoneum, and round peritoneal defects (looking like small holes in the peritoneal surface).[7] The biopsy must show the presence of endometrial glands, stroma, and some evidence of menstrual activity (such as tissue hemorrhage or hemosiderin laden macrophages), before the diagnosis can be made.

Staging

Once a diagnosis is made, some effort should be made to classify the severity of the endometriosis. This is essential so that an appropriate treatment is chosen (simple treatments will not work for severe disease and aggressive surgical treatment is not warranted in mild disease). It will also allow us to assess accurately later if the disease has responded to treatment. Unfortunately no classification system so far has received universal acceptance. The most popular is the *Revised American Fertility Society Classification of Endometriosis*. This attempt to score the severity of the disease is based upon how deep the peritoneal and ovarian endometriosis is, how badly the pouch of Douglas is obliterated by adhesions, and by how dense the adhesions are on each tube and ovary. This score then classifies the endometriosis as being minimal, mild, moderate or severe (Figure 11.1). In the absence of a formalized scoring system the clinician should at least document the laparoscopic findings at diagnosis in detail, so that future laparoscopies can identify if treatment has worked or if the disease has progressed.

Management and Prognosis

Endometriosis is difficult to treat because most treatments for it result in an eventual recurrence of the disease of up to 60%. There is no known cure. The single most effective treatment so far is to perform a total abdominal hysterectomy and bilateral salpingo-oophorectomy (TAH BSO).

Management options consist of watching for disease progression and doing nothing, medical treatments and surgical treatments. There are many possible medical and surgical treatment options and each of these is described in more detail at the end of the chapter. Before examining each treatment, however, we will look at how the clinician decides which management option to use. This depends upon the answers to three essential questions, which the clinician should have elicited during history taking. These are:

1. Is the patient infertile?

Patient's Name ——————————————— Date ————————————————

Stage 1 (minimal) - 1-5
Stage II (mild) - 6-15
Stage III (moderate) - 16-40
Stage IV (severe) - >40
Total

Laparoscopy ———— Laparotomy———— Photography————

Recommended treatment ————————————————

Prognosis ————

		< 1 cm	1-3 cm	> 3 cm
Peritoneum	Endometriosis	< 1 cm	1-3 cm	> 3 cm
	Superficial	1	2	4
	Deep	2	4	6
Ovary	R Superficial	1	2	4
	Deep	4	16	20
	I Superficial	1	2	4
	Deep	4	16	20

	Partial	Complete
Posterior cul-de-sac obliteration	4	40

		< 1/3 enclosure	1/3-2/3 enclosure	> 2/3 enclosure
Ovary	Adhesions	< 1/3 enclosure	1/3-2/3 enclosure	> 2/3 enclosure
	R Filmy	1	2	4
	Dense	4	8	16
	L Filmy	1	2	4
	Dense	4	8	16
	R Filmy	1	2	4
	Dense	4	8	16
	L Filmy	1	2	4
	Dense	4	8	16

*If the fimbriated of the fallopian tube is completely enclosed, change the pint assignment to16.
Denote appearance of superficial implant types as red (R), red, red-pink, flamelike, vesicular blobs, clear vesicles, white (W), opacifications, peritoneal defects, yellow-brown, or blank (B), hemosiderin deposits, blue. Denote percent of total described as R.........% and B...........%. Total should equal 100%.

Additional Endometriosis ————————————

Associated pathology————————————

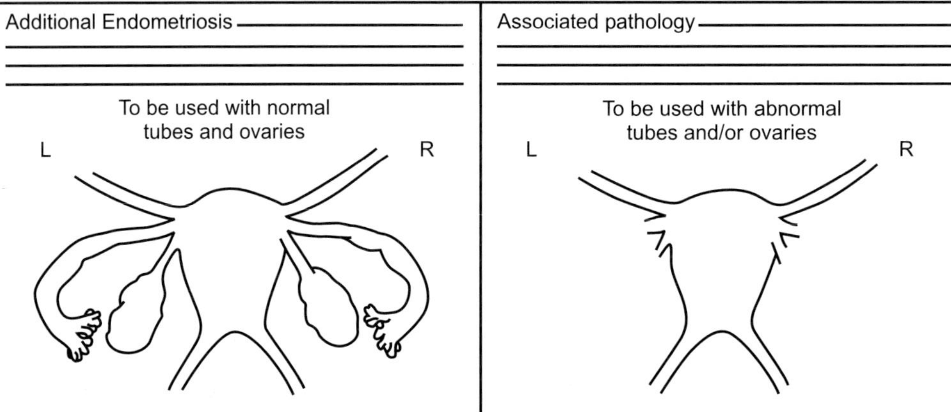

Figure 11.1: Modified American Fertility Society classification of endometriosis

2. Is the patient symptomatic?

3. How old is the patient?

These questions are considered in detail below and the most important points to note are summarized in Flow Chart 11.1.

Is the Patient Infertile?

If the patient is infertile, the aim is to investigate and treat the infertility as soon as possible. This is because the longer fertility treatment is delayed, the older the patient becomes, and the success rates of most fertility

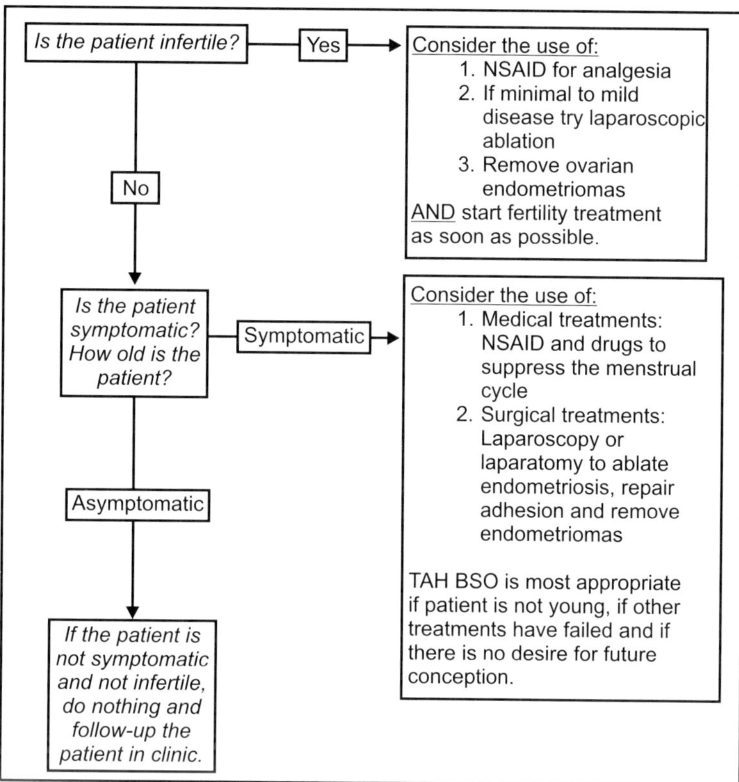

Flow chart 11.1: The management of endometriosis

treatments fall with advancing age. This is especially true if the patient is 35 years and over. This age factor is even more important in endometriosis because there is some evidence that *in vitro* fertilization pregnancy rates are even lower in endometriosis patients compared to other patients.[8]

Medical treatment options using hormonal drugs have been shown to have no beneficial effect on fertility rates in 13 randomized controlled trials (documented in the Cochrane Register of Controlled Trials).[9] The most effective medical treatment that can be used without interfering with fertility treatment is the use of nonsteroidal anti-inflammatory drugs (NSAIDs) for pain relief.

Laparoscopic ablation of minimal to mild endometriosis has been shown to improve fertility rates in a meta-analysis of nonrandomised controlled trials.[10] Because endometriosis can return within 12 months after laparoscopic ablation, fertility treatment should ideally be commenced immediately after such surgical treatment. Patients with ovarian endometriomas may also benefit

from having these removed or drained surgically prior to having fertility treatment. This is because most fertility treatments require the use of ovulation induction drugs to stimulate the ovaries to make eggs. An ovarian endometrioma will inhibit egg production in the affected ovary even with the use of such drugs. There is no evidence that more extensive surgical treatments for severe endometriosis will improve fertility rates, and they may even make conception more difficult (for example, repeated surgery can induce adhesion formation).

Is the Patient Symptomatic and How Old is the Patient?

Symptomatic patients warrant treatment to provide symptom relief. Both medical and surgical treatments have been shown to be effective in relieving symptoms, especially pain. Note, however, that a complete cure of the disease is unlikely. Most clinicians start with simple medical treatments (such as NSAID) before progressing to hormonal treatments aimed at suppressing the menstrual cycle and surgical treatments to ablate the endometriotic deposits. It is common to combine surgical and medical treatments (for example, laparoscopic ablation may be followed by 6 months of hormonal treatment).

If the endometriosis fails to respond to these treatments, and if the patient has no desire to conceive further, a TAH BSO is indicated. The patient's age is an important factor to consider when deciding if a TAH BSO is appropriate. If the patient is young, the aim is to try and avoid radical surgery. This is because if a TAH BSO is performed in a young patient, she is faced with requiring lifelong hormone replacement therapy (HRT) to prevent osteoporosis. HRT has its own attendent risks and a young patient would be exposed to these risks far longer than a menopausal patient taking HRT. There is also the rare possibility that the HRT itself may cause a recurrence of the endometriosis.

If the patient is neither symptomatic nor infertile, then no treatment is needed. Although it is known that some patients with minimal endometriosis may progress with time to a more severe stage of the disease, it has not been shown that early surgical or medical treatment will have any effect on disease progression. Many clinicians simply monitor such patients on a yearly basis and only consider treatment if symptoms occur. The closer the patient is to the menopause (the average age of menopause is 51 years), the more appropriate this 'wait and see' strategy is. This is because the majority of such patients will experience resolution of their disease once their menstrual cycles have stopped. Again, it should be noted that if the patients decide to use HRT; in some cases, their endometriosis might recur.

Surgical Treatments

Surgical treatments for endometriosis can be divided into conservative and radical options.

The aim of conservative surgery is to destroy all visible endometriotic deposits by vaporizing (using a laser), diathermising or excising the lesions. Usually, the degree of pelvic adhesions determines whether the procedure is done laparoscopically or via a laparotomy. If there are dense pelvic adhesions, it is safer to perform a laparotomy. Conservative surgery also aims to remove

adhesions and tries to restore the pelvic anatomy to normal. The ideal treatment for endometriomas is to excise them rather than simply puncturing and draining them. Drainage alone, even if followed by ovulation suppression drugs, is very likely to result in a recurrence of the endometrioma.[11] Because endometriotic deposits commonly occur on the uterosacral ligaments, a laparoscopic procedure to destroy the nerve supply to these ligaments can reduce the symptoms of dysmenorrhea. This procedure is called a Laparoscopic Uterosacral Nerve Ablation (LUNA). However, its efficacy has not been verified in large randomized trials.

Radical surgery aims to perform a TAH BSO as well as to destroy all visible endometriotic deposits on the pelvic sidewalls. Performing a TAH alone is insufficient because the endometriosis is likely to recur on the ovaries. Moreover, the removal of the ovaries causes a hypestrogenic state, which induces the endometriosis to regress (this is explained in detail in the next section). Many patients who are about to undergo a TAH for some other benign pathology, request the surgeon not to remove their ovaries provided they look normal. These patients must be counseled that endometriosis may be found incidentally at the operation, and if their ovaries are left *in situ*, they may get recurrent problems from ovarian endometriosis. In this case, it may be prudent to advise the patient that the ovaries should be left only if they look normal *and that there is no evidence of endometriosis in the pelvis.*

Medical Treatments

The first line medical treatment of endometriosis is to use an NSAID for pain relief. These drugs are very effective because many of them are prostaglandin synthetase inhibitors. Thus, they inhibit the formation of prostaglandins which (as explained in the patho-physiology section) are responsible for the main symptom of dysmenorrhea.

All other medical treatments for endometriosis aim to suppress the normal menstrual cycle. The principle here is that the ectopic endometrium proliferates and bleeds in response to ovarian hormone production just as normal endometrium in the uterus does. If the menstrual cycle is suppressed and the ovary stops making hormones, the patient's estrogen levels will fall dramatically. This is identical to what happens in menopausal women and women who have had their ovaries removed. The low estrogen levels in these women cause atrophy of the endometrium. Similarly, if an endometriosis patient has her menstrual cycles stopped, the resulting low estrogen levels will lead to atrophy of the uterine lining and atrophy of the ectopic endometrium. Because the ectopic endometrium usually consists of small superficial islands of endometrium, a few months without estrogen can cause these deposits to regress completely. However, the thick endometrial lining of the uterus will recover and proliferate once the hormone levels return to normal. Superficial endometriotic deposits are more likely to regress completely when exposed to a hypestrogenic state compared to deep endometriotic deposits. The latter may recur once the hormone levels return to normal. Thus, the aim is to use drugs to stop ovarian hormone production for a few months (creating a temporary 'artificial menopause' in the patient) in order to induce the superficial endometriotic deposits to atrophy and regress completely.

The medical treatments that do this consist of the combined contraceptive pill, progestogens, danazol, gestrinone and gonadotropin-releasing hormone agonists (GnRHa). They are all equally as effective as each other at pain relief.[12] So the decision on which treatment to use depends upon what the patient has tried before and the side effect profile of the individual drugs. Danazol, the combined contraceptive pill and GnRHa are the most widely used treatments for endometriosis. Danazol, gestrinone and GNRHa all have significant side effects so are never used as long-term treatments. Short courses of these drugs are given, which may be repeated at intervals should the patient's symptoms recur.

Symptom recurrence is common following medical treatment. For example, the cumulative recurrence rate after completing a course of GnRHa is 37% if the patient has minimal disease and 74% if the patient has severe disease.[13] Some patients may not respond to medical treatment. Severe cases of endometriosis may be best treated with radical surgery rather than medical treatment.

Progestogen treatment: Progestogens are synthetic drugs that mimic some of the actions of progesterone. Giving progestogens on a daily basis (or as a depot injection) will directly cause endometrial atrophy and will also suppress ovarian hormone production. The latter effect is mediated by high serum progestogen levels inhibiting follicle-stimulating hormone (FSH) and luteinizing hormone (LH) secretion from the pituitary gland (negative feedback). The side effects most commonly seen are breakthrough bleeding, weight gain, abdominal bloating, edema, acne and mood changes.

Combined oral contraceptive pill: The pill works primarily by inhibiting ovulation. It consists of a synthetic estrogen and a progestogen. The subsequent high serum estrogen and progestogen levels cause negative feedback to the hypothalamus and pituitary gland and inhibit FSH and LH production. Without FSH and LH production, the ovary will not produce a follicle. In the absence of a follicle there will be no oocyte to make estrogen and, therefore, no menstrual cycle will occur. Although serum estrogen levels are high, the pill suppresses endogenous estrogen production from the ovary, and the high progestogen levels antagonize the effects of the synthetic estrogen as well as directly stimulating endometrial atrophy. The last week of the pill packet either has no tablets or tablets containing no active drugs. Thus, the last week in a pill packet results in a dramatic fall in estrogen and progestogen levels, which in turn cause the shedding of the endometrial lining. This is called a withdrawal bleed (not a "normal" period) because it is caused by exogenous hormones and not by normal hormonal production from an oocyte in the ovary. In treating endometriosis, clinicians often prescribe the pill "back to back" for 3 to 12 months. This means that instead of having a pill free interval at the end of the pill packet, the patient takes active pills (containing hormones) continuously for those months. The rationale for this is that it prevents withdrawal bleeds from endometriosis in the pelvis and limits further development of the endometriosis by preventing retrograde menstruation. The side effects of the pill are covered elsewhere in this book.

Danazol: Danazol is a derivative of 17-alpha-ethinyl testosterone. Thus, like testosterone, it has strong androgenic and anabolic properties, which are responsible for its serious side effects. It has a very complex mechanism of action. It interferes with LH and FSH secretion, as well as directly suppressing ovarian hormone production. It is given as daily tablets for at least 6 months. The clinician aims to put the patient on a dose that will make her amenorrheic whilst still keeping the side effects tolerable. Because danazol is strongly androgenic, there is a possibility that if the patient gets pregnant with a female fetus while taking the drug, it may masculinize the fetus. To minimize this risk, danazol is started in the early part of the menstrual cycle (follicular phase) when an egg has not had the chance to develop. In addition, patients are advised to use barrier methods of contraception. The side effects for the patient are weight gain, acne, oily skin, fluid retention, muscle cramps, hot flushes, and mood swings. The patient must be counseled that if they start to develop hirsutism, a skin rash or deepening of the voice, they must stop the treatment immediately. Failure to do so may result in some of the androgenic changes becoming permanent.

Gonadotropin-releasing hormone agonists (GnRHa): GnRHa induce a hypoestrogenic state in the patient. Normally, pulsatile release of GNRH from the hypothalamus binds to cell membrane receptors on the anterior pituitary and results in secretion of FSH and LH. When a GnRHa is first given, it mimics the action of GNRH and causes an initial increase in FSH and LH. However, unlike GNRH release from the hypothalamus that is pulsatile, a GnRHa provides a continuous supply of proteins binding to the pituitary receptors. This has a dramatic negative effect on the pituitary receptors. After a few days, the excess concentration of GnRHa binding to receptors causes a loss in cell membrane receptors (they become internalized into the cell). This is called downregulation and is the main biological mechanism by which the activity of polypeptide hormones is limited. Continuous GnRHa release also causes desensitization (meaning the receptors become uncoupled from the secretory signal). This results in the pituitary gland being completely unable to respond to GNRH or GnRHa. Thus, no gonadotropins are produced by it and a hypoestrogenic state occurs. GnRHa achieves this effect within about ten days from first administration. Thus, symptomatic relief for the endometriosis patient is usually rapid. An additional advantage is that it can be given as a once monthly injection. Its side effects are all the symptoms of a hypoestrogenic state (the symptoms of the menopause), which include hot flushes, headaches, atrophic vaginitis and decreased libido. GnRHa also causes an increased urinary secretion of calcium so that after 6 months of use, there is a 3-5% loss in bone mineral density.[14] This osteopenic change is completely reversible provided the GnRHa is discontinued after 6 months. Because of this, GnRHa use is usually only maintained for just 3 to 6 months; and if longer treatment is required, the patient is also given daily low doses of progestogen with or without estrogen. This so-called "Add-back" therapy will prevent bone loss during GnRHa use.

Gestrinone: Gestrinone is a synthetic steroid that has androgenic and antigonadotropic properties. Its combined effect is to induce endometrial atrophy. Its androgenic side effects are similar to those of danazol. Although it has been shown to be effective in treating endometriosis, it has not been as widely used and validated as danazol and GnRHa.

ADENOMYOSIS

Adenomyosis is a condition characterized by the benign invasion of endometrium into the myometrium of the uterus. This is usually accompanied by a diffuse hyperplasia of the myometrium. The diagnosis can only be confirmed by a histological examination of the uterus after it has been removed at a hysterectomy (endometrial glands and stroma need to be identified within the uterine wall). Unlike endometriosis, it tends to occur in older multiparous women. The patient typically complains of increasingly severe menorrhagia, secondary dysmenorrhea and a distended abdomen. Examination reveals an enlarged and tender uterus. It is difficult to distinguish this clinically from uterine fibroids. However, a smoothly enlarged symmetrical uterus that is tender all over is more likely to be due to adenomyosis. Fibroids usually cause an irregularly enlarged uterus with tenderness absent or present only over one localized fibroid (if it is undergoing degeneration). The clinician should exclude a uterine malignancy, and bear in mind that a very rapidly enlarging uterus may be due to a leiomyosarcoma. Ultrasound scan shows that the myometrium is diffusely thickened. Endometriosis may coexist with adenomyosis in 15% of cases. Unlike endometriosis, the ectopic endometrium in adenomyosis is completely unresponsive to ovarian hormone fluctuations. Thus, medical treatments are limited to just using NSAID for analgesia. The treatment of choice is a hysterectomy. Removal of the ovaries is only indicated if other pathology is present (such as endometriosis).

PRACTICE POINTS

Endometriosis

Presentation: Causes dysmenorrhea, pelvic pain, dyspareunia, abnormal bleeding and infertility. Vaginal examination may reveal a fixed retroverted uterus, uterosacral nodules and palpable cysts.

Investigations: Ultrasound scan may detect an endometrioma. Visualizing powder burn lesions or an endometrioma at laparoscopy or laparotomy confirms the diagnosis.

Management: Treat infertility as soon as possible. Surgically ablate endometriotic deposits. Induce endometrial atrophy with progestogens, the combined contraceptive pill, danazol, gonadotropin-releasing hormone agonists or gestrinone. The best treatment is total abdominal hysterectomy and bilateral salpingo-oophorectomy.

Adenomyosis

Presentation: Causes menorrhagia, dysmenorrhea and a symmetrically enlarged tender uterus.

Investigations: Ultrasound scan shows a diffusely enlarged myometrium. Diagnosis is only confirmed by histology after a hysterectomy.

Management: Hysterectomy.

REFERENCES

1. Taylor JEA. Surgical considerations in gynecological endocrine disorders. Surgical Clinics of North America 1974; 54: 425-42.
2. Sampson JA. The development of the implantation theory for the origin of peritoneal endometriosis. American Journal of Obstetrics and Gynecology 1940; 40: 549.
3. Meyer R. Uber den Staude der Frage der Ademyosites Adenomyoma in Allgemeinen und Adenomyometitis Sarcomastosa. Zentralblatt fur Gynakologie 1919; 36: 745-59.
4. Muscato JJ, Haney AF, Weinberg JB. Sperm phagocytosis by human peritoneal macrophages: A possible cause of infertility in endometriosis. American Journal of Obstetrics and Gynecology 1982; 144: 503-510.
5. Meldrum DR, Shamonki IM, Clarke KE. Prostaglandin content of ascitic fluid in endometriosis. 25th Annual Meeting of the Pacific Coast Fertility Society, Palm Springs, California; 1977.
6. Koninckx PR, Meuleman C, Demeyere S, Lesaffre E, Cornillie F. Suggestive evidence that pelvic endometriosis is a progressive disease whereas deeply infiltrating endometriosis is associated with pelvic pain. Fertility and Sterility 1991; 55: 759-65.
7. Donnez J, Nisolle M, Clerckx F et al. Appearance of peritoneal endometriosis. In: IIIrd Laser Surgery Symposium, Brussels 1990.
8. Landazabal A, Diaz I, Valbuena D, et al. Factors that affect outcome of in-vitro fertilisation treatment. Lancet 1996; 348: 1402-06.
9. Hughes E, Fedorkow D, Collins J, Vandekeckhove P. Ovulation suppression versus placebo in the treatment of endometriosis (Cochrane Review). In The Cochrane Library 1999, Issue 3.
10. Adamson G D, Pasta D J. Surgical treatment of endometriosis-associated infertility: meta-analysis compared with survival analysis. Am J Obstet Gynecol 1994;171:1488-1504.
11. Vercellini P, Vendola N, Bocciolone L et al. Laparoscopic aspiration of ovarian endometriomas: Effect with postoperative gonadotropin-releasing hormone agonist treatment. Journal of Reproductive Medicine 1992; 37: 577-80.
12. In: The Investigation and Management of Endometriosis. RCOG Guideline No 24; 2000; Royal College of Obstetricians and Gynecologists, 27 Sussex Place, Regents Park, London, NW1 4RG.
13. Prentice A, Dreary AJ, Goldbeck-Wood S, Farquhar C, Smith SK. Gonadotropin-releasing hormone analogues for pain associated with endometriosis (Cochrane Review). In: The Cochrane Library 1999, Issue 3.
14. Henzl MR, Corson SL, Moghissi K, Buttram VC, Bergquist C, Jacobson C. Administration of nasal nafarelin as compared with oral danazol for endometriosis. New England Journal of Medicine 1988;318:485-89.

12.
Pelvic Inflammatory Disease (PID)

Siya Sharan Sharma
Pratap Kumar

INTRODUCTION

PID implies inflammation of the upper genital tract involving the uterine cavity, fallopian tubes and ovaries. The PID lesions are usually bilateral since infection is ascending or blood born; though at times, it may be unilateral. PID is caused by the microorganisms that colonize the endocervix or those that ascend the cervix from exterior to the endometrium and fallopian tube.

NATURAL BARRIERS TO PID

Before describing the etiological factors, the normal protective mechanism of female genital tract should be understood. Natural barriers that present pathogenic organisms from the vagina entering the fallopian tube include the following (Table 12.1):

Table 12.1: Natural barriers to PID

1. Intact hymen.
2. Acidity of vaginal secretions inhibits the growth of bacteria.
3. Narrow cervical canal with alkaline mucus plug.
4. Downward ciliary movement of endometrial and cervical lining discouraging the ascent of nonmotile organisms.

Vulnerability to PID

Factors and events that enable the genital tract more vulnerable to infection are given in Table 12.2 and organisms associated with PID are given in Table 12.3.

Table 12.2: Factors/events associated with PID

1. Menstruation, abortion and delivery.
   a. Widening of cervical canal and opening of internal os.
   b. Shedding of the protective epithelium of endometrium.
   c. Raw surface present in the uterine cavity.
   d. Vaginal pH is increased and become alkaline.
2. Intrauterine manipulations like dilatation and curettage
3. Manual removal of placenta
4. Insertion of intrauterine contraceptive devices (IUCDs) without strict asepsis.

Table 12.3: Organisms responsible for PID

Common
1. *Niesseria gonorrheae*
2. *Chlamydia trachomatis*

Occasional
1. *Gardenerella vaginalis*
2. *Mycoplasma hominis*
3. Tubercular bacillus
4. *Escherichia coli*

Rare
1. *Haemophilus influenzae*
2. Group B streptococci
3. Pneumococci

1. **STD organisms:** The most common (60-75%) cause of PID is sexually transmitted diseases (STDs). Commonly, PID is caused by *Niesseria gonorrhoeae* (30% of cases) and *Chlamydia trachomatis.*[1] These pathogens ascend along the mucosa and possibly with sperms to the pelvis and cause salpingo-oopheritis. Endogenous vaginal microorganisms such as *Gardnerella vaginalis* may cause PID.[2] The infection by anaerobic organisms is greatly favored by blood loss, anemia, and tissue damage as seen in septic miscarriage.

2. **Postabortal and postdelivery (puerperal) sepsis:** This is the second most common cause of the PID. The incidence of PID in about one third of all women is due to this factor. Illegal and septic abortions by untrained persons is the common factor. After delivery, manual removal of placenta may induce ascending infections in some cases.

3. **Operative procedures:** Minor surgical procedures such as dilatation and curettage, hysterosalpingography, and sonosalpingography, may cause acquired ascending infection resulting in PID.

4. **Intrauterine contraceptive device (IUCD):** IUCD users do not have higher incidence of PID. If aseptic and antiseptic procedures are followed during IUCD insertion, the incidence of PID is minimal.

PATHOLOGY (Figure 2.1)

Acute PID

Exterior of the fallopian tube (exosalpingitis): The fallopian tube is swollen, edematous, and congested or hyperemic with dilated vessels on the serosal surface.

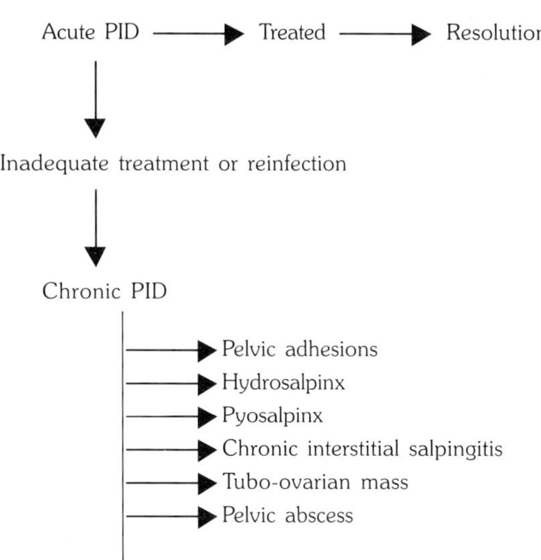

Figure 12.1: Sequelae of PID

Serous exudation is usually seen around the tube. Seropurulent discharge from the fimbrial end is the strongest feature in favor of salpingitis. Peritoneal surface may be congested in the pelvis.

Interior of the fallopian tube (endosalpingitis): In ascending infection the mucosa is the first one to be affected. The mucous membrane inflammation with edema, redness and deciliation takes place in the initial stage of salpingitis. Submucosa is infiltrated with leukocytes and plasma cells. The inflammatory exudate is discharged into the lumen. The inflammatory response leads to breach of mucosal surface and adhesions are formed between mucosal folds of the tube. This leads to narrowing and finally blockage of the tube resulting in infertility. The inflammation extends to the serosal surface in later stages.

In early part of this inflammatory process, fimbrial end remains open, and allows the seropurulent secretions to be discharged into the peritoneal cavity. The collection of this pus may lead to pelvic abscess. In later part of the disease, fimbria gets adherent to each other by fibrinous adhesions and fimbriae are drawn into the tube leading to closure of fimbrial opening. With continuous secretion of such exudates the ampullary portion of the tube is distended. The formation of retort shape pyosalpinx follows. Once ovaries are involved with tube, a tubo-ovarian mass is formed where both tube and ovary are entangled in adhesions. The pyosalpinx or tubo-ovarian mass becomes adherent to posterior surface of the uterus or broad ligament involving ovaries, sigmoid colon, and loops of small intestine. Tubal wall appears thickened and tense. In advanced stages and in untreated cases of PID, pelvic and general peritonitis may occur associated with paralytic ileus and rarely subdiaphragmatic and/or perinephric abscess and even septicemia.

Usually, infection through cervix and endometrium causes endosalpingitis affecting inner lumen of tube and fimbriae, leading to hydrosalpinx. In some women, after abortion or vaginal delivery, infection through cervix spreads via lymphatics to parametrium and broad ligament causing parametritis. This reaches the outer aspect of tube to cause exosalpingitis.

Chronic PID (Tubo-ovarian Mass)

This form of disease is the continuation of the acute form if the infection fails to resolve completely due to inadequate antibiotic treatment or reinfection. This may result in tubo-ovarian mass formation which may present as:

1. Hydrosalpinx
2. Chronic pyosalpinx
3. Tubo-ovarian mass
4. Chronic interstitial salpingitis

Hydrosalpinx: In PID hydrosalpinx which is bilateral, is the end result of previous acute salpingitis. Fimbrial end is closed and fimbriae are drawn into the tube. It is retort shaped with clear fluid collection in the ampullary part of the tube. Outer surface appears smooth, wall is thin and transluscent. Commonly, it is adherent to surrounding structures; but occasionally, if it is mobile. It may undergo torsion causing acute pain in the abdomen.

Pyosalpinx: Pyosalpinx is thick walled and surrounded by dense adhesions. The inner wall is replaced by a granulation tissue. Usually, it obliterates the pouch of Douglas (POD) where it is densely adherent.

Tubo-ovarian mass: In this condition the inflamed tube and ovary are matted together to form a mass, which may lead to an ovarian abscess.

Chronic interstitial salpingitis: The wall of fallopian tube is thickened and fibrotic, but there is no dilatation of tube due to pus or fluid. Usually, adhesions are present in the pelvis.

CLINICAL FEATURES OF PID

Pelvic inflammatory disease is common in young sexually active women (Table 12.4). Chlamydial infection remains asymptomatic or produces minimal symptoms, and therefore, the infection goes unnoticed and untreated, but the damage it causes to the tube is extensive leading to adhesions, fibrosis and tubal blockage.

Table 12.4: Summary of clinical criteria for the diagnosis of PID

Symptoms
    Not necessary for diagnosis

Signs
1. Uterine, cervical or adnexal tenderness
2. Leukorrhea and or mucopurulent endocervicitis

Additional/Laboratory investigations
1. Endometrial biopsy (not always done for fear of disseminating the infection, unless infected retained tissue is suspected) and culture and sensitivity showing evidence of endometritis.
2. Elevated C reactive protein or ESR
3. Temperature higher than 38°C
4. Leukocytosis
5. Positive test for gonorrhea or *Chlamydia*

Specific tests
Sonography of pelvic organs to search for tubo-ovarian mass or adnexal mass

One previous episode of PID predisposes the woman to another episode of PID in 12%, two episodes of PID increase the risk to 35% and three episodes to as much as 75%.[3]

Acute PID

Symptoms

1. The commonest symptom is acute abdominal pain. The pain is in lower abdomen and is difficult to pinpoint. Pain may be felt in the upper part of abdomen if peritonitis is present.
2. It is accompanied by high temperature and vomiting may occasionally be present.

3. There may be history of dyspareunia and vaginal discharge, especially in cases associated with STDs.
4. Menstrual problems include intermenstrual bleeding or menorrhagia which is due to endometritis and congestion of the pelvis.
5. In cases of pelvic abscess diarrhea may develop with passage of small loose stools due to rectal irritation.
6. In some women, associated urinary tract infection is present giving rise to increased frequency of micturation and dysuria.

Signs

1. She may appear ill with high temperature ranging between 38-40°C.
2. Tachycardia and tachypnea are associated findings.
3. Dehydration is present and tongue is dry and coated.
4. Abdominal examination reveals distention, tenderness, and rigidity, especially in lower abdomen. Direct or rebound abdominal tenderness may be present. Tubo-ovarian mass is difficult to palpate in acute stage of PID but may be felt in chronic disease. The mass observed in 20% of women is usually tender and fixed in the pelvis.
5. Speculum examination may show purulent discharge from the cervix.
6. On bimanual pelvic examination cervical movements are tender. This is due to the presence of peritoneal inflammation that causes pain when peritoneum is stretched by moving the cervix that causes traction of the adnexa on the pelvic peritoneum. Vaginal fornices are also tender. Tender pelvic mass may be felt which has restricted mobility. This mass is usually posterior and close to uterus. If pelvic abscess is present, there will be fluctuating tender swelling in the pouch of Douglas, bulging into the posterior fornix.

There are wide variations in symptoms and signs leading to difficulties in the diagnosis of acute PID. Many women with PID exhibit subtle or mild symptoms that are not readily recognized as PID. Consequent delay in diagnosis and therapy contributes to the inflammatory sequelae in the upper genital tract.[4]

Laboratory Investigations

1. **Blood:**
   a. Haemoglobin and PCV are usually within normal parameters.
   b. Total and differential leukocyte counts are increased and neutrophils are more in acute phase of infection while lymphocytes are increased in chronic infections.
   c. Erythrocyte sedimentation rate (ESR) is raised.
   d. C-reactive protein levels are elevated characteristically to 20-30 mg/dl or more.
   e. Blood urea and electrolytes.
   f. Test for gonorrhea and *Chlamydia* should also be performed.
2. **Wet smear microscopy:** Evaluation of high vaginal and endocervical secretions is important for the correct diagnosis of PID. In women with PID, an increased number of polymorphonuclear leukocytes may be detected in a wet mount of the vaginal secretions or in the mucopurulent discharge.[5]
3. **Culture and sensitivity:**
   a. Endocervical and high vaginal swabs are taken and cultured for both aerobic and anaerobic organisms.
   b. Urethral swab culture is done if gonorrhea is suspected.
   c. For chlamydial infection, endocervical swab is taken, this is inoculated on cyclohexidine-treated McCoy cells for culture.
   d. Endometrial biopsy is done in special circumstances and sent for culture and sensitivity to confirm the presence of endometritis.
   e. Blood culture if there are constitutional symptoms of high fever, peritonitis or septicemia.
4. Ultrasonography is useful in detecting tubo-ovarian mass or abscess in pelvis.

Chronic PID

Symptoms

1. The overall general health is poor and woman appears tired and exhausted.
2. History of previous pelvic infections is the clinching feature in the diagnosis.

3. Constant lower abdominal pain is the main complaint. This pain is worsened prior to and during menstruation.
4. Low backache and dyspareunia are accompanying features due to pelvic adhesions or mass in POD.
5. Occasionally, vaginal discharge may be present due to cervicitis.
6. Menstrual problems including menorrhagia, polymenorrhagia, and congestive dysmenorrhea are present due to pelvic congestion.
7. Infertility may be a complaint if tubes are blocked.
8. Rectal irritation and accompanying diarrhea are also seen in a few women due to pelvic abscess.

Signs

1. Discharge is seen coming through the external os. Cervical movement are tender.
2. Adnexal and forneceal tenderness and thickening are also present.
3. Uterus generally is retroverted with limited mobility. Sometimes it is difficult to define the uterus separately from adnexa or pelvic mass due to dense pelvic adhesions and fixity of the pelvic organs. This condition is known as "frozen pelvis".

Differential Diagnosis

1. *Acute appendicitis:* Pain is central around the umbilicus and later radiates to right iliac fossa. Vomiting is severe, but the temperature is not so high.
2. *Ectopic pregnancy:* Pain in the abdomen may be more on one side. Irregular uterine bleeding with or without amenorrhea. Movement of the cervix causes pain. Temperature is not high. Signs of internal hemorrhage may be present. Pregnancy test is positive.
3. *Twisted ovarian tumor:* Presents with sudden pain and vomiting but no fever. Uterus is normal in size and a tender adnexal mass is palpable.
4. *Ruptured ovarian cyst:* Though acute pain is present, there is no pyrexia or vaginal discharge.
5. *Septic abortion:* Mimics clinical features of PID. History of amenorrhea is significant.

6. *Degenerated fibroids:* Clinical findings like fixity and tenderness are similar if it is adherent to the pelvic organs.

TREATMENT

Broad-spectrum antibiotic regimens are the mainstay of PID treatment. Antibiotics should provide empiric, broad-spectrum coverage of likely pathogens including *Neisseria gonorrhoeae, Chlamydia trachomatis*, gram-negative facultative bacteria, anaerobes, and streptococci.

Sexual partners of women with PID should be evaluated and treated for urethral infection with *Chlamydia* or gonorrhea.

Acute PID

Mild: These women are treated on an outpatient women basis with the combination of antibiotics. It is convenient for the women and save time and money (Table 12.5).

Table 12.5: Outpatient antibiotic treatment

Regimen—A
Cefoxitin 2 gm intramuscularly Plus Probenecid 1 gm orally concurrently, or
Ceftriaxone or cephalosporin 250 mg intramuscularly
<Plus>
Doxycycline 100 mg orally 2 times daily for 14 days (For *Chlamydia*)
Regimen—B
Ofloxacin 400 mg orally BID for 14 days or Ciprofloxacin 500 mg single dose (For gonorrhea)
<Plus>
Clindamycin 450 mg orally qid, or metronidazole 400 mg orally tid for 14 days.
Or
Tetracycline 500 mg qid for 10 days/Erythromycin 500 qid for 7 days.

Moderate to severe: These women are treated in the hospital. Hospitalization is required to perform investigations and gives time to diagnose the disease (Table 12.6).

Indications for the Hospitalization in PID

1. When diagnosis is uncertain.
2. Pelvic abscess is suspected.
3. Clinical disease is severe, i.e. high temperature, adnexal mass, pelvic or general peritonitis.
4. Compliance with an outpatient's regimen is doubtful.

Table 12.6: Hospitalized women

Regimen – A
Cefoxitin 2 gm intravenously every 6 hours, or
Cefotetan 2 gm intravenously every 12 hours,
<Plus>
Doxycycline 100 mg intravenously or orally every 12 hours
IV Antibiotics are continued for at least 48 hours after the clinical improvement, later oral route is preferred, Doxycline 100 mg for 10-14 days.
Instead of Cefotetan other Cephalosporins such as Ceftizoxime, cephalotaxime and cepfriaxone can be used
Regimen – B
Clindamycin 900 mg intravenously every 8 hours
<Plus>
Gentamicin loading dose IV/IM 2 mg/kg body weight, followed by a maintenance dose of 1.5 mg /kg every 8 hours.
IV Antibiotics are continued for at least 48 hours after the clinical improvement. Later oral route is preferred; Doxycline 100 mg for 10-14 days or Clindamycin 450 mg orally five times a day for 10-14 days.

Indications for Discharge from the Hospital in those with PID[6]

1. When fever has settled (38°C for more than 24 hours).
2. Total leukocyte count has become normal.
3. Rebound tenderness is absent.
4. Repeat examination shows marked amelioration of pelvic organ tenderness.

Treatment Plans for Hospitalized Women

1. Rest: Women with PID are weak and they require bedrest till they feel stable.
2. Medical management with antibiotics, analgesics and intravenous fluids.
3. Minimal invasive surgery if required.
4. Major surgery may be rarely required.

Medical Management

Intravenous fluids: Required to correct dehydration because of vomiting and fluid loss and electrolyte imbalance. Ryle's tube aspiration is required in case of peritonitis and intestinal distention.

Analgesics: Antispasmodics and NSAID group to relieve the woman from pain.

Antibiotics: The antibiotic therapy should be instituted without waiting for culture and sensitivity reports, since a wait may worsen the situation. In most cases of PID the polymicrobial factors are responsible including aerobes and anaerobes. So it is wise to administer a combination of antibiotics to get the quick response of therapy and to prevent the permanent damage to the tubes. Initially, intravenous route is employed and once the patient becomes stable, oral therapy should be provided. Timely and appropriate change in antibiotics is required if therapy fails or culture and sensitivity report demands.

Treatment of PID

Surgical Treatment

Approximately 75% women with TO abscess will respond to antimicrobial therapy alone. Failure of medical therapy suggests the need for surgical exploration and drainage of the abscess.[7]

1. Drainage of pelvic abscess by colpotomy or colpocentesis.
2. Laparotomy:
   a. to drain peritoneal pus.
   b. to correct intestinal obstruction.
   c. in ruptured and twisted TO masses or abscesses.
3. Laparoscopy to drain TO abscess is indicated when:
   a. Size of abscess is less than 10 cm.
   b. No response to antibiotic treatment in 42-72 hours.
   c. Abscess ruptures.
   d. Pyoperitoneum
4. Ultrasound-guided abscess aspiration can be done vaginally, but success is limited.

Treatment of Chronic Pelvic Inflammatory Disease

Apart from medical management, these women require surgical intervention as this condition is the end result of acute PID. Surgical treatment depends on the age and parity of the women, symptoms and pelvic pathology.

In young women, conservative surgery like salpingectomy or salpingo-oophorectomy may be required. When extensive damage preclude conservative surgery or when the woman is old and multiparous, abdominal hysterectomy and bilateral salpingo-oophorectomy may be needed.

Tuboplasty: Women who have mild and adequately treated disease with minimal tubal damage require corrective surgery of the fallopian tube. Hysteroscopic falloposcopy or laparoscopic salpingoscopy is preferably performed to assess the damage before embarking on surgery. Adhesiolysis may be needed in cases where tube is blocked or anatomy is disturbed due to pelvic adhesions. Fluoroscopic tubal re-cannulation or hysteroscopic balloonplasty is advised if tube is blocked due to mild intratubal adhesions or cellular debris or plugs.

Uncommon Complications of Chlamydia and Gonorrhea

Both these infections may spread into the abdominal cavity and cause periappendicitis and perihepatitis.

Fitz-Hugh-Curtis syndrome: PID with perihepatitis has been known as "Fitz-Hugh-Curtis syndrome". These women present with right hypochondrial pain and tenderness and hyperpyrexia. This may be confused with cholecystitis. One has to look for other features of PID. If laparoscopy is performed in these women, fine 'violin string' adhesions are seen between the liver capsule and visceral peritoneum. The optimum treatment for this is to give an antibiotic course for three weeks.

Sexually acquired reactive arthritis (SARA): This occurs due to dissemination of *Chlamydia* to joints and is seen in less than 1% of PID women. There is usually an asymmetrical oligoarthritis, affecting large joints of the lower limb.

Reiter's syndrome: In this condition chlamydial arthritis is accompanied by uveitis and a rash that, if florid, may be similar to psoriasis.

Gonococcal arthritis: Disseminated gonococcal infection occurs rarely and presents as a septic oligoarthritis, usually affecting the small joints of the hand or wrist, with a scanty papular rash.

REFERENCES

1. Soper DE, Brockwell NJ, Dalton HP. Microbial etiology of urban department acute salpingitis: Treatment with ofloxacin. Am J Obstet Gynecol 1992;167:653-60.
2. Soper DE, Brockwell NJ, Dalton HP, Johnson D. Observations concerning the microbial etiology of acute salpingitis. Am J Obstet Gynecol 1994;170:1008-17.
3. Padubidari V, Daftary SN (Eds). Howkins and Bourne Shaw's Textbook of Gynecology, 12th edn, New Delhi: BI Churchill Livingstone Pvt Ltd, 2000; 106-114 and 351-366.
4. Hillis SD, Joesoef R, Marchbanks PA, Wasserheit JN, Cates W Jr, Westrom L. Delayed care of pelvic inflammatory disease as a risk factor of impaired fertility. Am J Obstet Gynecol 1993;168:1503-9.
5. Westrom J. Diagnosis and treatment of salpingitis. J Reprod Med 1983;28:703-8.
6. Soper DE. Pelvic inflammatory disease. Infect Dis Clin North Am 1994;8:821-40.
7. Reed SD, Landers DV, Sweet RL. Antibiotic treatment of tuboovarian abscesses: Comparison of broad spectrum beta lactum agents versus clindamycin-containing regimens. Am J Obstet Gynecol 1991;164:1556-62.

FURTHER READING

1. Berek J, Adashi EY, Hillard PA (Eds). Novak's Gynecology, 12th edn, Mary Land: Williams and Wilkins, 1996.
2. Campbell S, Monga A (Eds). Gynecology by ten teachers, 17th edn, London: ELTS with Arnold, 2000.
3. Padubidari V, Daftary SN (Eds). Howkins and Bourne Shaw's Textbook of Gynecology, 12th edn, New Delhi: BI Churchill Livingstone Pvt Ltd, 2000.

13.

Siya Sharan Sharma
Pratap Kumar

Sexually Transmitted Diseases

INTRODUCTION

The female genital tract is vulnerable to acquire infection from the external environment because of its anatomical location. The defense mechanisms are so protective that the organisms are not allowed access to the genital tract despite its anatomical vulnerability.

DEFENSE MECHANISM OF FEMALE GENITAL TRACT (Table 13.1)

Table 13.1: Defense mechanism of female genital tract

1. Vulva:
    a. Closure of the introitus by apposition of the labia protects entry of organisms.
    b. Secretion of the apocrine glands which is rich in undecylenic acid that is fungicidal.

2. Vagina:
    a. Closure by apposition of its anterior and posterior walls.
    b. Well developed and mature stratified squamous epithelium.
    c. Vaginal acidity: The normal vaginal pH is lower than 4.5 and is acidic. This is maintained by the production of lactic acid from epithelial glycogen by the lactobacilli.
    d. Vaginal flora – Doderlein's bacillus (lactobacillus) is normally predominant and by its lactic acid production, keep other organisms in check and maintains vaginal acidity. Vaginal defense is directly proportional to the relative number of bacilli.

3. Cervix: Functional closure of the cervix is affected by mucus which is also said to be bacteriolytic.

4. Uterus: Periodic shedding of surface endometrium during menstruation tends to eliminate any infection which may try to gain access.

Variations in the Efficiency of Defense Mechanisms

With Age

The defenses are imperfect during childhood and after the menopause when

a. The vagina has thin and vulnerable epithelium, its content of glycogen and Doderlein's bacilli is low, and the vaginal acidity is reduced.

b. The endometrium is also poorly developed or atrophied at these ages and does not undergo cyclical shedding.

With Menstruation

a. During menstruation the cervical plug is absent and vaginal acidity is lowered by the alkaline menstrual discharge.
b. Infection may ascend to the uterus and tubes at this time.

During Puerperium

In adult women the genital tract defenses are weakened during and immediately after miscarriage or delivery because:

a. There is raw placental site,
b. There are often breaks in the epithelial lining of the cervix and the vagina,
c. The tissues are bruised and devitalized,
d. The vulva, vagina, and cervix are wide open,
e. The discharge of liquor and lochia are alkaline so reduced vaginal acidity,
f. Degenerating blood clots and fragments of decidua offer a nidus for infections,
g. Patient's general resistance is lowered by pregnancy and possibly by anemia and malnutrition.

SEXUALLY TRANSMITTED DISEASES (STDs)

The incidence of STDs is increasing due to high promiscuity and multiple sex partners. Sexually transmitted diseases being common in all parts of the globe require a clear understanding of the etiology, clinical features, and treatment. The appropriate treatment is the key to the success in relieving the patients of their chronic and irritating symptoms and signs. Timely intervention in the disease processes will reduce the long-term adverse effects on the genital tract and on the psychology of the women.

STDs are responsible for infertility—due to blocked tubes and pelvic adhesions, ectopic gestation, and pre-cancer of cervix and vulva. Perinatal transmission of infection can cause miscarriage, preterm labor, intra-uterine fetal death, fetal anomalies, and neonatal diseases like ophthalmia.

Traditionally, only a few infections such as gonorrhea, syphilis, human papilloma virus (HPV), and chancroid, were considered STDs. In recent times some more diseases have been associated with sexual transmission (Fig. 13.1). These include trichomoniasis, candidiasis, herpes genitalis, chlamydial infection, genital warts, HIV, and hepatitis A

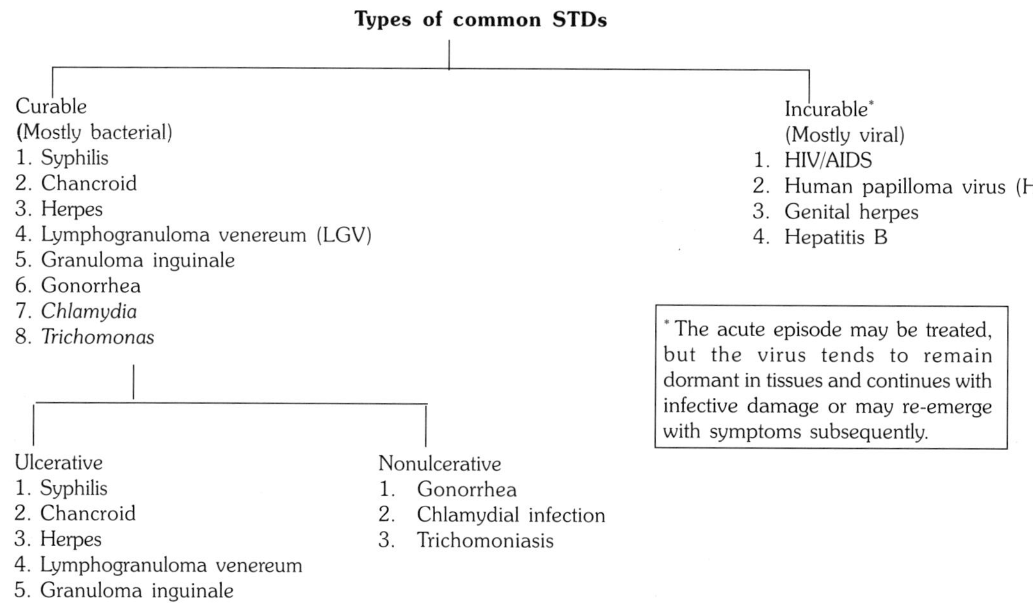

Figure 13.1: Types of common STDs

Table 13.2: Summary of STDs—organisms, mode of transmission and sequelae

Name of disease	Causative organism	Mode of transmission	Sequelae
A. Bacterial			
1. Gonorrhea	Neisseria gonorrhoeae	Sexually Transmitted Infection (STI)	Urethritis, epididymitis, cervicitis, salpingitis, endometritis, disseminated disease
2. Chlamydial infection	Chlamydia trachomatis	STI	Same as above and Reiter's syndrome
3. Syphilis	Treponema pallidum	STI	Vulval ulcers, lymphadenopathy, tabes dorsalis*, aortic aneurysm*
B. Viral			
1. AIDS	Human immunodeficiency virus (HIV)	STI, contaminated needles, transfusion of infected blood and blood products, mother to fetus	Multisystem infections Kaposi's sarcoma Death
2. Herpes	Herpes simplex virus (HSV)	STI	Genital herpes Neonatal herpes Aseptic meningitis CIN, Cancer cervix,
3. Condyloma accuminata	Human papilloma virus (HPV)	STI	Penile cancer
C. Protozoan			
1. Trichomoniasis	Trichomonas vaginalis	STI	Vaginitis, vulvitis
D. Fungal			
1. Candidiasis	Candida albicans	Contact, non-STI	Vaginitis, vulvitis

*Late manifestations

Table 13.3: Summary of STDs—diagnostic tests and treatment

Organism	Diagnostic tests	Treatment
Gonorrheae	Gram staining of smears from cervix and urethra Culture of discharge	Cefotaxime 500 mg single dose Ciprofloxacin single dose
Chlamydia	PCR	Doxycycline 100 mg oral, bid for 7 days
Syphilis	VDRL	Benzathine penicillin G 3-4 million units, single dose
Trichomonas	A drop saline with a drop of discharge— shows motile flagellate organism	Metronidazole 400 mg oral tid for 7 days
Bacterial vaginosis	Clue cells in wet smear	Metronidazole 400 mg oral tid for 7 days
Herpes genitalis	Fluid and scrapings from base of ulcer for special culture	Acyclovir 200 mg 5 times a day for 5 days
Candida albicans	A drop 10% KOH with a drop of discharge— shows mycelia	Clotrimazole vaginal tablet 500 mg single dose
Chancroid	Ito test	Erythromycin 500 mg oral qid for 7 days
PID	PV tenderness USG fluid in POD	Ciplox TZ 500 mg bid for 7 days
Non-specific vaginitis	Wet smear, Gram stain, culture	Teramycin vaginal tablets 100 mg bid for 10 days

PCR: Polymerase chain reaction
PID: Pelvic inflammatory disease
USG: Ultrasonogram
VDRL: Venereal disease research laboratories
PV: Per vagina
POD: Pouch of Douglas

Table 13.4: Differential diagnosis of vaginal infections

Criteria	Normal	Bacterial vaginosis	Candida vaginitis	Trichomonal vaginitis
Predisposing factors	None	Change in vaginal milieu Loss of lactobacilli Overgrowth of *Gardnerella, Bacteroides, Mycoplasma*	Diabetes Pregnancy Broad-spectrum antibiotics Oral contraceptive pills	Common during child-bearing age Sexually transmitted
Symptoms	None	Discharge, Bad odor after coitus	Itching, Burning discharge	Frothy discharge Bad odor Vulvar pruritus Dysuria
Signs	None	Fishy odor, Vaginal discharge	Discharge lightly adherent to vaginal wall, when tried to remove leaves multiple petechial hemorrhages	Swollen inflamed labia, introitus, multiple small punctate strawberry spots at vaginal vault and cervix
Characteristics of discharge	White, clear	Thin, homogeneous White to grey Adherent, Increased amount	White Curdy, like cottage cheese Increased	Yellow to green Frothy Adherent Increased
Vaginal pH	3.8-4.2	> 4.5	≤ 4.5	>4.5
Amine/Whiff test with KOH	Absent	Present	Absent	Fishy when BV is also present
Microscopic	Lactobacilli	Clue cells, Coccoid bacteria, No WBCs	Mycelia Budding yeast Pseudohyphae with KOH	Trichomonads WBCs >10/hpf

KOH: Potassium hydroxide
BV: Bacterial vaginosis
WBC: White blood cell count
hpf: high power field

and B. A few infections such as candidiasis are triggered by coitus although it colonizes in vagina normally. It is evident that STDs are caused by bacteria, viruses, fungi and parasites (Tables 13.2 to 13.4).

Chlamydial Infection

Chlamydia is the commonest bacterial sexually transmitted infection. About 10% of women of childbearing age are infected. Women under 25 years of age are more prone to develop this infection. Unfortunately, approximately 80% of women are asymptomatic though they have infection.

Organism

Chlamydia trachomatis is small, Gram negative, an obligate intracellular parasite bacterium. Commonly, it causes genital infections, but some strains are responsible for trachoma, conjunctivitis, and lymphogranuloma venereum (LGV).

Pathology

The infectious particle (the elementary body) infects columnar epithelial cells in genital tract. They gain entry to the cell by binding to the specific surface receptors. These appear as intracytoplasmic inclusion bodies. These reproduce inside the host cells by binary fission. After a 48 hours life cycle, elementary bodies are released from the cell surface. Heavily infected cells die, but it is the inflammatory response to infection that contributes most to damaging the epithelial surface.

Clinical Features

Chlamydia trachomatis causes cervicitis and pelvic inflammatory disease. It is present in cervix often without symptoms. *Chlamydia trachomatis* infect only the glandular epithelium and are responsible for mucopurulent endocervicitis[1] producing purulent endocervical discharge (mucus), generally yellow or green in color. Edema, erythema, and friability of glandular epithelium are present, especially when glandular epithelium is visible in cases of cervical ectropion. Touching the ectropion with a cotton swab can assess the friability or easily induce bleeding. Dysuria and frequency of micturition are the urinary symptoms of chlamydial infection. Infection may spread upwards to the tubes, causing chronic salpingitis, pelvic inflammatory disease (PID), and consequent infertility.

In pregnancy this infection may cause abortion, preterm labor and intrauterine growth restriction (IUGR). During delivery, ophthalmia neonatorum may be caused by *Chlamydia* derived from maternal cervix.

Investigations

1. *Culture and innoculation*: After cleaning ectocervix of its secretions with a swab, a small cotton swab is placed into the endocervical canal and the cervical mucus is extracted. It must be cultured by inoculation in suitable cells, in which inclusion bodies develop and can be recognized after staining.
2. *Serological tests:*
   a. Antigen detection: Immunofluorescent and enzyme-linked immunosorbent assay (ELISA) tests are used to detect specific antigens.
   b. Antibody detection: Microimmunofluorescence is used to detect serum antibodies.
3. *Detection of DNA:* To detect DNA of *Chlamydia*, polymerase chain reaction (PCR) and ligase chain reaction (LCR) are much more sensitive than all the above-mentioned tests. They are noninvasive methods.

Treatment

It is essential to treat the sexual partner(s) together. The treatment choices are as following:[2]
1. Doxycycline 100 mg orally, bid for 7 days and for 14 days in case of salpingitis. It is the most commonly used and effective drug.
2. Alternative options: Oral tetracycline or Clindamycin 500 mg, 6 hourly for two weeks.

In pregnancy:
a. Erythromycin sterarte, 500 mg 12 hourly for two weeks is the suitable alternative to tetracyclines.
b. Azithromycin 1 gm orally single dose is also equally effective.

Gonorrhea

Gonorrhea was described by Hippocrates as 'Strangury' as early as 400 BC. The present name was given in AD 130-200. This infection may occur at any age but common in reproductive young age when patient is sexually active. It is acquired during coitus. Most women are asymptomatic carriers.

Organism

This infection is caused by *Niesseria gonorrhoeae*. The intracellular Gram-negative cocci are kidney-shaped, seen in pairs (diplococci), with their long axes parallel.

Pathology

Glandular columnar epithelium, such as that of cervix, urethra, Skene gland, Bartholin's gland, or fallopian tube, is easily invaded. The infection spreads along the mucous membranes; thus, after infection of the cervix, it may ascend to the endometrium and fallopian tubes, causing acute salpingitis. It also ascends in a piggy-back manner attached to the sperms. Squamous epithelium of the adult vagina is resistant to infection by *Gonococcus*; but in children, the vaginal epithelium is thinner and less resistant, so vaginitis may develop.

There is intense inflammatory response in the mucosa of involved parts. Abscess may be formed in Skene or Bartholin's glands and if left untreated may rupture or become chronic in nature.

In salpingitis edema of stroma, swollen and adherent plicae, and exudation of pus in the tubal lumen are present. Chronic infection leads to tubal blockage resulting in infertility. Occasionally, pyosalpinx, hydrosalpinx, tubo-ovarian mass, pelvic abscess, or peritonitis may develop.

Incubation Period

The initial symptoms usually are seen 2-7 days after exposure.

Clinical Features

A patient may harbor gonococci, and transmit the infection, without having any symptoms. About 50% of women have chronic asymptomatic infection.

In young patients it causes vaginitis and vulvitis with clinically evident discharge without the involvement of upper genital tract.

Acute Gonorrhea

Symptoms and signs of gonorrhea in women are relatively mild in comparison to men. In acute phase, patients may have involvement of lower or upper genital tract alone or both.

Lower Genital Tract

1. *Urethritis and cystitis*: Little micturition discomfort with slight yellowish purulent urethral discharge is present.
2. *Bartholinitis and Skeinitis*: The Bartholin's glands are inflamed and the patient complains of tender swelling. If the gland is compressed, a bead of pus is seen at its opening on the inner surface of the labia minora. Bartholin's abscess may rupture through the skin or vaginal mucosa.
3. *Vaginitis and vulvitis*: Not common but at times the patient may have swelling of labia.
4. *Cervicitis*: Increased mucopurulent cervical secretion which is yellowish green in color is the characteristic. The cervical hyperemia and erosions may be seen.
5. *Proctitis*: About one third of patients may have rectal discharge, discomfort during defecation, and rectal bleeding. It is frequent in women who have anal intercourse.

Upper Genital Tract Infection (Pelvic inflammation)

Salpingitis may produce severe symptoms of pelvic inflammatory disease (PID) which includes lower abdominal pain, low backache, dysmenorrhea, and fever. It may cause pyosalpinx, hydrosalpinx, or tubo-ovarian mass.

Chronic Gonorrhea

This is difficult to diagnose since the signs and symptoms cannot be distinguished from those of non-gonococcal genital and pelvic infections. In such situations the past history of any STD or PID in patient herself or in her partner, is important. The common complaints are backache, vaginal and cervical discharge, bartholinitis, mild chronic urethritis, and proctitis. Patients are chronically ill. Patients may give history of recurrent attacks of backache, low-grade fever, and dyspareunia in cases of salpingitis and pelvic infections. Uterus is retroverted and fixed. Adnexal swelling due to pyo-salpinx, hydrosalpinx, or tubo-ovarian mass may be felt.

Investigations

1. *Microscopic smear examination*: The most likely place to obtain pus or discharge containing the *Gonococcus* are the urethra and the cervical canal. First wipe away gross discharge, then urethral and cervical discharge is taken. Gram staining reveals the presence of an increased number of neutrophils (> 30/high-power field). The presence of intra-cellular gram-negative diplococci leads to the diagnosis of gonococcal infection.
2. *Culture*: The inoculum must be incubated imme-diately. The *Gonococcus* is grown on blood agar or Thayer-Martin media in an atmosphere of 5-10 percent carbon dioxide.
3. *Gonococcal complement fixation test*: It is the standard test for the presence of antibody. This test is positive only after some weeks from the onset of infection.

Treatment

Gonorrhea is treated with one of the following modalities:

1. *Penicillins*: Penicillin is the drug of choice.
   a. Procaine penicillin, a single dose of 4.8 mega units IM gives cure rate of 90%.
   b. Amoxycillin or ampicillin (oral/IM), a single dose of 3 gm with oral probenecid 1 gm is equally effective.
2. Patients allergic or resistant to penicillin respond to macrolides or cephalosporins.
   Macrolides:
   a. Spectinomycin 2 gm single dose intramuscular injection which is preceded by oral 1 gm pro-benecid.
   b. Azithromycin 1 gm orally as a single dose.

Cephalosporins: Cefotaxime 1 gm intramuscular injection which is preceded by oral 1 gm probenecid.

3. *Gonococcal PID* (e.g. salpingitis) is treated after hospitalizing the patient.
   a. Benzyl penicillin intramuscularly 1 mega units six hourly for three days to be followed by,
   b. Procaine penicillin 600,00 units, IM, daily for seven days.

   After 7 days, repeat the serological tests. Permanent cure is assumed only after 3 negative smears at weekly intervals. The patients are advised not to have coitus till test becomes negative. All sexual contacts are treated.
4. *Surgery*: A Bartholin's or other abscess requires drainage and marsupialization along with antibiotic course.

Trichomonas vaginalis Vaginitis

It is the disease of childbearing period, but even young girls and postmenopausal women are not immune. This infection is sexually transmitted, but it can be transmitted due to poor hygiene and by using the infected person's bath towels or clothes. Poor immune resistance and high pH (5-6) of vagina favor this infection as seen during menstruation. It accounts for about 20-30% of cases of vulvovaginitis. About 70% male partners contract the disease after a single exposure to an infected woman and this transmission rate is even higher from male to female.

Organism

Trichomonas vaginalis vaginitis is caused by the sexually transmitted, flagellated, actively motile anaerobic parasite, *Trichomonas vaginalis*. It exists only in trophozoite form.

Clinical Features

Clinical symptoms and signs range from asymptomatic to mild to severe forms depending on the amount of parasitic load apart from individual's immune resistance.[3]

Vaginal discharge is greenish yellow, thin, profuse, purulent, malodorous and characteristically frothy. The pH of vaginal secretions is usually higher than five.

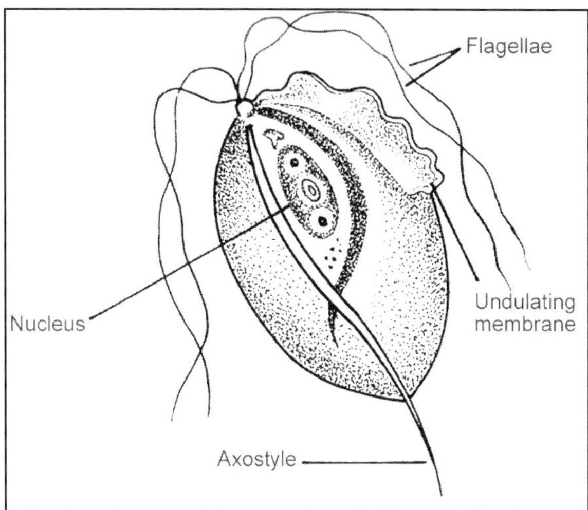

Figure 13.2: Trichomonad

Discharge causes intense itching and inflammation of the vulva, which may extend up to the perineum. Patchy erythema and hemorrhagic punctations give the appearance of "strawberry cervix". Strawberry spots may also be seen on vaginal wall.

Urinary symptoms include dysuria and frequency of micturation and a low-grade urethritis may be revealed on examination. Abdominal pain, low backache and dyspareunia may sometimes occur.

In pregnancy *Trichomonas vaginalis* vaginitis increases the risk of premature rupture of the membranes and preterm delivery.

Investigations

1. *Wet smear*: Wet smear is prepared by mixing 1-2 drops of vaginal discharge with normal saline on a slide. Motile trichomonads and increased number of leukocytes are visualized under microscopic examination. The sensitivity of this test in detecting the microorganism is 60%. Motile organism is identified from its shape and four flagellae. Its constant motion distinguishes it from pus cells.
2. *Culture*: Culture can be carried out on Feinberg-Whittington medium. Antibiotics are added to the medium to suppress the growth of other organisms. The reliability of culture is up to 96%.

Treatment

Both the sexual partners should be treated simultaneously. Both partners are advised to avoid the coitus during the therapy or to use the condom. These drugs are avoided in first trimester of pregnancy.

1. Metronidazole is the drug of choice for the effective treatment of *Trichomonas vaginalis* vaginitis and 95% cure rates are achieved with Metronidazole in the dose of 400 mg thrice daily for 7 days. Equally effective cure rate is achieved with single dose therapy with 2 gm orally. This is convenient to take and has better patient compliance.

   If the initial therapy is not effective, these patients should be treated for seven more days. If repeated treatment is not yet effective, the patients should be treated with a single 2 gm dose Metronidazole once daily for 3-5 days.

2. Secnidazole in a single dose of one gram is also good alternative.

Vulvovaginal Candidiasis (Moniliasis)

This is the commonest infection of the female genital tract, experienced by over 75% women at least once in their lifetime and about half the women will experience two or more episodes per year.[4]

Organism

Gram-positive fungus *Candida albicans* is responsible for 85-90% of vaginal fungal infections (Fig. 13.3). It grows in an acid medium with an abundant supply of carbohydrates. *Candida* are dimorphic fungi existing as blastopores and mycelia. Blastopores are responsible for transmission and asymptomatic colonization, and mycelia, which result from blastopore germination,

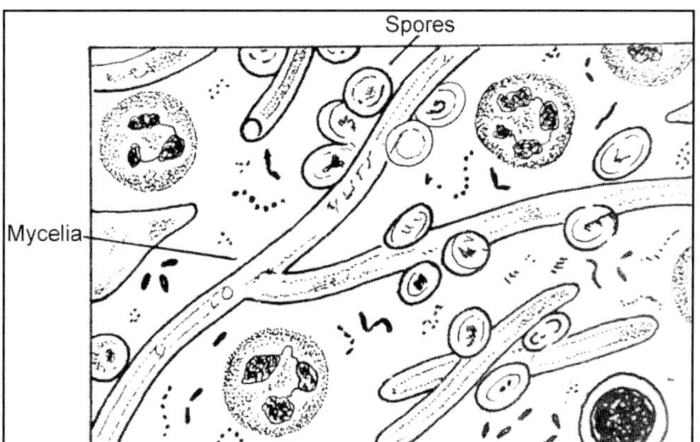

Figure 13.3: Mycelia and spores of *C. albicans*. Note the presence of leukocytes

enhance colonisation and facilitate tissue invasion. The organism is carried in the vagina, under the nails, and on the skin.[5]

Predisposing Factors

1. Pregnancy: Pregnancy predisposes to infection because of the increased vaginal acidity and high glycogen content. Also, there is qualitative decrease in cell-mediated immunity.

2. Hormonal oral contraceptive pills also predispose to monilial vaginitis for the same reasons.

3. Antibiotic use: Normally, lactobacilli prevent the overgrowth of opportunistic fungi. Antibiotics decrease lactobacilli concentration and thus allow the overgrowth of fungi.

4. Diabetes mellitus: Rich supply of glucose and a qualitative decrease in cell-mediated immunity lead to a higher incidence of vulvovaginal candidiasis.

5. Sexual contact is not important in the transmission of this infection, but the possible trauma caused by the coitus may be sufficient to trigger an attack in a predisposed individual.

Clinical Features

The classical symptoms of vulvovaginal candidiasis consist of vulvar pruritis, and a profuse vaginal discharge that typically resembles cottage cheese or curds, and it smells like yeast. During micturition, inflamed vulvar and vestibular epithelium come in contact to urine causing external dysuria which is known as "splash" dysuria.

Examination reveals erythema and edema of the labia and vulvar skin. Often, there is excoriation from scratching. Discrete pustulopapular lesions may also be seen. The whitish discharge is adherent to vaginal walls, which on separation leaves behind the petechial oozing surface. Typically, cervix appears normal. The pH of vagina in patients with vulvovaginal candidiasis is usually normal or lowered (<4.5).

Investigations

1. *Wet smear:* A drop of vaginal discharge is taken on a slide and a drop of 10% KOH is added, mixed and placed on a slide with a coverslip. KOH dissolves all the cellular debris. In about 80% of patients,

either budding yeast forms or mycelia are observed under the microscope.

2. *Culture*: Culture of vaginal fluid on Saborauds's medium can grow the fungi and reveal rounded colonies 1-2 mm in diameter within 48-72 hours. The growth of fungus has yeast-like odor.

Treatment

1. Patients are advised to maintain strict genital and perineal hygiene, avoid synthetic undergarments, and avoid scratching the vulva with finger nails.
2. Predisposing factors if present should be treated accordingly.
3. Antifungal medication: The symptomatic relief is seen after 2-3 days. The usual duration of therapy is for 7 days, but duration can be decreased to 1-3 days by increasing the concentrations of the antifungal agents. Topical use is better since it reduces the side effects.

Tropical azole group antifungal:
  i. Clotrimazole:
    a. Vaginal tablets:
      — 100 mg vaginal tablet for seven days.
      — 200 mg vaginal tablets for three days.
      — 500 mg vaginal tablet, single dose only.
    b. Cream:
      — 1% cream 5 gm intravaginally for 7-14 days.
  ii. Miconazole:
    a. Vaginal tablets:
      — 100 mg vaginal suppository for 7 days.
      — 200 mg vaginal suppository for 3 days.
    b. Cream 2% cream 5 gm intravaginally for seven days.

Oral antifungal agents: Fluconazole is used in a single 150 mg dose. This therapy protocol appears to have equal efficacy like topical application, in the treatment of mild to moderate vulvovaginal candidiasis.[6]

Chronic Vulvovaginal Candidiasis

A small number of women develop chronic or recurrent vulvovaginal candidiasis. These patients experience persistent irritative symptoms of the vulva. Burning replaces itching as the prominent symptom in patients with chronic vulvovaginal candidiasis.

Treatment

The treatment of patients with chronic vulvovaginal candidiasis consists of inducing a remission of chronic symptoms with daily Ketoconazole 400 mg or fluconazole 200 mg until symptoms resolve. Patients should then be maintained on prophylactic doses of these agents (ketoconazole 100 mg/daily, fluconazole 150 mg /weekly) for 6 months.[7]

Genital Ulcerative Diseases

See Figure 13.4 and Table 13.5.

Herpes Genitalis

Organism

Genital infections are caused by two main types of DNA containing herpes simplex virus (HSV). HSV II is the usual cause of herpes genitalis. HSV I usually causes herpes labialis; but occasionally, it may cause herpes genitalis through orogenital contact. This virus enters the cell by invasion and reproduces itself in large number in the cell resulting into the disruption of the cell.

Clinical Features

Primary herpes: First symptom attack, appear in less than seven days of the sexual contact, incubation period

Sexually transmitted genital ulcers

Common	**Rare**
1. Herpes simplex virus (HSV)	1. Lymphogranuloma venereum (LGV)
2. Syphilis	2. Granuloma inguinale (donovanosis)
3. Chancroid	

Figure 13.4: Sexually transmitted genital ulcers

Table 13.5: Comparative clinical presentations of genital ulcers suggestive of specific diagnosis

Ulcer	Syphilis	HSV	Chancroid	LGV	GI
Number	Single	Multiple and grouped	One to three	Single	Multiple and discrete
Appearance	Circular, shallow, well-defined edges	Small, shallow, with grouped vesicles	Small, shallow, irregular outline, undermined, greenish slough	Shallow, gradually deepens	Beefy-red granular, clean sharp margins,
Pain and Tenderness	Painless	Painful	Painful	Painless	Painful
Lymphadenopathy	Rubbery, discrete, painless, mobile	Enlarged, tender	Tender, soft, fluctuating,	Tender, hard, form sinuses over skin	Tender, hard, form sinuses over skin

HSV: Herpes simplex virus
LGV: Lymphogranuloma venereum
GI: Granuloma inguinale

ranges between 3-6 days. In a few infected individuals, lesions are not noticed, but there may be complaints of tingling and burning in the genital region.

Lesions: Small and extremely painful vesicles appear on an erythmatous base on clitoris, labia, and vestibule, but they may also occur on the vaginal wall and cervix. These vesicles soon break down to form small painful shallow ulcers, and within a few days scab appears over the ulcer. Grouped vesicles mixed with small ulcers are almost pathognomonic of genital herpes. Virus is shed from the lesions until healing is complete in about a fortnight to three weeks. Inguinal lymph nodes are enlarged and tender.

In some women, micturition may be painful. About 30% patients suffer from fever, malaise, and headache.

Recurrent Herpes

Following the primary herpes, virus colonizes the neurons in the dorsal root ganglia causing latent infection. In some patients, the virus remains dormant; but in others, recurrent attacks occur at irregular intervals. Acute infection occurs intermittently when virus particles are produced and track down the axons to the skin. Although recurrent attacks may be milder and shorter than the primary attack, they cause much discomfort and misery to both partners. The signs and symptoms last for 7-10 days.

Pregnancy with Herpes

In early pregnancy the primary attack may cause an abortion. During the last weeks of pregnancy, the primary attack may be responsible for transplacental spread of the virus to the fetus, where it subsequently may cause damage to the central nervous system with a high neonatal mortality rate. Surviving babies may show evidence of neurological deficit. If there is evidence of recurrent active lesions in the vagina or vulva in the last weeks of pregnancy or at the onset of the labor it is advisable to deliver her by cesarean section to avoid contamination of the baby in the birth canal.

Investigations

1. *Direct smear:* Microscopic examination of smear, from the ulcer shows giant multinucleated cells with characteristic intranuclear inclusion bodies.
2. *Culture:* The serum is obtained from the vesicle or a sterile culture swab is rubbed over the ulcer. Culture is most sensitive and specific test; sensitivity approaches 100% in the vesicle stage and 89% in the pustular stage and drops to as low as 33% in patients with ulcers.

Treatment

1. Saline baths relieve the local pain.
2. Primary episode of genital herpes should be treated with Acyclovir, 200 mg orally 5 times daily, for 7-10 days or until clinical resolution is attained.

3. Recurrent infection: Daily suppressive long-term therapy, 400 mg orally twice daily, reduces the frequency of HSV recurrences by at least 75%. Suppressive treatment with oral *acyclovir* does not totally eliminate the potential for transmission.

Follow-up

Patients and their partners should be informed and warned that they are infectious whenever they have any evident lesions. Women should have annual cervical smears for the follow-up since HSV may cause precancerous lesions of the cervix.

Syphilis

Organism

It is caused by a spirochete *Treponema pallidum*, it replicates slowly.

Clinical Presentation

Syphilis presents in three stages of its clinical course.

Primary syphilis: A minute abrasion of the skin, on contact allows the organism to reach the subcutaneous tissue where they multiply. The incubation period is 9-90 days. The continuous multiplication of the spirochete gives rise to a lesion, which usually ulcerates, and is termed a chancre. The ulcer is the typical of the first stage of syphilis.

- *Syphilitic ulcer (Chancre):* Syphilitic ulcer usually is single, painless, circular and indurated, with an eroded base. There is marked edema of the surrounding tissue. It may not be noticed by the patient and will heal spontaneously in 3-10 weeks, leaving a very slight scar. The most common site of the chancre is the cervix, but it may occur on the labia.

  The chancre first takes the form of a raised papule with an indurated base, and later it breaks down to form a shallow punched out ulcer with well-defined edges and a smooth shiny floor. It exudes a serous discharge, unless secondarily infected when the discharge is more purulent. About a week after the chancre appears, the related lymphatic glands enlarge and in 3-6 weeks, they become rubbery, but remain painless, discrete, and mobile.

These glands do not suppurate until septic secondary infection occurs.

A cervical chancre is less friable, has less tendency to bleed on touch, and has the sharp outline of the ulcer than the cervical cancer.

Secondary syphilis: Skin rash: After two months of the appearance of the chancrem the first evidence of dissemination of the spirochaetes occurs in the form of a nonirritating extragenital rash, which is usually symmetrical. This is a coppery-colored maculopapular rash on the trunk and limbs. It can also appear on the face and forehead (corona veneris). In addition, there may be anemia, slight pyrexia, headache and occasional alopecia. Some patients may develop sore throat and 'mucus patches' within the mouth, which are whitish areas on the inner aspects of the lips, cheek and palate.

- *Condylomata lata:* Another form of manifestation which occurs soon after the appearance of the rash is the formation of the condylomata lata in moist areas like around vulva and anus. They appear as raised plaques which may be bilaterally symmetrical. They tend to become macerated, and so appear as raised discs with a flat or slightly indented top which is covered by grayish exudate (sodden white areas).

Tertiary syphilis: Gummata: In the later stage of the disease, perhaps many years after the chancre has healed, lesions occur due to end-arteritis. These lesions are firm elastic tumors and may be seen on skin, mucous surfaces, bones, and viscera, although they are very rare in the female genital organs.

- *Neurosyphilis:* It includes meningovascular disease with focal lesions, tabes dorsalis and general paralysis of insane.
- *Cardiovascular lesions:* These include aneurysm of the aorta and other large arteries.

Syphilis in Pregnancy

Sometimes the disease is discovered as the result of a routine serological test during an antenatal visit. If the patient becomes pregnant soon after acquiring the syphilis, the fetus may die, usually in the second half of pregnancy, and spirochaetes may be found in its liver or in the intima of the umbilical cord. If untreated, subsequent pregnancies may proceed nearer to term until a child is born alive with signs of congenital syphilis.

Investigations

1. *Microscopy:* To demonstrate the presence of spirochete, the edge of the lesion (primary syphilis) is gently wiped with a swab dipped in normal saline until serum, but not blood, exudes. The serum is transferred to a glass slide and examined under dark ground illumination. Under the oil immersion lens the treponemata appear as mobile white corkscrew-shaped organisms against the dark background. The examination is repeated on three successive days.

2. *Serology:* Confirmation by serological reaction on the patient's serum is obtained 4-6 weeks after the appearance of the chancre. Serological reactions are strongly suggestive of syphilis, but the final diagnosis should never be made only on the basis of one type of test. While the tests are almost completely reliable in the secondary stage, they do not become positive for 4-10 weeks after the infection.

    a. *Nonspecific antigen tests* include non-treponemal rapid plasma reagin (RPR) test, or venereal disease research laboratory (VDRL) test for antibody.

    b. *Specific and confirmatory tests* for treponemata include the fluorescent treponemal antibody absorption (FTA ABS) test and the treponemal pallidum hemagglutination (TPHA) test. These tests may remain positive for many years, even after the disease has been effectively treated. The best combination for screening is to use the VDRL and TPHA tests.

Treatment of Syphilis

Sustained treponemicidal levels of antibiotics are needed for a minimum of 12 days in early syphilis.

Penicillins

1. Procaine penicillin 1.2 million units in aqueous solution, intramuscular, daily for at least 10-12 days.
2. Alternatively, *Benzathine penicillin* G, 2.4 million units intramuscularly in a single dose, is the recommended treatment for adults with primary, secondary, or early latent syphilis. The same dose should be repeated after 7 days.
3. For neurosyphilis, intravenous procaine penicillin 2.4 million units daily with probenecid 500 mg four times a day, for 10-12 days, is the effective regimen.
4. In penicillin sensitive patients:
    a. Tetracycline 500 mg 6 hourly for 21 days, or
    b. Erythromycin 500 mg 6 hourly for 14 days may be given.

If the infection has been there for more than a year, treatment is extended to 21 days for penicillin regimens and for 28 days for other regimens.

Latent syphilis is defined as those periods after infection with *Treponema pallidum* when patients are seropositive but show no other evidence of disease. Patients with latent syphilis of longer than 1 year's duration or of unknown duration should be treated with Benzathine penicillin G, 7.2 million units total, administered as three doses of 2.4 million units intramuscularly each, at 1 week intervals.

Patients treated in early pregnancy may expect a healthy child, but mother and child must be treated until they become seronegative and then observed for at least two years. During this period, the serological reactions must remain seronegative, and a final cerebrospinal fluid examination must also be negative before declaring complete and certain cure. Mother is advised to have further treatment during each subsequent pregnancy.

Chancroid

Organism

This condition, commonly known as soft sore, is caused by sexually transmitted infection with *Haemophilus ducreyi* (Ducrey's bacillus). It is gram-positive bacilli.

Clinical Features

The incubation period is 3-5 days. Small shallow ulcers occur on the vulva and vagina. The ulcers are multiple and painful, and may be surrounded by a zone of hyperemia. They are irregular in outline with under-mined edges. Their bases are covered with greenish slough which is contagious.

The lymphatic glands in groin become enlarged and known as "bubo". They are tender, soft, and fluctuating in some, thus differing from syphilis, in which the glands are discrete, firm and painless. Frequently, the suppuration of these lymph glands is observed, as secondary infection with pyogenic organisms is common.

The sore tends to heal spontaneously if kept clean, but if secondary pyogenic infection occurs, there may be considerable destruction of tissue and consequent scarring.

Chancroid is distinguished from primary syphilis by the short incubation period, the multiplicity of lesions, and the inguinal lymph nodes's characteristics.

Investigations

1. *Gram staining*: It is Gram-positive bacilli, arranged like fish in a streak of mucus.
2. *Culture*: Bacilli can be cultured on Rabbit's serum.
3. *Ito test*: *H. ducreyi* vaccine, 0.3 ml is injected intradermally, and appearance of an area of erythema 8 mm across at 24 hours is considered positive.

Treatment

1. Cotrimoxazole (trimethoprim 80 mg plus sulfamethoxazole 400 mg) two tablets twice daily for seven days, or
2. Erythromycin base, 500 mg qid for 7 days.

Three to seven days after initiation of therapy, the gradual resolution of the genital ulcer is seen and it completely heals within 2 weeks unless it is large.

Lymphogranuloma Venereum (LGV)

This is caused by a sexually transmitted strain of *Chlamydia trachomatis* which belongs to lymphogranuloma-pistacossis group. The incubation period is 7-21 days. From the point of entry, the agent is disseminated via the bloodstream and lymphatics to result in a chronic inflammatory disease.

Clinical Features

The earliest genital lesion is a vesicopustular eruption which becomes a painless, shallow ulcer, which gradually deepens and extends. The inguinal bubo is a hard cutaneous induration, reddish blue in color and it is seen bilaterally in about 10-30 days after inoculation. The enlarged inguinal nodes may break down to form multiple sinuses. Secondary infections of these ulcers may cause severe pain. Systemic symptoms such as fever, headache, arthralgia, chills and abdominal cramps are seen in the later part of the disease. Ulcers eventually heal, leaving irregular scars, and characteristic 'windows' in the labia minora where the tissue has been destroyed. As the edema and subsequent ulceration cause fibrosis, the urethra may also be destroyed; and the involvement of rectum causes stenosis, sometimes with a rectovaginal fistula. After some years, epithelioma may develop in the involved skin.

Investigations

1. *Complement fixation test*.
2. *Frei's test*: Antigen (0.1 ml) is inoculated intradermally on forearm. In positive response there is inflammatory nodule at the site of test in 2 days, it may reach to maximum size of 7 mm in 4-5 days. This test is positive in 2-6 weeks after the infection and remains positive for several years.
3. *Microimmunofluorescence test*.
4. *Culture*.
5. Detection of inclusion bodies in the smear from urethra and vaginal ulcer.

Treatment

1. Tetracycline 500 mg orally six hourly for 7-14 days. The treatment may have to be repeated after a week.
2. Surgical treatment may be required if the urethra is destroyed or there is a rectal stricture.

Granuloma Inguinale

Organism

It is caused by *Calymmatobacterium granulomatis* and is sexually transmitted.

Clinical Features

This is a chronic ulcerative granulomatous disease that develops in vulva, perineum and inguinal region. The incubation period is 8-12 weeks.

The disease begins as discrete papules, which break down to form painful ulcers, with a beefy-red granular zone with clean sharp edges. Ulceration may extend over the vulva, perineum and groins, and the vaginal epithelium or rectal mucosa may be involved.

The ulcer may develop into chronic ulcer with satellite lesions, enlarged lymph nodes with superadded infection resulting in an inguinal swelling (bubo). This bubo may show redness, ulceration, or formation of granulation tissue. A chronic inflammatory exudate comprising lymphocytes, giant cells and histiocytes exudes from these bubos. Healing is followed by dense fibrosis, and there may be extensive swelling of the vulva (pseudoelephantiasis). Epithelioma may occur in the damaged skin.

Investigations

1. *Gram staining*: Smear from the ulcer shows gram-negative bipolar rods within leukocytes which are called "Donovan bodies."
2. *Biopsy*: The diagnosis is made by discovery of Donovan bodies in a biopsy. It may show granulation tissue infiltrated by plasma cells and large macrophages with rod-shaped cytoplasmic inclusion bodies (Miculicz cells).

Treatment

1. Tetracycline 500 mg orally six hourly for 2-3 weeks is the drug of choice. Erythromycin can also be used.
2. *Surgery*: Residual fibrosis may require surgical treatment.

Genital Warts (Condyloma Acuminata)

Organism

Genital warts are caused by human papilloma virus (HPV) infection. Amongst the various types of HPV, the nononcogenic HPV types 6 and 11 are usually responsible for genital warts. Occasionally, HPV types 16 and 18 which cause cervical precancer, may also cause genital warts. It is advised to screen all the patients with past and present HPV warts by cervical cytology.

Clinical Features

The incubation period is three months. The warts tend to occur in areas most directly affected by coitus, namely the posterior fourchette and lateral areas on the vulva. Less frequently, warts can be found throughout the vulva, in the vagina, and on the cervix. Minor trauma associated with coitus can cause breaks in vulvar skin, allowing direct contact between the viral particles from an infected male and the breached skin of female sexual partner. Infection may be latent or may cause viral particles to replicate and produce a wart. On dry areas of skin, the warts are usually flat and small, although on warm moist areas, they may be much larger. Exophytic genital warts are highly contagious; more than 75% of sexual partners develop this manifestation of HPV infection when exposed.

Treatment

The aim of treatment is removal of warts since it is not possible to eradicate the viral infection. Treatment is most successful when warts are small and that have been present for less than 1 year. Selection of specific treatment regimen depends on the anatomic site, size, and number of warts, as well as expense, efficacy, convenience, and potential adverse effects. Recurrences more often result from reactivation of subclinical infection.

Specific treatment consists of the local application of 10-25% podophyllin in spirit. This should be washed away 4-6 hours after the application to prevent local skin ulceration. This therapy may need to be repeated several times before the warts disappear. If this therapy fails to remove the warts, cutting diathermy, cryotherapy, laser therapy, or interferon can be used.

REFERENCES

1. Kiviat NB, Paavonen JA, Wolner-Hanssen P, Critchlow CW, Stamm WE, Douglas J et al. Histopathology of endocervical infections caused by *Chlamydia trachomatis*, herpes simplex virus, *Trichomonas vaginalis*, and *Neisseria gonorrhea*. Hum Pathol 1990; 21:831-7.
2. Centers for Disease Control. The Sexually Transmitted Diseases Treatment Guidelines. Washington DC: Centers for Disease Control, 1993:1-102.

3. Wolner-Hanssen P, Krieger JN, Stevens CE, Kivlat NB, Koutsky L, Critchlow C et al. Clinical manifestation of vaginal trichomoniasis. JAMA 1989; 261:571-6.
4. Hurley R. Recurrent Candida infection. Clin Obstet Gyanecol 1981; 8:208-13.
5. Sobel JD. Vulvovaginal candidiasis. In Pastorek J (Ed): Obstetric and Gynecologic Infectious Disease. New York: Raven Press, 1994:523-36.
6. Brammer KW. Treatment of vaginal candidiasis with a single oral dose of fluconazole. Eur J Clin Microbiol Infect Dis 1988; 7: 435-60.
7. Sobel JD. Management of recurrent vulvovaginal candidiasis with intermittent ketoconazole prophylaxis. Obstet Gynecol 1985; 65: 435-60.

FURTHER READING

1. Berek J, Adashi EY, Hillard PA (Eds). Novak's Gynecology, 12th edn, Mary Land: Williams and Wilkins, 1996.
2. Campbell S, Monga A (Eds). Gynecology by ten teachers, 17th edn, London: ELTS with Arnold, 2000.
3. Padubidari V, Daftary SN (Eds). Howkins and Borne Shaw's Textbook of Gynecology, 12th edn, New Delhi: BI Churchill Livingstone Pvt Ltd, 2000.

14.

Siti Zawiah Omar
V Sivanesaratnam

HIV in Obstetrics and Gynecology

INTRODUCTION

Human immunodeficiency virus (HIV) infection is currently a leading threat to the health of women and children in the world today. By the end of the last decade, there were a total of about 35 million people living with HIV/AIDS worldwide, 50 percent of whom were women.[1] The primary modes of transmission of HIV are through sexual activity, parenteral exposure to blood and perinatally from mothers to infants.

There is no evidence of transmission through casual contact, water, food or environmental surfaces. Heterosexual transmission is the most common mode of HIV transmission for women worldwide.

AIDS is also a significant contributor to childhood mortality. Today, there are about 2 million children under 15 years of age living with HIV/AIDS. Mother-to-child transmission (MCT) is recognized as the main mode of acquisition of the disease.

PATHOPHYSIOLOGY

HIV is a retrovirus (RNA virus) that can be incorporated into the host genome.[2] It preferentially infects cells with the CD4+ antigen, particularly helper lymphocytes, but also macrophages, cells of the central nervous system, and according to certain evidence, cells of the placenta. The characteristic immunological abnormality is a depletion of CD4 lymphocytes. As a consequence, HIV infection leads to progressive depletion of predominantly cell-mediated immunity, rendering the individual susceptible to opportunistic infections (e.g. *Pneumocystis carinii*, central nervous system toxoplasmosis) and neoplasias (e.g. Kaposi's sarcoma) that rarely afflict patients with intact immune systems. An HIV-infected patient with one of several specific opportunistic infections, neoplasia, dementia, encephalopathy, or wasting syndrome is diagnosed as having AIDS.[3]

At the time of initial infection, an individual may be asymptomatic or may develop an acute mononucleosis-like syndrome that may be accompanied by aseptic meningitis. Antibodies can be detected in most individuals 6-12 weeks after exposure; but in rare circumstances, this latent period (the so-called "window phase") can be longer.[4] After seroconversion has occurred, an asymptomatic period of variable length usually follows. The mean time from infection to development of AIDS is over 10 years. Evidence of immune dysfunction may be followed by clinical conditions ranging from fever, weight loss, malaise, lymphadenopathy and central nervous system dysfunction to infections such as herpes simplex virus or oral candidiasis. These nonspecific conditions are usually progressive and are a prelude to an opportunistic infection that is diagnostic of AIDS. Studies of infected-individuals have noted that 5 years after infection was confirmed, up to 35% had progressed to AIDS.

It is important to note that patients with AIDS make up a small minority of the HIV-infected population. For each patient with AIDS, there are at any given time many more asymptomatic infected individuals who presumably remain infected for life and who will, it is believed, eventually develop AIDS.

HIV IN GYNECOLOGY

Several aspects of gynecologic care, including contraception, gynecologic infections and gynecologic malignancy, have particular relevance to HIV-infected women.[5]

Heterosexual transmission is the most common mode of HIV transmission for women worldwide and accounts for 75-85% of transmissions.[6] Although female-to-male transmission can occur, male-to-female appears to be much more efficient. Several factors, including a higher estimated quantity of HIV in semen compared with vaginal secretions, as well as the relatively larger inoculum delivered with ejaculation account for the latter to be more efficient. Retention of HIV-infected semen in the vagina, an environment in which the virus remains viable, and traumatic mucosal injury during intercourse further increase the risk of transmission.[7] The presence of genital ulcers from concurrent sexually transmitted diseases and a friable cervix also enhance HIV transmission. Women who engage in anal intercourse are at increased risk of HIV transmission, most likely as a result of trauma to the rectal mucosa. Likewise, intercourse during menses has been shown to increase female-to-male HIV transmission.

There is little information pertaining to hormonal function in women with HIV. On multivariate analysis, HIV infection was independently associated with an approximately three-fold risk of amenorrhea, which was also more frequent in women infected with HIV with lower CD4+ cell counts.[8]

Sexually Transmitted Diseases

HIV and other sexually transmitted diseases (STDs) may interact in a variety of ways.[9] The presence of STD can facilitate shedding of HIV in an HIV-infected person. In an HIV-uninfected person, STD can increase susceptibility to HIV infection by recruiting HIV-susceptible inflammatory cells (CD4+ T cells, Langerhans cells, macrophages) to the genital tract or by disrupting mucosal barriers to infection. Both ulcerative and nonulcerative STDs have important interactions with HIV. There is a two to five-fold increased risk of HIV infection among persons who have ulcerative and nonulcerative STD. In Cohort studies of women infected with HIV, the incidence of specific sexually transmitted diseases diagnosed were syphilis (3-20%), *Neisseria gonorrheae* cervicitis (2-7%), *Chlamydia trachomatis* cervicitis (12%), herpes simplex virus genital ulcers (4-18%), and trichomoniasis (9-27%). Complete evaluation of ulcerative lesions in women infected with HIV should include dark-field examination or direct immuno-fluorescence test for *T. pallidum*, HSV culture or antigen tests, *H. ducreyi* culture, and possibly biopsy to exclude invasive squamous carcinoma. Approximately 20% of genital ulcers are because of infection with multiple agents. Coinfection should be considered as a possible cause of treatment failure.

Management of STDs using standard therapeutic agents is successful for most women infected with HIV. Careful follow-up evaluation is needed for detection of treatment failure, that requires retreatment with another agent.

Candidiasis

Recurrent vaginal moniliasis is the most common gynecologic infection in HIV-infected women. Several studies conducted in the late 1980s and early 1990s found recurrent or chronic vaginal moniliasis in 7-89% of HIV-infected women. These studies also suggested that chronic or recurrent vaginal moniliasis often was the first HIV-associated opportunistic infection in the affected women. Women with recurrent candidal vaginitis often have near-normal CD4+ lymphocyte counts. As the HIV infection progresses, *Candida infections* of the oropharynx and esophagus become more prevalent, especially when CD4+ lymphocyte counts drop below 50 cells/mm^3.

Vaginal moniliasis presents in much the same way in immunocompromised individuals as it does in immunocompetent patients: pruritis, a white curd-like discharge, dyspareunia, dysuria, and vulvar erythema. The curd-like discharge is easily visualized on vaginal speculum examination, and a potassium hydroxide preparation of the discharge will reveal characteristic pseudohyphae and spores.

The causative organism is *Candida albicans* (most common); others include *C. glabrata, C. tropicalis,* and *C. parapsilosis.* Several other factors, including hormonal changes, antibiotic use, and diabetes mellitus can also contribute to recurrent infection.

Candida vaginitis can be treated with either topical antifungal agents (e.g. miconazole, clotrimazole, or terconazole) or with oral fluconazole. Although single-dose fluconazole (150 mg) is used for the treatment of vaginal candidiasis, immunocompromised women often require a longer course (5-7 days) to eradicate the infection. Studies have found that treatment of male sexual partners or aggressive attempts to clear the fungus from the gastrointestinal tract do not significantly reduce the incidence of reinfection. The use of fungal prophylaxis to reduce frequent or severe episodes of vaginitis is controversial.

Pelvic Inflammatory Disease (PID)

Unlike vaginal candidiasis, PID may present differently in HIV coinfected women. In immunocompetent women, PID typically presents with marked leukocytosis, pelvic pain, fever, cervical motion tenderness, and an adnexal mass. In HIV-infected women with PID, abdominal pain and leukocytosis may be less prominent. Similar type of organisms have been cultured: *Neisseria gonorrheae, Chlamydia,* anaerobes, and *Mycoplasma hominis.* Also, HIV-infected patients tend to be on various antibiotic therapies that may alter cervical culture results. It has been suggested that immunocompromise per se is sufficient justification for the inpatient management of pelvic inflammatory disease and it seems prudent to follow that recommendation in the HIV-infected patient.

Herpes Simplex Virus (HSV)

Recurrent HSV is a common problem among HIV-seropositive women. As immune dysfunction progresses, patients often experience more prolonged and severe outbreaks. Chronic lesions may become quite large and atypical in appearance, causing significant local destruction and erosion. Immunosuppressed patients are also at higher risk of developing disseminated skin involvement and visceral involvement with HSV, including pneumonitis and esophagitis.

HIV-infected individuals may require higher-than-usual dosages of antiviral medication. Acyclovir, 400 mg 3 to 5 times per day has been found to be useful. Therapy should be continued until clinical resolution of the lesion occurs. Intravenous acyclovir (5 mg/kg) every 8 hours may be required in severe cases. Famciclovir has recently been approved for the treatment of recurrent genital HSV and is an alternative to acyclovir with the advantage of improved oral absorption.

Human Papilloma Virus (HPV)

HIV-infected women are much more likely to show signs of HPV infection than non-HIV-infected women, and this risk increases dramatically as the CD4+ cell count declines. HPV is the etiologic agent of anogenital warts (condylomata acuminata). Thus, multifactorial factors are implicated; behavioral patterns of the partners (multiple sexual partners, concurrent STDs, etc) may put them at higher risk for HPV infection, while immunosuppression from HIV inhibits the body's immunologic defense mechanisms and attenuates defenses against infection and tumor surveillance.

The high prevalence of HPV infection among HIV-infected women is of particular concern because HPV is strongly associated with cervical dysplasia, pre-invasive disease (cervical intraepithelial neoplasia) and invasive carcinoma. HPV serotypes 16, 18, 31 and 35 are considered the oncogenic strains. Concurrent infection with HPV and HIV dramatically increases the risk of malignant transformation.

Cervical dysplasia rates of 15-40% have been reported among HIV-infected women from Pap smears. The severity of dysplasia appears to be inversely proportional to the degree of immunosuppression, i.e. the decline in CD4+ cell count. These patients are at high risk of progressing to widespread involvement— including endocervical, vulvar, vaginal and anal intraepithelial neoplasia. Short-term recurrence rates of 40-60% are cited with standard therapy (cryotherapy, laser therapy, cone biopsy, loop excision) for pre-invasive disease. Topical 5-fluorouracil treatment, recently, has been found to be efficacious for prevention of recurrence after ablative therapy for cervical intraepithelial neoplasia and vulvovaginal intraepithelial neoplasia.

Pap smear test: The current recommendations for *Pap smears* for HIV-infected women are as follows: a baseline Pap smear and comprehensive gynecologic examination upon diagnosis. If the initial smear result is normal, the Pap smear should be repeated after 6 months. If the second examination is normal, then Pap smears should be repeated annually. For women who have a CD4+ cell count below 200 cells/mm^3 or a prior history of HPV, continued biannual exams should be strongly considered. If the initial Pap smear shows inflammation with reactive squamous cellular changes, any identified aetiology should be treated and the Pap smear repeated after 3 months. If the initial Pap smear shows dysplastic changes or atypical squamous cells of undetermined origin (ASCUS), the patient should be referred for colposcopy.

Invasive Cervical Cancer

Invasive cervical carcinoma in the HIV-infected women is characterized by high-grade tumors, lymph node involvement, and often metastatic spread at the time of diagnosis. The clinical course of the neoplasia also tends to be more aggressive, with high recurrence rate and poor response to therapy. Radiation and chemotherapy may be used, but poor response to radiation therapy alone together with suppressed number and function of T-cell lymphocytes may lead to poor outcomes. Women will most often succumb to cervical cancer than the HIV disease.

Contraception

There are several important issues to consider in making recommendations for contraceptive use by women infected with HIV.[10] These include whether the contraceptive will cause an increase in HIV/STD transmission, the effect on the course of HIV infection, and whether the method is acceptable to the woman and her sexual partner.

Condoms (male and female) offer the best method of protection against acquisition of sexually transmitted infections including HIV. Hormonal contraceptives can impact regulation of humoral and cell-mediated immunity. Cervical ectopy, which is common in oral contraceptive pill users, may be an important factor in HIV acquisition/shedding.

Other contraceptive methods available including vaginal microbicides/spermicides do not seem to be useful in protection against HIV transmission.

HIV AND PREGNANCY

The increasing HIV infection rates in women and the overall high fertility rates, especially in those areas of Sub-Saharan Africa where HIV is most prevalent, have resulted in increasing infant morbidity and mortality.[1,11] Every year, more than half a million children get infected with HIV, representing some 10 percent of the total number of newly infected persons each year. Over 90 percent of these infections occur through mother-to-child transmission (MCT). Estimates of MCT vary from 14-39 percent in different regions.

Mother-to-child transmission of HIV: Most HIV infections worldwide are HIV-1; infection with HIV-2 is less common. Transmission of HIV-2 from mother to child occurs less often than transmission of HIV-1. MCT transmission of HIV-1 can occur prenatally, at the time of delivery, or postnatally through breastfeeding.[3,12-15] The frequency of transmission is as follows:

- — *In utero*   : 23-35%
- — Intrapartum   : 65-75%
- — Postpartum   : 12-29%

Evidence for early transmission was documented by the detection of the HIV-1 virus in fetal specimens and by the presence of p24 antigen in fetal serum.

Transmission occurring at the time of delivery was first based on observations from a study based on twins, which found that the first born twin had a two-fold higher risk of contracting HIV-1 than the second born twin. Exposure of the fetus to the virus from the cervicovaginal secretions was thought to play a role, although the same phenomenon was observed for twins delivered by cesarean section. In addition, recent reports have indicated that the mode of delivery may affect the MCT rate. Cesarean section whether elective or emergency has been shown to decrease the risk of transmission and prolonged rupture of membranes (more than four hours) to increase the risk of transmission. Postnatal transmission through breastfeeding may explain the higher transmission rate seen in Africa.

Lack of manifestations of HIV-1 infection at birth and the finding that HIV-1 is detected in the first week of life in 50% children later proven to be infected—shows that transmission is highest at time of delivery.[8,15]

The risk of MCT of HIV-1 is higher in women with clinical, immunological or virological markers of advanced HIV-1 infection. A high viral load has been associated as a key factor in MCT of HIV-1.[16] In addition, the phenotype of the mother's virus, low CD4+ count and immunological factors such as the presence of neutralizing antibodies may play their role in transmission.

Effect of HIV infection on pregnancy: In the few studies in which infected pregnant women have been compared with infected nonpregnant women,[3,7] little or no difference has been observed in the rates of clinical and immunologic deterioration. HIV-infected women, however, still need to be monitored closely. Low CD4 cell counts have been shown to be predictive of the development of serious infections during pregnancy, just as they have been shown to have prognostic significance for nonpregnant individuals. Rates of preterm birth, low birth weight and pregnancy complications in asymptomatic HIV-infected women have not differed significantly from those in matched controls.

Interventions to Reduce MCT of HIV

The first and basic aspect of preventing MCT is informing pregnant women and their partners about HIV/AIDS and the possibility of MCT. Information and education are crucial to enable people to prevent getting infected themselves and passing it on to their children. Emphasis and introduction of universal precautions is crucial not only in HIV-infected individuals, but it should be applied to all patients.

Studies of intervention to reduce the risk of transmission include elective cesarean delivery,[17] disinfection of the birth canal, Vit-A prophylaxis, antiretroviral (ARV) therapy, formula feeding and passive/active immunization.[12] The last approach is in the trial stage (Table 14.1).

Long course antiretroviral agents: Antiretroviral therapy may decrease viral load and/or inhibit viral replication in the infant. The PACTG 076 randomized placebo-controlled study looked at reduction of MCT of HIV with Zidovudine (ZDV).[13,15]

- During pregnancy—ZDV 100 mg 5 times daily started between 14-34 weeks of pregnancy (currently given as 300 mg twice daily),
- During labor—intravenous ZDV.
- Infants—oral ZDV 2 mg/ kg 6 hourly for the first 6 weeks of life.

All women who had CD4+ cell counts of more than 200 per mm^3, were symptom-free and were not on

Table 14.1: Guidelines for use of ARV in pregnancy

No prior use of ARV	*On ARV when became pregnant*	*No prior Rx at the time of delivery*
• Consider ARV > 14 weeks • Add AZT during pregnancy • Use appropriate combination for patient	• Counsel • Continue existing Rx, if effective • Add AZT (d4T-stavudine-add intrapartum and postpartum only) • If discontinuing Rx prior to 14 weeks, stop all Rx and restart again >14 weeks	• AZT during labor • AZT to neonate • Modify regimen after delivery, as clinically indicated

ZDV therapy. The first interim analysis on 356 mother-infant pairs demonstrated a rate of MCT of 25.5% in the placebo group and 8.3% in the ZDV group. Treatment with ZDV achieved a 67.5% reduction in transmission risk. The drug was well tolerated in both the pregnant women and the neonates. The results from the PACTG076 trial as yet have shown no evidence of teratogenicity or short-term adverse effects of ZDV in the fetus or newborn, but long-term follow-up is still required.

In 1999, a randomized clinical trial confirmed the results from European prospective studies that an elective cesarean-section delivery decreases the risk of vertical transmission of HIV infection by more than half compared with vaginal delivery.[17]

Short course antiretroviral agents: Other antiretroviral regimens[18,19] include:

- Short course ZDV treatment, 300 mg 12 hourly from 36 weeks pregnancy plus oral ZDV 300 mg every 3 hours during labor.
  50% efficacy in a non-breastfeeding population in Thailand
  37% efficacy in a breastfeeding population in Cote d'Ivoire at 6 months postpartum.
- Short course 300 mg ZDV and 150 mg lamivudine twice daily from 36 weeks of gestation till delivery; additional 200 mg ZDV provided every 3 hourly during labor. Postpartum twice-daily ZDV and lamivudine was resumed for a week and the infant given 5 mg/kg ZDV and 2 mg/kg lamivudine in syrup form every 12 hours for a week. Efficacy rate was 53% (PETRA-A study). Therapy using similar doses only during labor and continued postpartum give an efficacy rate of 38% (PETRA-B study).
- Nevirapine (a non-nucleoside reverse transcriptase inhibitor) regimen consisted of a single 200 mg oral dose given to women at onset of labor and a 2 mg/kg dose given to neonates within 72 hours of birth. Compared with ZDV given at onset of labor, intrapartum and to neonates till one week old, nevirapine decreased transmission by 47.0% at age 14-16 weeks. The regimen was well tolerated and seems to be the most cost-effective regimen, especially in low-resource settings.

- Other combination regimens such as using didanosine (ddI), *etc.* are being studied.

Modification of obstetric practice: Obstetrical procedures that may increase MCT should be modified. The following will help reduce the risk of intrapartum infection.

- Reducing the rate of artificial rupturing of membranes, thereby preventing prolonged rupture of membrane.
- Usage of vaginal lavage with chlorhexidine in women whose membranes have ruptured for more than 4 hours.
- Reducing the duration of labor/second stage of labor.
- Reducing the number of episiotomies.
- Minimizing the use of assisted deliveries—forceps/vacuum.
- Wiping bloody secretions from neonates—decrease exposure to infected bloody fluids.
- Minimizing vigorous nasogastric suctioning of neonates that damages oral mucosa.

Information regarding a doubling the risk of HIV transmission through *breastfeeding*[20] should be stressed, and postnatal care for both mother and baby should be provided. In many situations, particularly in developing countries, exclusive formulae feeding is not possible; an alternative in these situations is pasteurization of breast milk. Contraceptive advice and in some settings (e.g. South Africa, Thailand) subsidizing infant formula may be considered.

HIV TESTING AND COUNSELING

Identification of HIV-infected women during pregnancy allows for several beneficial interventions, including the possible introductions of strategies to reduce transmission.[14]

Disadvantage of perinatal HIV screening:
- Psychological problems in seropositive clients
- Social stigma and discrimination
- Possible loss of job, housing, etc.

Advantages of perinatal HIV screening for seropositive cases:
- Opportunity to decide whether to continue/terminate pregnancy

- Mother and child can be closely monitored
- Possibility to reduce MCT
- Decision making on reproductive issues
- Partner notification for VCT
- Prevention of further horizontal transmission.

Factors enhancing the benefits and minimizing the adverse effect of HIV testing:

- The test should be voluntary
- Pre- and post-test counseling have to be provided
- The test should be strictly confidential
- AIDS education should be offered to all hospital personnel including doctors, nurses, maids and other hospital workers in order to decrease negative attitude towards seropositive patients.

REFERENCES

1. UNAIDS/WHO Working Group of Global HIV/AIDS and STD Surveillance in collaboration with the National AIDS Program. Report on the Global HIV/ AIDS Epidemic. Geneva: WHO; December 2001.
2. Lifson AR, Rutherford GW, Jaffe HW. The natural history of human immunodeficiency virus infection. Journal of Infectious Diseases 1988; 158:1360-67.
3. Human Immunodeficiency Virus infections: ACOG Technical Bulletin Number 169- June 1992. International Journal Gynecology Obstetrics 1993; 41: 307-19.
4. Ranki A, Valle SL, Krohn M, Antonen J, Allain JP, Leuther M et al. Long latency precedes overt seroconversion in sexually transmitted human-immunodeficiency-virus infection. Lancet 1987: 2: 589-93.
5. Larkin J et al. HIV in women: Recognising the signs. Medscape Women's Health 1996;1(11).
6. Royce RA, Sena A, Cates WJr, Cohen MS. Current concept: Sexual transmission of HIV. New England Journal of Medicine 1997; 336: 1072-78.
7. Shaheen F, Sison AV, McIntosh L, Mukhtar M, Pomerantz RJ. Analysis of HIV-1 in cervicovaginal secretions and blood of pregnant and non-pregnant women. Journal of Human Virology 1999; 2: 154-66.
8. Korn AP. Gynecologic Care of women infected with HIV. Clinical Obstetrics and Gynecology 2001; 44(2): 226-42.
9. Young MA, Clark RA. Selected issues in the treatment of women infected with HIV. Clinical Obstetrics and Gynecology 2001; 44(2): 167-81.
10. Daly CC, Helling-Giese GE, Mati JK, Hunter DJ. Contraceptive methods and the transmission of HIV: Implications for family planning. Genitourinary Medicine 1994; 70: 110-17.
11. Brocklehurst P, French R. The association between maternal HIV infection and perinatal outcome: A systematic review of the literature and meta-analysis. British Journal of Obstetrics and Gynecology 1998; 105: 836-48.
12. Shapiro DE, Sperling RS, Mandelbrot L et al. Risk factors for perinatal human immunodeficiency virus transmission in patients receiving zidovudine prophylaxis. Pediatric AIDS Clinical Trials Group protocol 076 Study Group. Obstetrics Gynecology 1999; 94: 897-908.
13. Connor EM, Sperling RS, Gelber R et al. Reduction of maternal-infant transmission of human immunodeficiency virus type 1 with zidovudine treatment. Pediatric AIDS Clinical Trials Group protocol 076 Study Group. New England Journal of Medicine 1994; 331: 1173-80.
14. Fiscus SA, Adimora AA, Schoenbach VJ et al. Trends in human immunodeficiency virus (HIV) counseling, testing, and antiretroviral treatment of HIV-infected women and perinatal transmission in North Carolina. Journal of Infectious Diseases 1999; 180: 99-105.
15. The International Perinatal HIV Group. The Mode of Delivery and the Risk of Vertical Transmission of Human Immunodeficiency Virus Type 1—a Meta-Analysis of 15 Prospective Cohort Studies. New England Journal of Medicine, 1999; 340: 977-87.
16. Mofenson LM, lambert JS, Stiehm ER et al. Risk factors for perinatal transmission of human immunodeficiency virus type 1 in women treated with zidovudine. New England Journal of Medicine 1999; 341: 385-93.
17. The European Mode of Delivery Collaboration. Elective Caesarean-section versus vaginal delivery in prevention of vertical HIV-1 transmission: A randomized clinical trial. Lancet, 1999; 353: 1035-39.
18. Shaffer N, Chuachoowong R, Mock PA et al. Short-course zidovudine for perinatal HIV-1 transmission in Bangkok, Thailand: A randomized controlled trial. Lancet 1999; 353: 773-80.
19. Guay LA, Musoke P, Fleming T et al. Intrapartum and neonatal single-dose nevirapine compared with zidovudine for prevention of mother-to-child transmission of HIV-1 in Kampala, Uganda: HIVNET 012 randomised trial. Lancet 1999; 354: 795-802.
20. Nduati R, John G, Mbori-Ngacha D et al. Effect of breast-feeding and formula feeding on transmission of HIV-1: A randomized clinical trial. JAMA 2000; 283: 1167-74.

15.

Benign Lesions of the Genital Tract

Jayakrishnan

INTRODUCTION

This chapter will be confined to discussion of the benign lesions of the female genital tract. The emphasis is on the common and important lesions of vulva, vagina, uterus and ovaries. The intention is to provide a sound and thorough framework upon which to build the advanced knowledge.

CLASSIFICATION

Benign Lesions of the Vulva

Patients with vulval symptoms are met frequently in general practice. A systemic approach, appropriate treatment and reassurance of benign pathology should alleviate the symptoms. There has been confusion over the terminology 'vulvar dystrophies'. This includes Lichen sclerosus, squamous cell hyperplasia and other dermatoses.

Lichen Sclerosus

This is the commonest condition found in elderly women complaining of vulval itch. It may also be seen in children. The exact cause is not known, but it may be associated with autoimmune disorders.

The affected skin looks thin and crinkled. The contour of the vulva disappears and labial adhesions form. The diagnosis can be made clinically but biopsy should be performed whenever possible. About 4 percent of women with lichen sclerosus develop vulval cancer.

If the patient is asymptomatic, no treatment is needed. Mild itching may be helped by bland creams like aqueous cream or 1 percent hydrocortisone ointment. Applied three times a day. More potent steroids may be required for short periods. Some women benefit from 2 percent testosterone ointment which should be applied 2 or 3 times daily for 6 weeks. Thereafter, frequency can be reduced to once or twice a week.

Squamous Cell Hyperplasia

Squamous cell hyperplasia is when there is histological evidence of hyperplasia without any other clinical features to account for the lesion.

The lesion is mainly confined to labia majora, minora and introitus.

Histology: The characteristic histological features include elongation of rete pegs, hyperkeratosis and dermal inflammation.

Clinical features: Pruritus vulvae is the main complaint. If cracks develop, secondary infection may result. The margins are well defined.

Prognosis: Histology is mandatory. Atypia is present in 8 to 10 percent of cases. If atypia is present, the chances of malignancy is much high.

Treatment: Hydrocortisone cream 2% can be effectively applied locally. If atypia is present considering the risk of development of malignancy simple vulvectomy may be advised, especially in cases of severe atypia and in cases where regular follow-up cannot be relied.

Other Dermatoses

This includes allergic dermatitis, psoriasis, intertrigo and lichen planus. These problems are usually seen by dermatologist, but knowledge of their existence will help to identify these patients who should be referred.

Vulval Ulcers

The causes of benign vulval ulcers are:
- Aphthous ulcers
- Herpes genitalis
- Primary syphilis
- Crohn's disease
- Behçet's disease
- Lipschutz ulcer
- Lymphogranuloma venereum
- Chancroid
- Donovanosis
- Tuberculosis

Aphthous ulcers: This is analogous to those seen in the oral cavity. Mainly seen as small painful yellow ulcers with yellow base on labia majora. This is self-limiting.

Herpetic ulcers: They are extremely painful vulval ulcerations. General symptoms like malaise, fever and lymphadenopathy may be present. Recurrent attacks are possible. Topical acyclovir is recommended.

Crohn's ulcer: This ulcer looks like clean knife cuts on the vulva. This often precedes the appearance of intestinal symptoms.

Behçet's disease: It is a chronic condition characterized by oral, genital and ocular ulceration. Vulval lesions can be very erosive. They often last for several months and leave extensive scarring. No specific treatment is available. Estrogen dominant oral contraceptive pills are said to have a beneficial effect and topical steroids are also used.

Lipschutz ulcer: It affects mainly the labia minora and the introitus. No cause is found but could be due to Epstein-Barr virus.

Lymphogranuloma venerum: It is a tropical infection due to certain subtypes of *Chlamydia trachomatis*. It causes a painless vulval ulcer which heals after 3 to 4 weeks. Inguinal lymphadenopathy develops a few weeks later.

Chancroid: This infection is due to *Haemophilus ducreyi*. Common in tropical parts of the world.

Donovanosis: This can cause chronic, spreading ulcers and is most common in South-East Asia and India.

Tuberculosis: This is rare but important cause of vulval ulceration and inguinal lymphadenopathy.

Benign Tumors of the Vulva

Cystic Lesions

Epidermoid and sebaceous cysts are possible. Treatment is by excision. Mucinous cysts may arise from the minor vestibular glands, whereas mesonephric cysts are found on the labia majora. Cysts may arise around the urethra in Skene's ducts or in the suburethral glands.

Bartholin's Cyst

These cysts are from the ducts of Bartholin's gland, which lies in the subcutaneous tissue below the lower third of labia majorum. This is a retention cyst. Patients usually present after infection and abscess formation. Incision and marsupilisation of the abscess and antibiotic therapy give good result. Gonococcal infection needs to be ruled out by sending the pus for culture.

Nonepithelial Tumors

This includes lipoma and fibromas. Treatment is by excision.

Benign Lesions of the Vagina

Vaginal cysts are rare because there is no gland in the mucous layer. The common cysts are Gartner's cyst and inclusion cysts.

Gartner's Cyst

Usually situated in the anterolateral wall of the vagina. The cyst is lined by low columnar cells and secretes mucinous material. Treatment is by surgical excision.

Inclusion Cysts

This arises from vaginal epithelium buried under the mucosa during healing from trauma mainly following childbirth. The lining epithelium is stratified squamous. Treatment is by excision.

Benign Lesions of the Cervix

Cervical (Erosion)

The squamous epithelium of the ectocervix is replaced by columnar epithelium in this condition. It could be congenital or acquired.

Cervical Ectropion

A condition wherein endocervical area is exposed due to bilateral cervical tears.

Congenital

This is due to the maternal estrogenic effect on the newborn. It is self-limiting. It can reappear at or soon after puberty under the influence of estrogen.

Acquired

During pregnancy and pill conception, the squamous epithelium of ectocervix can be replaced by columnar epithelium. This usually returns back to normal after three months of delivery or withdrawal of pill.

Cervical Cyst

Nabothian cysts: These are retention cysts produced by blockage of openings of the cervical glands. The lining epithelium is columnar. These cysts are usually multiple.

Mesonephric cysts: Usually situated on the outer side of the cervical stroma. This is lined by cuboidal epithelium. They are asymptomatic. Treatment is by excision.

Endometriotic cysts

These are situated in the portio vaginalis part of the cervix. Usually, they are small and reddish in color. Symptoms include intermenstrual bleed, postcoital bleed, dysmenorrhea and deep dyspareunia. Treatment is destruction by cauterization and rarely by excision.

Benign Lesions of the Uterus: Fibroids (Myomas)

Uterine fibroids are the commonest benign tumors, which arise from the uterine myometrium and less commonly from the cervix.

Incidence: At least 20 percent of women of reproductive age group have got fibroids in their womb. The incidence of symptomatic fibroid is only 3 percent. In black women, the incidence is very high and are more common in nulliparous.

Classification and Pathophysiology

Macroscopically, fibroids are round and firm in consistency with a characteristic whorled appearance on cross section. They may be single or multiple with varying sites and sizes. Four clinical subgroups are described (Fig. 15.1).

Intramural, Subserosal, Submucosal and Cervical

Intramural: They lie within the uterine wall separated from the adjacent normal myometrium by a thin layer of connective tissue, which forms the false capsule. Small nutrient arteries penetrate this capsule. Large intramural fibroids enlarge and distort the uterine cavity.

Subserosal: This project outward from the uterine surface covered with peritoneum. As growth is unrestricted by surrounding myometrium, they may attain a very large size. These fibroid can become

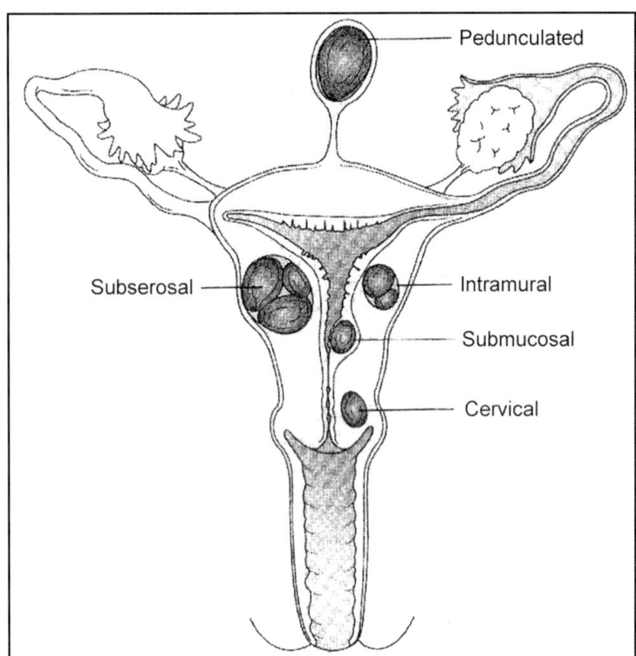

Figure 15.1: Fibroids are named on the basis of their position within the muscles

pedunculated. Sessile subserosal fibroid projecting from the fundal region may become separated from the uterus forming a so-called 'parasitic' fibroid. Subserosal fibroid arising from the lateral wall may lie in between the layers of broad ligament and can displace the ureters laterally. These broad-ligament fibroids (otherwise called false broad-ligament fibroid) are different from true broad-ligament fibroid which have no attachment to uterine wall, but have their origin in smooth muscle fibers within the broad ligament.

Submucous fibroid: These are less common comprising about 5 percent of the total fibroids. They project into the uterine cavity covered by endometrium and distort the uterine cavity. Pedunculated submucous fibroids on a long stalk may prolapse through the cervix. These can produce intermenstrual bleeding or become ulcerated and infected.

Cervical fibroids are relatively uncommon, but give rise to great surgical difficulty by virtue of their relative inaccessibility and close proximity to the bladder and ureters.

Microscopic Appearance

Microscopically, fibroids are composed of smooth muscle cell bundles, also arranged in whorl-like patterns (Fig. 15.2). admixed with variable amount of connective tissue. The center of the fibroid is relatively poor in blood supply. Hence, they can undergo changes. Hyaline degeneration results in a homogeneous consistency and may become cystic. Fatty change or calcification also can happen. Red degeneration happens almost exclusively in pregnancy. The symptoms are pain and tenderness and mimick an acute abdomen. Fibroid in this condition is reddish and with a peculiar fishy smell. Very rarely sarcomatous changes can happen.

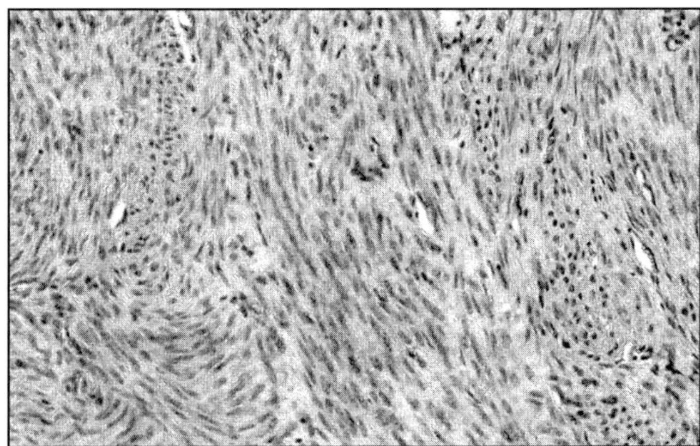

Figure 15.2: Leiomyomas consist of whorled fascicles of uniform smooth muscle cells, as shown in this histological section

Etiology: The etiology is unknown. The growth of the fibroid is dependent on ovarian hormones. Fibroids are unknown before menarche and it will regress after menopause.

Symptoms: Between 30 and 50 percent of women present with excessive bleeding during menstruation. It can even produce anemia. Fibroids will not usually cause intermenstrual bleeding other than when there is ulceration or it is a submucous or cervical fibroid. Hence, any disruption of normal cyclicity should not be attributed to fibroids without first excluding other causes. The mechanism of hemorrhage is due to various reasons. They are ulceration of endometrium overlying submucous fibroids, increase in the surface area of the endometrium and due to venous congestion.

The next major symptom is pelvic pain and other pressure symptoms. Acute torsion of a pedunculated fibroid or degeneration is the cause for pain. If the submucous fibroid is trying to get expelled through the cervix, it will produce pain similar to labour pains. Rarely this can cause inversion of uterus. Large fibroids can produce bladder symptoms in the form of increased frequency and retention, especially with cervical fibroid.

There is an association between subfertility and fibroids. The mechanism is either due to the cornual block or due to distortion of the cavity thus preventing implantation. Alterations in the local blood flow and increase in the binding of steroids to fibroids may create unfavorable factors in the local environment, which prevent implantation.

Diagnosis and investigations: General examination may reveal varying degree of anemia. If the fibroid is more than 14 weeks, it may be palpated through abdomen. It is firm in consistency, with a well-defined margin. Bimanual examination shows the uterus to be enlarged. It may be regular or irregular enlargement. Uterus is not felt separate from the swelling and cervix moves with the movement of the swelling. In a subserous fibroid it may feel separate from the uterus, especially if it is pedunculated.

Ultrasound will confirm the diagnosis. Ultrasound cannot differentiate a pedunculated subserous fibroid from a solid ovarian tumor. Diagnostic laparoscopy is helpful in this situation. Hysterosalpingography or hysteroscopy will help to detect submucous fibroids, especially in cases of unexplained infertility and repeated miscarriage. Hysteroscopy and endometrial biopsy is indicated in cases of irregular or intermenstrual bleeding to exclude the presence of coexisting endometrial pathology.

Differential diagnosis: These are pregnancy, full bladder, adenomyosis, ovarian pathology or tubo-ovarian mass.

Treatment: Recent advances in medical and surgical methods of treatment have increased the potential range of therapeutic options for women with fibroids.

Expectant Management

If the fibroids are asymptomatic, smaller than 12 weeks size, and its nature can be confirmed by ultrasound active treatment is unnecessary. The risk of sarcomatous change is 1 in 1000, making prophylactic removal of fibroid unjustified. Annual pelvic examination for assessing the growth of the fibroid supplemented with ultrasound is enough to manage these cases.

Hysterectomy: This is the definitive treatment for symptomatic fibroids. Due consideration is given to factors like women's wish to preserve reproductive function. Conservative surgical management of myomectomy, i.e. removal of fibroids, is done in those desiring to conserve the uterus. In most cases total abdominal hysterectomy will be the procedure of choice. Preoperative treatment with GnRH analogues can shrink the fibroids and make vaginal hysterectomy possible.

Endoscopic surgical management: Most submucous fibroids protruding through the os can be removed vaginally with cautery or ligation of the pedicle. If the fibroid is very large, piecemeal removal is necessary. In order to reduce the bleeding in these cases preoperative treatment with GnRH analogue is recommended.

Medical Management

Two main objectives of medical management are relief of symptoms and reduction of the size of fibroids. It will not disappear completely by medical management. For this reason, medical management has got its own limitations.

Progestogens: Progestogens are widely used in the management of DUB but are not effective in the reduction of bleeding with fibroids. They may be specifically indicated in perimenopausal women with fibroid where bleeding is of anovular dysfunction type rather than a direct consequence of the fibroid.

Androgenic steroids: Androgenic steroids such as danazol or gestrinone are useful in reducing menstrual blood loss by virtue of their direct effect on the endometrium and negative feedback inhibition of pituitary gonadotropin release. A small reduction in the size of fibroids has been reported. It is used only for short-term waiting for the operation or to raise the hemoglobin level before operation.

Prostaglandin synthetase inhibitors: These may be used in relieving the pelvic pain in women with fibroid.

LHRH analogues: Agonist analogues of LHRH are currently available and reliably relieve the symptoms of uterine fibroids and also cause a significant reduction in their size. However, their effect is lost on stopping the treatment. LHRH analogue will downregulate the pituitary and thus reduce estrogen level. Women can develop vasomotor symptoms, vaginal dryness, etc. Long-term treatment is not possible because of these side effect and bone loss. After 6 months of treatment, the fibroid may be halved in size. This treatment is advocated in medically unfit women, obese women and in those known to have severe pelvic adhesions, where surgery is not a safe option.

Benign Tumors of Ovary

Benign small cysts of the ovary are asymptomatic and often disappear spontaneously. The major role of the doctor is to rule out malignancy and not to produce undue morbidity.

Benign ovarian tumors can be broadly classified into functional or physiological and pathological cysts.

Physiological Cysts

These are large versions of the cysts, which form in the ovary during normal ovarian cycle. Because of the easy availability of the ultrasound, this is often found incidentally. They are mostly seen in young women. The common cysts are follicular cysts and corpus luteum cysts. The features of the functional cysts are:
- They are rarely complicated in appearance
- They are related to hormonal changes
- Usually, they do not exceed more than 5 cm in diameter
- They are mostly unilocular and contain clear fluid.

Follicular cyst: This cyst is lined by granulosa cells, and this is the commonest benign ovarian tumor. A follicular cyst may persist for a long time and they can become huge in size. This needs follow-up every month for three months. If symptoms develop or they do not resolve, they need intervention in the form of ultrasound-guided aspiration, laparoscopy or laparotomy. Combined steroidal contraceptive can be prescribed for a short duration to suppress cyst formation.

Corpus luteal cyst: This is less common than follicular cysts. This is mainly due to the overactivity of corpus luteum. It can be associated with pregnancy and usually disappears around 12 weeks. The cyst can enlarge and continue producing progesterone and the menstrual period can get delayed. One complication is cyst rupture that produces intraperitoneal bleeding and acute abdomen. With a delayed period and intraperitoneal bleed, this can mimic a ruptured ectopic pregnancy. If features of acute abdomen appear, laparocopy or laparotomy may be needed to arrest bleeding and to enucleate the cyst.

Pathological Cysts or Benign Ovarian Neoplasms

The classification of this is as follows:
- Benign germ cell tumors:
  - Mature teratoma
  - Dermoid cyst
- Benign epithelial tumors:
  - Serous cystadenoma
  - Mucinous cystadenoma
  - Endometroid cystadenoma
  - Brenner tumor
- Benign sex cord stromal tumors:
  - Granulosa cell tumor
  - Theca cell tumor
  - Fibromas
  - Sertoli-Leydig cell tumor

Benign germ cell tumor: This is the commonest ovarian tumor seen in women less than 30 years of age. Malignant tumors are usually solid.

  i. *Mature teratoma*: These are rare tumors and contain mature tissues just like dermoid with minimal cystic areas. Immature teratomas are malignant and this should be identified and proper therapy instituted.

  ii. *Dermoid*: This is the common benign germ cell tumor. It is bilateral in around 12 percent of cases. It is usually a unilocular cyst and can become big.

It contains a variety of tissues like skin, appendages, fat, bone, nervous tissue, etc. They contain sebaceous material and hair. These cysts are usually heavy because of the presence of bone and cartilage and is prone to torsion. This can rupture and slow leak of the content can produce chemical peritonitis. Most of the other cysts occur in women above 40 years.

Benign epithelial tumors: The majority of ovarian tumors both benign and malignant are epithelial in origin.

i. *Serous cystadenoma*: These are the most common benign tumors and are bilateral in 10 percent of cases. Usually, they are unilocular with papillary projections into the cavity. The cavity is lined by cuboidal or columnar cells and may have cilia. The fluid inside the cyst is thin and serous.

ii. *Mucinous cystadenoma*: 25% of the tumors are constituted by this. Usually, unilateral, large and multiloculated. The cyst will have a smooth surface. The cavity is lined by mucous secreting columnar cells. The cyst fluid is very thick and glutinous.

iii. *Endometroid cystadenoma*: Benign endometroid cysts are difficult to differentiate from Endometriotic cysts and most of these are malignant.

iv. *Brenner tumor*: These account for 1-2% of the tumors. They arise from the surface epithelium. The tumor consists of nests of transitional epithelium in a dense fibrotic stroma. Most of them are benign. Majority are less than 2 cm in size.

Benign sex cord stromal tumors: These constitute only 6% of ovarian tumors. These occur at any age and produce hormones.

i. *Granulosa cell tumors*: Most of these are malignant and not all produce estrogens.

ii. *Theca cell tumors*: Almost all are benign and unilateral. Many produce estrogens and produce systemic effects such as precocious puberty, endometrial hyperplasia, endometrial cancer and postmenopausal bleeding. They rarely cause ascites.

iii. *Fibromas*: Most frequent around the age of 50 years. They are not common, are hard in consis-

tency, mobile and lobulated with a glistening white surface. Ascites occurs with many of the larger fibromas, Meig's syndrome is ascites and pleural effusion in association with fibromas and is seen in only 1% of cases.

iv. *Sertoli-Leydig tumors*: These are usually of low-grade malignancy. Many produce androgens and thus virilization is possible. Some produce estrogens. They are usually small and bilateral.

Clinical Features

Presentation of benign tumors are as follows:
1. Asymptomatic
2. Pain
3. Abdominal swelling
4. Pressure effects
5. Menstrual disturbance
6. Hormonal effect

Many tumors are found incidentally. Ovarian tumors can undergo torsion, rupture, hemorrhage and infection producing acute abdomen. The patient may come with a visible enlargement of abdomen, especially in mucinous tumors. Pressure from the tumor can produce bowel or bladder symptoms. In extreme cases it can produce edema of the legs, varicose veins and hemorrhoids. Menstrual disturbance is associated with hormone-secreting tumors.

Differential Diagnosis

1. Full bladder
2. Pregnancy
3. Ectopic gestation
4. Appendicitis
5. Pelvic inflammatory disease
6. Fibroids.

Investigations

The patient presenting to the casualty ward may require emergency surgery. Pelvic examination will show an adnexal mass and the uterus is felt separate from the mass. The mass is usually mobile. Abdominal examination may show the swelling if it is large enough. Ultrasound can demonstrate the presence of ovarian mass with reasonable sensitivity and fair specificity. Chest X-ray is taken to rule out secondaries. Intravenous urogram to rule out pressure effects is also advised in relevant situations. A raised CA125 is strongly suggestive of carcinoma.

Management

Management will depend upon the severity of the symptoms. In older women nothing is achieved by conservative management, especially if the tumor is more than 5 cm. Surgery is advised. In younger women if the cysts are above 10 cm, they are unlikely to disappear spontaneously. Laparoscopy or laparotomy is indicated. Patients with symptoms definitely require treatment. In pregnancy the tumor can undergo torsion and laparotomy is advised irrespective of gestational age if they present with symptoms. If asymptomatic, then they are advised to wait until 14-16 weeks are completed when the chance of torsion is greater and chances of miscarriage will be less.

Surgery

Ovarian cystectomy or oophorectomy is done. In a young woman with no children and with bilateral ovarian cysts, bilateral ovarian cystectomy (removal of only the cyst leaving behind normal ovarian tissue) is done; whereas with one-sided ovarian cyst, an ovariotomy is done (removal of the whole of the diseased ovary). In a perimenopausal woman, total hysterectomy with bilateral salpingo-oopherectomy is done. A bimanual examination is always done at the time of catheterization prior to surgery to confirm the presence of the tumor.

REFERENCES

1. Aharoni A, Reiter A, Golan D, Paltiely Y, Sharf M. Patterns of growth of uterine leiomyomas during pregnancy. A prospective longitudinal study. British Journal of Obstetrics and Gynecology 1988;95:510-13.
2. Buttram VC, Reiter RC. Uterine leiomyomata: Aetiology, symptomatology and management. Fertility and Sterility 1981;36: 433-45.
3. Campbell S, Bhan V, Royston P, Whitehead MI, Collins WP. Transabdominal ultrasound screening for early ovarian cancer. British Medical Journal 1989;299:1363-67.
4. Friedrich EG. Vulvar disease, 2nd ed. Saunders, Philadelphia, 1983.
5. Novak ER, Woodruff JD. Myoma and other benign tumors of the uterus. In: Novak's gynecological and Obstetric pathology, 8th edn. WB Saunders: Philadelphia, 1979; 260-79.
6. Nezhat C, Winer WK, Nezhat F. Laparoscopic removal of dermoid cysts. Obstetrics and Gynecology 1989;73:278-81.
7. Ridley CM. The vulva. Churchill Livingstone, Edinburgh, 1988.
8. West CP, Lumsden MA. Fibroids and menorrhagia. Bailliere's Clinical Obstetrics and Gynecology 1989;2: 689-709.

16. *Contraception and Sterilization*

Noor Azmi bin Mat Adenan

INTRODUCTION

This chapter describes the methods of contraception currently available and practiced. The basic mechanism of action, their advantages and disadvantages will be highlighted. Some controversial issues will be explored. A practical approach of selecting the most appropriate and acceptable type of contraceptive method for a particular patient or couple will be presented.

Health is no longer defined as free from any physical illnesses or being cured from one. It also includes the mental, social and family happiness. Prevention has been the norm, rather than curative. Ability to decide when to become pregnant, to avoid an unnecessary pregnancy and to determine the family size are examples of how preventive medicine helps to achieve these. This allows women to pursue their career, to breastfeed their children and avoid undesired short- and long-term complications of pregnancy[1] and to avoid an unwanted pregnancy resulting in a termination of pregnancy, either done legally or illegally.

During our practice in prescribing a contraceptive method to a patient, we must be sensitive to the cultural, moral and religious issues of that person. A Catholic would not use any hormonal or related methods.[2] A Muslim might not agree for sterilization, although in reality Islam is very flexible and allows contraceptive methods in an appropriate circumstance.[3]

METHODS AVAILABLE

Abstinence

This is either no sexual encounter altogether or practicing ways of receiving and giving sexual pleasure without vaginal penetration. There is no possible encounter of the sperm and the ovum; therefore, there is no chance of pregnancy. This is suitable for anyone who can live without intercourse for a defined period. It is cheap and could still achieve sexual pleasure. It also avoids transmission of sexually related diseases, provided that no contacts with body fluid occur, such as during oral-genital or anal intercourse. It is suitable for teenagers who can say NO, but supply of condom or access to emergency contraception should be made available in case they change their mind at the height of passion.

Rhythm or Calendar Method, Basal Body Temperature Method, Ovulation (Billing's) Method, Symptothermal Method or Ovulation Predictor Test

These methods are suitable for those women who have regular menstrual cycles and based on the fact that ovulation usually occurs 14 days from the next menses. Secondly, this method assumes that the sperm is able to survive for about three days in the female genital tract and the ovum is viable for about 24 hours. The women will check their previous cycles about the timing of her ovulation using any or combination of the above-mentioned methods. The women should avoid coitus at least three days before and three days after the average ovulation day. In order to increase the effectiveness, an extra day can be added on each side.

The failure rate for this method depends on the accuracy of determining the exact ovulation days. Since ovulation can be influenced by any emotional upset, illness and stress, it is not surprising that the failure rate can be as high as 10 to 15% per 100 women years. The advantages are that there are no drugs being used and, therefore, devoid of any side effect. Any act of coitus during the fertile period needs other methods of contraception. These natural methods are very popular amongst certain religious groups.

Coitus Interruptus or Withdrawal Method

This is one of the oldest and widely practiced method. Success depends entirely on the ability of the male partner to recognize the sensation of pre-ejaculation and to withdraw the penis in time.

It is free and has no medical side effect. However, it interrupts the sexual act and may not be acceptable to all couples. Further, there are reports that the pre-ejaculate secretion may contain enough sperms to cause pregnancy or sexually transmitted diseases.[4] It needs a committed and determined couple to have any success and even then the failure rate is about 10 to 30%.

Barrier Method

This method can further be divided into male and female types.

The male type is more popular and easily available. It involves the application of the condom onto the erect penis, taking care not to leave an air bubble at the tip which could result in a condom bursting during ejaculation. It may also slip off during coitus. Therefore, it may disturb the act of coitus and needs determination to use it correctly. Failure rate is generally in the range of 3 to 5% and depends on correct usage, the quality of the condom and concurrent use of spermicide such as nonoxynol-9. Use of male condom should be encouraged as a second protection towards pregnancy but most importantly in minimizing sexually transmitted diseases.[4,5]

The female barrier methods can be in the shape of the diaphragm, cervical cap, vaginal condom or sponge. They can be inserted early when coitus is anticipated and, therefore, may not really interfere with the act of coitus. Insertion is more complicated and needs to be learnt. The female condom is like the male condom, and is meant for single use. The diaphragm and sponge can be left up to several hours and permits repeated coitus, provided extra spermicide is used. They should not be removed until 6 hours after intercourse but should not be left within the vagina for more than 24 hours to avoid toxic shock syndrome (TSS). The cervical cap can be left in place for 24 to 48 hours for the next coitus. The female barrier methods, offer some degree of protection against sexually transmitted diseases but are not as good as the male condom, as the vaginal wall is still exposed to the male seminal fluid. The vaginal condom is the best in this respect.

Lactational Amenorrhea Method

This method which is usually practiced during the puerperium, depends on the presence of high level of circulating prolactin hormone during lactation that will inhibit ovulation. The women must not have any menses yet and remains in amenorrhea and observes exclusive or almost exclusive breastfeeding. The method is only reliable for about six months. An additional method of contraception is necessary after this initial period or if supplementary feeding is being given to the infant.

Hormonal or Steroidal Contraceptives

This is widely used and amongst the most reliable methods. The exact choice depends on the local availability and preference of the prescribing doctors, patient profiles and accessibility to medical care. There are varieties of hormones being used, but these can be classified as:

- Monophasic combined oral contraceptive pill (COCP)
- Sequential (biphasic or triphasic) combined contraceptive pill
- Progestogenic-only pill (POP)
- Injectable depot
- Hormonal impregnated devices
- Implant

Combined Oral Contraceptives Pill (COCP)

Usually contains ethinyl estradiol or mestranol as the estrogen component in the lowest possible effective dose to minimize side effects. It used to be 50 micrograms, but now-a-days, the dose per tablet is usually in the region of 20 to 30 micrograms only.

The progestin component varied from the traditional (ethynodiol), the second generation (levonorgestrel and norethisterone) and the newer third generation (desogestrel, gestodene and norgestimate). There are also those which contain cyproterone acetate as its progestin component (Diane 35); the latter has anti-androgenic effect and suitable for those with symptoms of excessive testosterone production as in polycystic ovarian syndrome (PCOS).

Mechanism of action: Combined OCP contains synthetic hormones that are at a higher dose than the physiological level. Therefore, they cause the negative feedback on the endogenous gonadotropin (FSH and LH) production by the hypothalamo-pituitary-ovarian (HPO) axis. This prevents ovulation and, is thus, an effective contraception with failure rate 0.1 to 0.5%. The progestogen component helps by causing the endometrium to be thinned and unfavorable to implantation. It also thickens the cervical mucus to reduce sperm and other microorganism penetration.[4,5] It should be stressed, however, that oral contraceptive DO NOT prevent sexually transmitted diseases.

These drugs need to be taken fairly regularly daily for 21 days to confer protection. During the first two weeks, if she misses taking one tablet, she needs to take both the forgotten one and the current due when she remembers. If she forgets to take it for two consecutive days and remembers only on the third day, she needs to continue with the rest of the tablets, BUT use other contraceptive method for the subsequent days. However, if she forgets to take a tablet in the third week (days 15 to 21), she needs to take the two tablets (the forgotten and the one due) when she remembers, AND also use other contraceptive method for seven days and start with a new pack immediately. The women should not be pill free more than seven days in a row during or between the packs as this will cause escape ovulation in 10% of cases.

Drugs interaction: COCP is mainly metabolized by liver enzymes and enter the enterohepatic circulation, involving the normal gut flora. Therefore, any drugs that interfere with these pathways will influence the serum level of COCP and its effectiveness. The common drug interactions are:

- Liver enzyme inducers, such as anticonvulsants (except sodium valproate), rifampicin and griseofulvin.
- Broad-spectrum antibiotics change the gut flora and increase estradiol metabolite excretion.

Women should be advised to take extra precaution when they are taking these medications as the lower serum level of contraceptive may not prevent ovulation and result in method failure.

The WHO *contraindications* for the use of oral contraceptives (category 4, refrain from using) in certain situations, include:

- Cardiovascular:
  - Previous arterial or venous thromboses
  - Ischemic or severe heart disease or pulmonary hypertension
  - Hypercoagulable tendency
  - Previous cerebral hemorrhage
  - Severe hypertension
- Hepatic disease:
  - Cholestatic jaundice in pregnancy
  - Hepatoma
- Pregnancy

- Estrogen-dependent tumors such as active breast cancer
- Diabetes with complications
- Age >35 and smokes >20 sticks per day
- Major surgery with immobilization

The biphasic and triphasic types are not many and are not very widely available. They contain the least amount of steroid hormones and are, therefore, associated with less side effects.

Major side effect of oral contraceptive

- *Myocardial infarction and stroke*

  These are related to the estrogen component. The risk increases slightly in current users and persist for about 10 years after cessation. However, women less than 35 years old, non-smokers, non-diabetics and normotensive are only minimally at risk.[4,5] A long-term study in, UK showed a 1.9 relative risk (RR) of death from cerebrovascular event, 2.5 RR of cervical cancer and 0.2 RR of dying from ovarian cancer. This is true for current and recent users (within 10 years), but the risk ceases after 10 years of cessation.[5]

- *Venous thromboembolism*

  The newer generation is associated with less androgenic side effect and thus less weight gain, acne and breast discomfort. However, there were reports about the apparent increase of deep vein thromboses with them.[5] This was later found to be not entirely true.[4,5,7,8] Since the second generation is as effective as the newer generation, it is prudent to start on them, unless there is problem with weight gain and provided there is no history of thromboembolism in the past.

  All of them increase the risk of thromboses and should be stopped 4 to 6 weeks prior to a major surgery. The risk for COCP users is 1% compared to 0.5% in nonusers. The women should be advised on other contraceptive method during this period. However, to routinely stop COCP and/or using prophylaxis for deep vein thromboses alone in an otherwise low risk-case (who has minor procedure) is debatable.

- *Common side effects*

  These include nausea, headache, breasts tenderness, weight gain, irregular menses and depression.

COCP and Cancer

- *Breast cancer*

  Development of breast cancer is multifactorial and involves genetic, natural endogenous hormones, environment and increasing age. Most studies showed inconsistent results. However, recent data suggest that there is relative risk of 1.24 of developing breast cancer on current users (of at least six months) compared to never user. This risk returns to normal after 10 years of cessation, irrespective of family history, parity, ethnic, dose and length of usage. The pills may act as a promoter rather than as a carcinogenic agent in this aspect.[9,10] However, in long-term users who start before 20 years of age, the risk remains elevated. Any previous history of breast cancer, therefore, is a contraindication for oral contraceptive containing estrogen.[4]

- *Ovarian and endometrial cancer*

  Most studies showed a risk reduction of 40 to 60% for ovarian and endometrial cancer in users compared to nonusers. A minimum of three months and a year of treatment are required to get these protective effect respectively. Protection probably due to suppression of ovulation in the ovaries and progestin effect on the endometrium. The protection conferred continues for 10 to 15 years after cessation of COCP.[10,11] However, similar protection was not shown by the sequential regime. In those with BRCA 1 or 2 gene carriers, the effect of parity confers more protection than length of COCP use.[12]

- *Cervical cancer*

  COCP was initially thought not to cause increase risk, but they are at increased risk due to the sexual exposure and lifestyle of the user herself. These women tend to start sex early, have multiple partners and more unlikely to use barrier method.[10] Recent work also suggests that COCP may promote the activity of the human papillomavirus infection.[11]

- *Liver tumor and hepatobiliary system*

  Certain rare malignant and benign tumors have been reported in COCP users. The exact mechanism is unknown.[10]

Progestogen-only Pill

The progestogen-only pill suppresses ovulation in about 60% of users. Generally, it depends on its atrophic effect on the endometrial lining and cervical mucus changes for its efficacy. Therefore, the failure rate is slightly higher than the combined pill. However, they do not cause suppression of lactation and have minimal metabolic changes. They are, therefore, more suitable to the lactating mothers, those with history of venous embolism, those who cannot tolerate COCP side effects and diabetic mothers. It must be taken at a more regular time of the days (usually within 4 hours) to maintain effectiveness, compared to about 8 hours for COCP. It also can be used to reduce menstrual bleeding, cramp and lower the risk of pelvic inflammatory diseases, ovarian and endometrial cancer like the COCP.[4] Users need additional contraception for 48 hours if one pill is missed and also during the first month of starting.

The side effects include amenorrhea or irregular period in certain women and may cause development of functional cyst in the ovary.

Depo or Injectable Progestogens

These include the Depo Provera 150 mg 3 monthly and the norethisterone enantate 200 mg 2 monthly. They are highly effective contraceptive methods with failure rates about 0.3 to 0.5%. They act by preventing ovulation, thicken the cervical mucus as well as making the endometrium hostile for implantation. They, therefore, confer protection against endometrial and ovarian cancer.

However, some irregular bleeding for the first few months can occur followed by a period of amenorrhea. Proper consultation and advice about these need to be emphasized to prevent discontinuation and inappropriate anxiety. Other side effects are weight gain and breasts tenderness.[4]

Implant

The most popular one was the Norplant. It contains 6 matchstick-sized rods containing Levonorgestrel that need to be inserted subcutaneously under local anesthesia, usually at the forearm. It provides effective protection like any injectable Progestin for up to five or six years or until it is taken out.

The Norplant 2 contains two rods and protects up to three years. The rods need removal, again under local anesthesia.[4]

Newer preparations like Implanon used single rod containing etonorgestrel have been developed and provide protection for three years.[13]

In general, failure rate is about 0.05 to 0.1%. Failure rate is higher in obese women. Side effects are the same as for progestin-only injectable like irregular periods, weight gain, breasts tenderness and possible infection at implant site.

Intrauterine Contraceptive Device (IUCD)

This method has been used since the days of the Prophet when the migrating businessmen inserted pebbles into the uterus of their camels to prevent pregnancy during their long journey across the desert. The knowledge has been applied to human beings and varieties of materials have been tried before, such as inert plastic in variable shapes. Now-a-days, the material used is copper (e.g. Multiload Cu250; Copper T devices). It acts by causing some degree of local inflammation on the endometrium, making implantation for the oncoming fertilized ovum almost impossible on the hostile surrounding. The copper content may even be toxic to the sperm and immobilize them and reduce their capacity to fertilize.

It is suitable for parous women who are in a stable monogamous relationship. It is not recommended for the nullipara whose cervical os is tightly closed, as it may cause trauma and cervical infection and possible infertility problem. Even in parous women, it is usually inserted during the last few days of menses because during these few days, pregnancy is unlikely, the cervical canal needs no dilatation and slight bleeding associated with the insertion will not cause unnecessary anxiety to the patient. The failure rate is about 0.1 to 1.5%.

In case of method failure to prevent a pregnancy, the risks of ectopic pregnancy would be 4 to 8% (more than the background 1% for the general population), but the majority of the pregnancies will still be in the uterine cavity. The IUCD is effective in preventing all pregnancies, more so for an intrauterine than an extra-uterine pregnancy. Therefore, if pregnancy does occur with an IUCD *in situ*, the risk of an ectopic pregnancy in that user is slightly higher than if she is not on an IUCD.

In the rare cases of intrauterine pregnancy occurring with the IUCD in place, it is advisable to remove the device immediately. Leaving it in place increases the chance of miscarriage by 50% and taking it out reduces this chance by 25%. Moreover, there is increased risk of severe infection and also of prelabor rupture of membrane if it is left *in situ*.[14]

The side effects for copper IUCD are heavier and painful menses, slightly increased risk of pelvic infection with possible tubal infertility, failure due to expulsion and uterine perforation during insertion.[4,14]

A newer type of intrauterine device uses inert plastic material coated with progestogen (e.g. Mirena with Levonorgestrel). The progestogen enhances its efficacy by causing an atropic endometrium. It may prevent ovulation in certain percentage of patients and also thickens the cervical mucus causing difficulty for sperm and other microbials to invade the uterine cavity. It is slightly bigger in size and has a slightly different technique of insertion, but can be used for 6-8 years and does not cause heavy flow. It is used to reduce menstrual flow in selected patients with menorrhagia and for endometrial protection in women on hormone replacement therapy.

Sterilization

This can be divided into male and female sterilization. The commonest one being performed is the **female sterilization**, either in the immediate postpartum or as an interval procedure. There are various methods available such as the Pomeroy, Uchida and fimbriectomy during laparotomy or minilaparotomy; or laparoscopically using Filshie clips, Fallop ring and so on. There is not much difference in term of minor or major surgical morbidity by using the minilaparotomy or the laparoscopic approach.[14] Newer technique using hysteroscopically directed tubal embolization has been reported. The main aim is to cause blockage along the tubes to prevent the meeting of the ovum and the oncoming sperm. The failure rate varies but in general is less than 1%. Even though reversal is possible,[4] this

is a permanent method and is not meant to be temporary. Failure can be due to sterilization at the time of an undiagnosed early pregnancy, slippage of the occlusion material, recanalization or fistula formation between the two ends. In case of failure to prevent pregnancy, the chance of an ectopic pregnancy is higher; and this is largely due to the development of a tuboperitoneal fistula.

Male Sterilization

It is a simple procedure where the vas deferens is identified and transected bilaterally, either under local or general anesthesia. Preoperative counseling usually include:

Emphasizing that it is a permanent method. Although reversal is possible, but there is no guarantee of success. Semen or sperm may be cryopreserved before vasectomy if necessary. The patient must provide seminal fluid for analysis of post procedure, till it shows two to three reports of azoospermia; and alternative contraception is needed till then. There is small 1% risk of recanalization and 3% risk of post-procedure scrotal haematoma and pain, which usually resolves spontaneously. Although it is more easily accessible than female fallopian tubes, it is less acceptable to the general male population due to certain myths about it. Only small percentage develop sperm antibody. It does not reduce libido and there is no evidence linking it to increased rate of prostate cancer.[16]

Male hormonal methods and vaccines for reversible contraception are currently being developed and will increase the options for the male.

NONCONTRACEPTIVE BENEFIT OF COMBINED ORAL CONTRACEPTIVES

The oral contraceptive can be prescribed for different indications, in addition to contraceptive effect. The added advantages are:

- To reduce menstrual bleeding and thus reduce iron deficiency anemia.
- Reduce menstrual pain or cramps (dysmenorrhea)
- Reduce Mittelschmerz (ovulation) pain by inhibiting ovulation

- Thickened cervical mucus helps to reduce pelvic inflammatory disease
- Protects against ovarian cancer in current users and for 10 to 15 years later
- Protects against endometrial cancer in current users and for 10 to 15 years later
- Protects against benign breast diseases
- Helps to regulate an abnormal menstrual cycle
- Treatment of acne and hirsutism (cyproterone acetate)
- Treatment of endometriosis
- Reduces ectopic pregnancy.

PRACTICAL CONSIDERATION IN PRESCRIBING CONTRACEPTION

The use of contraceptive methods needs to be individualized. Various factors need to be considered such as moral, religious, and cultural issues as well as availability and accessibility to medical services. In general, the following factors should be considered:

- Age
- Parity
- Length of protection required, for spacing or permanent
- Future plan for pregnancy
- Previous contraceptive experience
- Nursing mother
- Existing medical problems like diabetic, hypertension
- Lifestyle—smoking, social activity
- Related gynecology disorders (dysmenorrhea, menorrhagia, irregular period, etc)
- Compliance
- The importance of preventing pregnancy/degree of protection needed.

Contraception for the Elderly

Women over 40 years old either normally have completed their family or are advised against pregnancy for fetal or maternal reasons. Contraception is still needed because at 40-44 years and 45-49 years age groups, the annual risk of pregnancy are 10% and 2-3% respectively, until they are truly in menopause.[5,19]

In general, they can use all the different methods available. The low-dose contraceptive pill is safe in the above 40 years age provided they are healthy, non-smoker, have no hypertension and are not diabetic. Smoking and oral contraception increase the risk of cardiovascular events. Although the risk increases with age, this is not too high compared to nonusers of similar age group. This is balanced by the benefit of regular menses, increase in bone density, reduction of climacteric symptoms and the other noncontraceptive benefits.[5,19]

Progestin-only pill can be used safely as it has less cardiovascular effect, but may confer less protection with some irregular bleeding.

Those with irregular menses need to be investigated to rule out cervical and endometrial cancers. An intra-uterine device is not the best choice for them, except the Mirena as advised by the WHO scientific group 1994 in Geneva.[19] For those with regular menses, any device is acceptable.

Barrier methods if used properly are reliable. The low effective rate should be seen together with the reduced frequency of intercourse and low fecundity rate.

Sterilization can be offered for those interested. In the female, this has added advantage of visualizing the ovaries and may confer some protection against ovarian cancer.

Contraception for the Teenagers

Teenagers have the tendency to indulge in sexual acts without realizing the immediate and long-term complications. Advice about abstinence or outercourse and the risk of sexually transmitted diseases should be given. Nevertheless, too much preaching will only turn them away. Therefore, contraceptive advice is necessary.

Compliance to oral contraceptives is normally poor after some minor side effects. Therefore, incorrect myths about oral contraceptive need to be rectified. Other noncontraceptive benefits should be explained and can help to improve compliance.[5] Early start on oral contraceptives with long-term breast and cervical cancer risks have to be balanced with the risks of unplanned and unwanted pregnancy.

Condom is highly advisable as a second protection, as well as the main method to minimize sexually transmitted diseases.[4,5]

An IUCD is not an appropriate choice as the risk of pelvic inflammatory disease is high due to their promiscuity behavior.

Understanding and access to medical advice and emergency contraception should be made more freely available to them. Confidentiality and whether to involve their parents are two issues that need proper judgement by the medical practitioner.

Postcoital/Emergency Contraception

This has an important role in cases of possible failure of technique, rape or incest cases, unscheduled unprotected intercourse and so on. This is important when sexual act occurs around the midcycle and pregnancy is highly likely. The subject must also present early to reap the full benefit of the treatment. Therefore, it should be noted that not all unprotected intercourse need emergency contraception. There are several methods that can be used.

* *High-dose oral estrogen*
  Not popular now-a-days due to nausea and thrombotic effect.

* *Yuzpe method*
  This involves taking orally 100 to 120 micrograms of ethinyl oestradiol within 72 hours of coitus and repeat the dose in 12 hours. It is about 4 tablets of the ordinarily available oral contraceptive. It can be nauseating; and if vomiting occur within half an hour of ingestion, the dose needs to be repeated with an antiemetic as well, and the second dose at 12 hours later. It confers protection in about 75 to 85% of cases.[4,5] It works by delaying ovulation or causing the endometrium to be out of phase.

* *High-dose progestogen*
  Commonly used is the levonorgestrel (LNG). A dose of 0.75 mg of LNG should be taken within 72 hours of the coitus and repeated 12 hours later. It has been found to be less nauseating and is thus more acceptable to patients.[17,18] Protection rate is comparable to the Yuzpe method. Newer regimes using lower doses have been tried and results are encouraging with almost similar protection rate but with much lower side effects. It also works by delaying or preventing ovulation.

* *IUCD insertion*
  Suitable to be used in parous women who also wish for further protection. It should to be inserted within 72 hours of coitus and acts by causing local inflammation and a hostile environment for implantation. Protection rate is about 80 to 90%.

* *Antprogestogen (Mifepristone—RU 486)*
  This drug is not widely available. It is an anti-progestogen and therefore highly effective either as a contraceptive or as an abortifacient. The dose used is 600 mg and can disrupt a cycle considerably.[17] It can be used within 7 days of coitus and gives protection against pregnancy in almost all cases.

TERMINATION OF PREGNANCY

This is not a contraceptive method by definition. However, in countries where abortion is legal, it can be used if there is failure of the above-said methods. This can be achieved by medical means using the abortifacient such as RU 486 (Mifepristone) with or without Misoprostol, or using surgical evacuation procedure. A properly conducted procedure will have a 100% success rate. Complications are rare but include infection with future subfertility, especially if performed illegally by a less experienced operator.

REFERENCES

1. A Conde-Agudelo, J M Belizan. Maternal morbidity and mortality associated with interpregnancy interval: Cross sectional study. British Medical Journal, 2000;321:1255-59.
2. N Tonti-Filippini. The pill: Abortifacient or Contraceptive? A literature review. Linacre Quarterly, February 1995:5-10. (Medline).
3. A Aghajanian, AH Merhyar. Fertility, contraceptive use and family planning program activity in the Islamic Republic of Iran. International Family Planning Perspectives June 1999; Vol 25(2).
4. T Nordenberg. Protecting against unintended pregnancy: A guide to contraceptive choices. FDA Consumer, April 1997.
5. S L Cerel-Suhl, B F Yeager. Update on Oral Contraceptive pills. American Family Physician 1999; 60: 2073-84.
6. H Jick, J A Kaye, C Vasilakis-Scaramozza, S S Jick. Risk of venous thromboembolism among users of third generation oral contraceptives compared with users of oral contraceptives with levonorgestrel before and after 1995: Cohort and case-control analysis. British Medical Journal, 2000;.321:1190-95.

7. LA J Heinemann, MA Lewis, M Thorogood, WO Spitzer, I Guggenmoos-Holzmann, R Bruppacher. Case-control study of oral contraceptives and risk of thromboembolic stroke: Results from international study on oral contraceptives and health of young women. British Medical Journal 1997;315:1502-04.

8. V Beral, C Hermon, C Kay, P Hannaford, S Darby, G Reeves. Mortality associated with contraceptive use: 25 year follow up of Cohort of 46000 women from Royal College of General Practitioners' oral contraception study. British Medical Journal 1999;318:96-100.

9. E Hemminki. Editorials. Oral contraceptives and breast cancer. British Medical Journal 1996; 313:63-64.

10. Cancer Facts: Oral Contraceptives and Cancer Risk. National Cancer Institute July 2000 (Medline).

11. DCG Skegg. Editorials: Oral contraception and health. British Medical Journal 1999;318:69-70.

12. B Modan, P Hartge, G Hirsh-Yechezkel et al. Parity, oral contraceptive and the risk of ovarian cancer among carriers and noncarriers of a BRCA 1 or BRCA 2 mutation. The New England Journal of Medicine, 2001; 345 (4):235-40.

13. JE Edwards, A Moore. Implanon: A review of clinical studies. British Journal of Family Planning 1999; 4:3-16.

14. Understanding IUDs. Contraception and Information Center of The Journal of the American Medical Association 2000.

15. Kulier R et al. Minilaparotomy and endoscopic techniques for tubal sterilization. Cochrane Database of Systemic Reviews. Issue 2, 2002.

16. Jon L Pryor, Douglas A Schow. Vasectomy. Chapter 57, in Glenn's Urologic Surgery 5th edn, Lippincott-Raven, 1998; 487-92.

17. A Webb. Emergency Contraception: Is it time to change method? Editorials British Medical Journal, 1999; 318: 342-43.

18. SM Strayer, RL Couchenour. Combined OCPs vs levonorgestrel for emergency contraception. Lancet 1998; 352:428-33.

19. Contraception and the late premenopause. Progress in Human Reproductive Research 1996; 40 (Medline).

17.
Psychosexual Problems and Sexual Dysfunction

O Tamizian
Sabaratnam Arulkumaran

INTRODUCTION

Sexual problems within a relationship are not uncommon and more women and men now feel able to seek advice about them. Inhibitions about sexuality and values about sexual behavior are based on a person's religious beliefs, upbringing and values obtained from parents. The recognition of a problem as a psychosexual disorder will be influenced by the expectations of society and the individual or couples concerned, as well as, by those of their professionals. Thus, although there may be an underlying organic basis, the presentation and prognosis are usually highly dependent on the expectation of the individual and the society in which she lives. The prevalence of sexual dysfunction in a study of 4000 randomly selected patients in four general practices was reported to be 44% among men and 36% among women. There is no doubt, however, that the prevalence varies according to how people are surveyed and what definition of sexual dysfunction is adopted.

PHYSIOLOGY OF HUMAN SEXUAL FUNCTION

The physiology of human sexual response was described in the 1960s by studies carried out by Masters and Johnson, who described the five phases of human sexual response as sexual desire, sexual arousal or excitement, plateau, orgasm and resolution. The physiological changes observed during sexual response are mediated by psychic and/or physical sexual stimulation but can be inhibited to a greater or lesser extent by subconscious influences.

i. *Sexual desire*: This is stimulated by the thought, sight, smell or touch of another person. It may be suppressed or merge into the arousal phase.

   Arousal or excitement phase: This is the initial response to sexual stimulation—physical or psychological. This phase is characterized by reflex vasodilatation in the genitalia. In the male this manifests as penile erection resulting from filling of the corpora cavernosa as a consequence of neurologically mediated vasodilatation. In the female, the increased vaginal wall blood flow produces a lubricating transudate. The labia and lower part of the vagina become congested and the clitoris increases in width becoming more sensitive to touch. There is also associated ballooning of the inner 2/3rds of the vagina, along with engorgement of the breasts and nipples becoming erect. There is an associated systemic component characterized by rise in pulse, respiratory rate and blood pressure.

Arousal at this stage remains vulnerable to distracting influences (thoughts, noise) and may also be affected by fatigue, alcohol or worry.

ii. *Plateau phase*: During this phase the changes in the arousal phase are consolidated and further enhanced as is the sexual pleasure and the partner's desire for penetrative intercourse. Lower genital tract and breast changes reach a maximum during this phase while continuing stimulation may build up sexual excitement to the intensity required to achieve orgasm.

iii. *Orgasm*: Orgasm provides an intense feeling of pleasure associated with the discharge of sexual tension built up in the preceding phases. In both sexes it is associated with rhythmic contractions of the genital muscles. In 90% of women, the thrusting of the penis in the vagina or digital or oral stimulation of her clitoral area leads to orgasm. Half the sexually active women achieve orgasm when the clitoral area is directly stimulated (finger or tongue) while a quarter reach it during penile thrusting in the vagina. One in six women is able to achieve multiple orgasms while one in ten is unable to achieve orgasm.

Following ejaculation, the male experiences a refractory period which may vary in length and increases from a few minutes in the teenager to several hours in the elderly. During this refractory period further stimulation not only does not produce a response but may also cause discomfort. Many women and a minority of men do not have a refractory period with further stimulation leading to further orgasms in this group.

iv. *Resolution*: Following orgasm, the body returns to the nonarousal state unless stimulation is continued. In the initial moments after orgasm the penis and clitoris are exquisitely sensitive but this is very transient with rapid decongestion of the tissues in the lower genital tract in both sexes.

The phases of sexual response leading up to orgasm are mediated by the parasympathetic nerves which lead to vasodilatation and vasocongestion of the genital organs. Failure of sexual arousal and, therefore, of these changes to occur results in erectile failure in a man and general dysfunction in a woman. The orgasmic phase is mediated by the sympathetic nerves, stimulation of which leads to the clonic muscle contractions of the pelvic floor and other muscles. Where the sympathetic component fails to occur in an orderly fashion, there is premature or retarded ejaculation as a result. The feeling of pleasure experienced by both sexes appears to have its origin in the sex center in the thalamic and limbic areas of the old cortex. Failure of achieving orgasm in women is often a result of failure of sensations invoked in the clitoris and vagina being transmitted to the brain.

ASSESSMENT OF THE PATIENT

Obtaining a Sexual Problem History

One of the main difficulties encountered is the embarrassment and discomfort felt by both the patient and clinician in trying to obtain a sexual problem history. This is partly because at an undergraduate level there is little or often no formal education or training in human sexuality. Thus, most health professionals learn about sexuality from reading and experience but their background, upbringing and prejudices influence their interaction with patients.

A good fundamental knowledge of human sexual functioning as well as experience in interviewing and counseling skills is paramount. Problems may be presented openly in response to a direct question, or may be hidden behind a variety of 'opening gambits'. Sexual difficulties underlie many cases of vague ill health in women, which defy diagnosis until repeated attempts at communication are made. Lack of energy, backache and irritability along with anxiety and depression may be the presenting symptom. Similarly, patients may present in family planning clinics focusing their problems on contraception but where the hidden agenda is 'permission' or 'approval' that sexual intercourse is respectable when the aim is pleasure and love rather than procreation. Each and every one of basic gynecological symptoms may be wholly or partially determined by organic pathology or psychogenic distress.

It is essential to be guided by the patient, using this information to focus on establishing what the current problem is rather than taking a more general sexual history. Once the main problem has been defined, then a history of the development and progression of the problem should be obtained. This information should include the duration, nature of onset, whether improving or deteriorating, whether situational (for example, in one relationship but not another, one position and not another) and any factors with exacerbate or ameliorate the problem. It is also helpful to explore the patient's own assessment of the cause of the problem. The clinician must always bear in mind that one of the goals of his consultation, is also to exclude or elucidate any possible underlying organic factor. By the completion of the consultation it is important to have determined whether the problem is primary or secondary, by ascertaining when the problem started and whether it is causally associated with any other event occurring at the time of the onset of the problem. Furthermore, it is important to determine whether there are relationship or environmental contributory factors by enquiring whether the problem always occurs or only occurs under certain circumstances or with particular individuals. Finally, it is essential to determine what prompted the patient to present now.

Clinical Examination

The role of clinical examination is to exclude developmental abnormalities which may interfere with sexual function and detect potential causes of dyspareunia, as well as evidence of other medical conditions that may interfere with sexual function. Vaginal atresia and imperforate hymen in the female and undescended testes or hypospadias are amongst causes that would be identified on clinical examination. In cases of dyspareunia, a clinical assessment is imperative. Spasm of the pubococcygeus muscle may be detected during pelvic examination leading to a possible diagnosis of vaginismus while deep pelvic pain elicited on bimanual examination may be similar to discomfort experienced on intercourse. Acute infections such as candidiasis, herpes and trichomoniasis along with acute or chronic inflammation of the Bartholin's gland or vestibular glands may lead to vulvovaginal irritation and superficial dyspareunia. Pelvic examination may detect evidence of PID or endometriosis as a cause of deep dyspareunia. A normal anatomical variant of a retroverted uterus and ovaries prolapsing into the pouch of Douglas may be a further cause of deep dyspareunia. Medical conditions such as respiratory or cardiac disease may interfere with sexual activity as would osteoarthritis and limited mobility of the hips. Loss of sensation or reflexes in the perineal area, associated with multiple sclerosis (MS) or damage to pelvic nerves through extensive pelvic surgery and associated scarring are also other causes that may interfere with sexual function. Any investigations should be guided by what the suspected underlying pathology is but great care should be taken not to ascribe the cause of a sexual problem to an incidentally discovered abnormality.

SEXUAL DYSFUNCTION IN THE FEMALE

The majority of sexual dysfunctions do not have an organic basis to them. Many stem from poor relationship with partner, low or mismatched sexual drive between partners, ignorance about sexuality or sexual technique and performance anxiety. Changing age also affects sexual drive, desire and response. Illness or treatment side effects, along with fear that sex may aggravate an existing condition further contribute to sexual dysfunction along with depression and excess alcohol.

The main sexual dysfunctions in women can be viewed under the headings of:
- Inhibited sexual desire
- Failure to achieve orgasm
- Dyspareunia
- Apareunia/Vaginismus

Inhibited Sexual Desire

Also described as hypoactive sexual desire disorder or general sexual dysfunction and may have a prevalence as high as 10% affecting women more than men. It is characterized by the absence of sexual fantasies and desire for sexual activity. It may have its onset at puberty or may occur some months or years after normal sexual activity. Inhibited sexual desire may be a manifestation of clinical depression or of a deteriorating relationship but may present as a mismatch between the sexual desires of the partners. Although the woman may not be aroused by or reject her partner's sexual advances, she derives little or no enjoyment from them. A variety of factors may contribute to this lack or loss of desire. These include guilt about sexual activity through upbringing, fear of pregnancy or infection or injury, for example, following surgery or a myocardial infarction. Relationship difficulties and boredom of a routine along with pressures of life and work may all have detrimental effects on sexual desire.

Management of inhibited sexual desire needs to involve both partners as the heart of the difficulties may be poor communication between the couple. Intensive therapy involves some level of compromise between the psychoanalytic and behavioral approaches and is loosely based around the work of Masters and Johnson (1970), Annon (1976) and Kaplan (1974, 1979). One of the most commonly used approaches is the use of graded 'tasks' the couple perform at home in a relaxed atmosphere. These tasks are divided into three phases. During the first phase, the couple set aside 30 minutes each day over the course of a week, where they indulge in mutual nongenital pleasuring (massaging, caressing, fondling). The next phase is embarked on only if the couple have satisfactorily progressed through the first phase. This second phase involves mutual genital pleasuring, each partner taking turns and may take the form of touching, massaging, kissing or licking each others bodies and genitals. The third and final phase is reached when the couple feel confident that they have enjoyed the second phase. When the third phase is reached, the couple progress fairly swiftly through the first two phases and attempt sexual intercourse. Their progress is monitored by the therapist at intervals and any problems may be aired or discussed.

Failure to Achieve Orgasm

Orgasmic dysfunction may be associated with a general inability to become aroused or alternatively may be a failure to climax after normal arousal and plateau phases. Most experts would agree that inability to achieve orgasm by intercourse alone is sufficiently common not to constitute a dysfunction if the woman is able to achieve climax by masturbation or oral/finger stimulation by her partner. Despite this, in the lay public, the common but erroneous belief is that unless a woman reaches orgasm during penile thrusting preferably simultaneously with the man, she is sexually dysfunctional. A number of techniques are available for a woman who wishes to achieve orgasm. The most successful of these is masturbation and learning to achieve orgasm by masturbation supplemented by discussion and counseling from a trained practitioner often cures anorgasmia.

Dyspareunia

Dyspareunia is defined as recurrent or persistent pain during or after intercourse. It is traditionally divided into superficial (when the pain is solely at the vaginal introitus) or deep (when the pain is felt deep in the pelvis). There may be an organic component to the pain and, therefore, organic causes need to be excluded before it can be classed as psychosomatic. It is important to elicit whether the pain is sufficient to prevent intercourse, whether it is continuous or intermittent and whether it persists after attempts at intercourse have ceased. It is essential to enquire about the basic features that are assessed with any pain in general such as onset, duration, radiation, associated feature, ameliorating and exacerbating features. Organic causes of superficial dyspareunia include vulvovaginal infections, atrophic changes of the lower genital tract and conditions such as lichen sclerosus and painful episiotomy scars. Atrophic changes of the lower genital tract along with inadequate lubrication and sexual stimulation are other causes. Deep dyspareunia may be associated with PID, endometriosis, ovarian cysts and pelvic tumors along with a retroverted uterus and ovaries prolapsing in the pouch of Douglas. At total hysterectomy, where a vaginal cuff has been removed, deep dyspareunia is more common due to thrusting against a scarred vault, which no longer has the capacity to balloon on arousal. Furthermore, a hysterectomy in a proportion of women results in earlier than usual ovarian failure and continued sexual enjoyment may well require estrogen replacement therapy. Vaginal repair operations for prolapse may also result in vaginal narrowing and dyspareunia.

Psychosomatic disorders are more likely to be longstanding. The causes of psychogenic dyspareunia may include lack of sexual knowledge, guilt about sexuality, childhood sexual abuse or history of sexual assault. Patients who have undergone gynecological cancer treatment (surgery and/or radiotherapy) may well have an organic and psychosomatic component to sexual dysfunction. Thus, libido may be affected by depression occurring as part of the illness process or the reaction to the diagnosis while radical surgery may be mutilating leading to deterioration of body image and consequently of sexual relationships. Radiotherapy, especially in the setting of cervical cancer may lead to cervical stenosis, reduced lubrication and soreness and, therefore, is best prevented by the prophylactic use of lubrication and dilators.

VAGINISMUS/APAREUNIA

In apareunia the woman is unable to have penetrative intercourse. This is usually as a result of involuntary spasm of the pubococcygeus muscle surrounding the introitus and lower one third of the vagina. Attempts at penetration cause pain in the clenched muscle, thus aggravating the situation. In its most severe form the patient is even unable to tolerate the examiner's finger in the vagina due to the marked muscle spasm. Vaginismus may affect up to 3% of women of reproductive age group. In the majority of cases the problem is psychosomatic but organic causes such as vaginal atresia, vulvovaginal infection and erectile failure in the man need to be excluded. Occasionally, vaginismus may be traced to a sexual assault during childhood or a painful or brutal initial experience of sexual intercourse or simply an inadequate or faulty sex education. Primary vaginismus is usually due to fear and as such is similar to a phobic disorder.

Management evolves around identifying and if possible, treating any underlying physical cause. If a treatment is not possible, then alternative techniques may be suggested to enable her to enjoy her sexuality. A therapist may be able to 'educate' the patient to relax her perineal muscles and reinforce to her that there is no physical abnormality and that 'structurally she is normal and not small made'. A series of graded exercises such as inserting a lubricated finger in the vagina progressing gradually to two and three fingers may be helpful. Alternatively, metal or glass dilators may serve the same purpose. Once three fingers can be introduced with comfort and without muscle spasm occurring, the patient may be ready to attempt penetrative intercourse in small steps. Initially, she may sit above her partner and whilst controlling his penis, allow it to touch the vaginal entrance, gradually allowing him to enter deeper on separate occasions before permitting him to thrust and finally allowing him to be on top.

SPECIAL CIRCUMSTANCES

Sexual Assault

Defined as 'carnal knowledge of a woman without her consent by force, fear or fraud', it includes rape and incest. The epidemiology of rape suggests that while only fewer than one third of rapes get reported, in three quarters of cases the perpetrator is known to the woman. Furthermore, about one woman in 200 has been raped or suffered attempted rape in the preceding year. Women who have been subjected to rape need to be listened to non-judgementally and sympathetically, addressing both emotional and physical issues. Physical examination will need to be performed and the significance and nature needs to be discussed with the woman. During the examination, careful documentation needs to be made of all findings including scratches and bruise on the arms and legs. The vulva and vagina need to be inspected for evidence of bruising, blood or seminal staining, while a vaginal smear is examined for spermatozoa. Screening is also offered for sexually transmitted diseases and postcoital contraception offered if there is a risk of pregnancy. Counseling also needs to be offered.

Pregnancy

During pregnancy, there is a wide variation between couples with regard to interest and responsiveness to sexual activity. In general there is a trend towards reduction in frequency and satisfaction as pregnancy advances. Postnatally, dyspareunia is common but under reported with a recent survey indicating that 58% had painful intercourse at 3 months with the problem persisting in almost 30% at nine months. Vaginal dryness may also be a problem, especially in the breastfeeding group.

Menopause

The time of the menopause can be a time when sexual difficulties arise and are often attributed to hormonal changes. However, the menopause often occurs at a time when a number of other life events may be also taking place such as adolescent children at home or leaving home as well as 'losses' such as parents, job, youthfulness. It is, therefore, essential to consider the overall picture and evaluate treatments such as hormone replacement therapy and/or testosterone for their effectiveness; and if the desired effect is not achieved, explore issues further as appropriate.

CONCLUSION

The management of sexual dysfunction is by obtaining a comprehensive general and sexual history, with particular attention to physical and psychiatric problems. It is important to identify the problem and rule out the presence of physical or pharmacological factors as well as exclude psychological factors (sexual fears, shame, guilt, fear of injury). It is necessary to look out for hidden clues in the history whilst exploring the patient's attitudes to her sexuality and responses. There is no possibility of offering treatment for everyone experiencing sexual difficulties or dissatisfaction and thankfully there is neither a necessity nor an expectation from patients of this to be done. In a proportion of cases, all the patient wishes to achieve as a result of a consultation, is to 'check' whether an aspect of their sexual life is acceptable; for example, being less sexually active in the puerperium or postmenopausally. In other cases, patients may need more information about normal sexual response and how this may be affected by; for example, during pregnancy, puerperium or peri- and postmenopausally. They may have misconceptions about 'normal sexual response' believing that multiple orgasms are the norm; whereas in actual fact, most women achieve orgasms more reliably by masturbation, partner stimulation or oral sex than by intercourse. A proportion of patients will benefit from experimental sex therapy such as sensate focus, supplemented and reinforced by discussion with the therapist. The patients' ability to share their sexual problems will to some extent depend on the attitude of the clinician. Therefore, sexual dysfunction is often best managed in a special setting other than a busy gynecology outpatients clinic.

18.
Pelvic Organ Prolapse

Pralhad Kushtagi

General Gynecology

DEFINITION AND INCIDENCE

A prolapse is downward or forward displacement of one of the pelvic organs from its normal location. Traditionally, prolapse is referred to displacement of the bladder, the uterus, or the rectum. The problem of pelvic organ prolapse excluding true rectal prolapse will be described in this chapter.

Of the common gynecological complaints one comes across in clinical practice, the problems related to pelvic support disorders are common and account for almost 400,000 surgical procedures annually for women in the United States, which is nearly 60 percent of major gynecological surgeries a year[1] and 101,907 hospitalizations due to prolapse and/ or stress urinary incontinence in the reproductive age group.[2] The development of effective operations to alleviate uterovaginal prolapse was one of the key factors that led to the establishment of gynecologic surgery as a separate specialty.

CLASSIFICATION

Pelvic organ prolapse can be classified etiologically into congenital (neonatal)—which is a rare event found at birth in some neonates and disappears soon, unless it is associated with spinal cord defects; acquired—due either to childbirth or any kind of injury; and nulliparous— where childbirth injury to the supports is not the cause.

Prolapse is commonly classified on the basis of anatomical structure that is protruded or prolapsed, namely:

- anterior vaginal wall: bladder   — cystocele
  urethra   — urethrocele
- central or cuff: uterus   — uterine prolapse
  — vault prolapse
- posterior vaginal wall: small bowel   — enterocele
  rectum   — rectocele

These descriptive terms have been in use since time immemorial, but they tend to prejudge the true nature of any prolapse by focusing attention on bladder, rectum, or uterus rather than focusing on the specific defects that are responsible for alteration in vaginal support.

Normally, the cervix or vaginal cuff is supported at or above the level of ischial spines. Pelvic organ prolapses have usually been graded on a scale of 0-3 (or 0-4), the grade increasing with increasing severity of prolapse, with 0 referring to no prolapse and 3 (or 4) referring to total prolapse (procidentia) with reference to vagina and introitus (Table 18.1).

Since introitus is an ill-defined and imprecise term, hymen is preferred as landmark to evaluate prolapse, even though plane of hymen is somewhat variable depending on the degree of levator ani dysfunction.[3] In the latter system of evaluation, consideration is given to anterior and posterior vaginal walls descent (Table 18.2).

Table 18.1: Uterine descent

Degrees	Description
1°	Cervix below ischial spines
2°	Cervix up to the introitus
3°	Cervix outside introitus[?]
4°	
(Procidentia)	All of the uterus outside the introitus[?]

[?]some workers combine 4° with 3° prolapse

Table 18.2: Halfway system for grading each site of pelvic relaxation

Grade 0: Normal position for each respective site
Grade 1: Descent halfway to the hymen
Grade 2: Descent to the hymen
Grade 3: Descent halfway past the hymen
Grade 4: Maximum possible descent for each site

Notes for using the grading system:
1. Prolapse is graded at each site (cystocele, uterine prolapse, vault prolapse, rectocele, enterocele) with patient straining maximally. The upright position may also be used.
2. When choosing between 2 grades, choose the higher grade.

Data from Baden and Walker.[3]

However, the International Continence Society has adopted a site-specific descriptive system, taking hymen as a fixed point of reference and measurements are taken from that point on the anterior and posterior vaginal walls and to the vaginal apex. In addition, the genital hiatus width of perineal body and total vaginal length are measured and recorded on a grid form.[4] This suggested system is complex and needs to be popularized since it describes patient characteristics, helps to develop effective treatment protocols, and to assess surgical outcomes.

ETIOLOGY

The etiology of pelvic floor disorders is more likely to be multifactorial. All pelvic prolapse conditions and urethral hypermobility result from pelvic floor relaxation.

The etiopathology is often attributed to childbirth injury. Prolonged labor and high forceps delivery, particularly if prolonged traction is required, have always been blamed as etiological factors in the development of genital prolapse. Considerable stresses imposed on the pelvic floor during a 'squatting' labor might increase the risk of subsequent prolapse, but return to physical activity soon after labor may be protective.[5] 'Bearing down' before full cervical dilatation puts a tremendous strain on the uterine supports and contribute to an increased risk of prolapse. Fundal pressure was a recommended method of placental delivery, but it could lead to gross stretching of the uterine ligaments and has now been abandoned in favor of patience, maternal effort and judicious controlled cord traction. Neuromuscular damage to the pelvic floor is associated with development of pelvic organ prolapse.[6] The function of the levator ani muscle can be compromised in two ways. First, there can be direct mechanical injury to the muscle. Second, damage to the nerve supply leading to their inability to contract, even though they themselves remain intact. The direct nerve supply from the sacral plexus to the levator ani is placed under great stretch during parturition resulting in transient neuropraxia and repeated childbirth could further injure such patients and ultimately produce symptoms of prolapse and incontinence as the muscular supports are progressively damaged. A prolonged second stage and heavy fetal weight are associated with neural damage.[7]

Previous pregnancy is not a required precondition for prolapse, because it can occur in nulliparous women, especially when the cervix is congenitally elongated. Women with congenital defects like overt sacral abnormalities such as spina bifida, or those with defects of pelvic floor muscles as in exstrophy of the bladder or those with primary myopathies, such as muscular dystrophy, have a striking propensity to develop uterine prolapse, often before pregnancy and at remarkably early age. Syndromes such as Ehler-Danlos syndrome characterized by fascial and connective tissue weakness have significantly higher prevalence of genital prolapse.

An underlying abnormality of connective tissue in pelvic floor ligaments and fascia is also believed to be the cause of pelvic support disorders. This may be due to an intrinsic abnormality of collagen synthesis (e.g., abnormal collagen, imbalance between synthesis and degradation, imbalance between collagen types) that leads to pelvic support disorders regardless of outside stressors. A second mechanism might be mildly abnormal fascia and ligaments that can withstand normal pressures, but with excessive strain (e.g., high parity, chronic straining, or loss of pelvic floor contraction) develop genitourinary prolapse. In these individuals, the abnormality might be errors in repair of damaged ligaments and fascia, or lack of remodelling in mature collagen.[8]

The tendency to prolapse is more likely to manifest after the menopause, when the ovarian steroidogenesis ceases and genital support tissues are no longer affected by estrogen. Although inherent tissue weakness and childbearing are among the most common causes of vaginal prolapse, an additional cause is a prior hysterectomy. If the vaginal vault was not sufficiently resuspended and the cul-de-sac was not obliterated, vault prolapse and/or enterocele are common sequelae.

The greatest forces that affect the pelvic floor come from increased intra-abdominal pressure and the weight of the abdominal organs in a woman with some weakness induced by childbirth trauma or inherent connective tissue weakness or aging and menopausal hypoestrogenism. Chronic intra-abdominal pressure from pulmonary disease or lifting, chronic straining during bowel movements, ovarian tumor, ascites, and fibroid uterus contribute to aggravation of the prolapse condition.

ANATOMY OF THE PELVIC FLOOR

Understanding the anatomy of structural components that support uterus and pelvic floor is essential to understand the problems of the pelvic floor and in planning surgical correction.

The top layer of the pelvic floor is the endopelvic fascia, which attaches the pelvic organs, especially the vagina and uterus to the pelvic walls, thereby suspending the pelvic organs. Support of the pelvic organs is provided by a group of muscles referred to as the levator ani.

Viscero-fascial Layer

The fascial layer of the pelvic floor is a combination of the pelvic viscera and endopelvic fascia. Hence, it is referred to as viscero-fascial layer. On each side of the pelvis, the endopelvic fascia attaches the uterus and vagina to the pelvic wall. It forms a continuous sheet-like mesentery. It runs continuously from uterine artery at its cephalic margin to the point at which the vagina fuses with the levator ani muscle below. The part that attaches to the uterus is called the parametrium, and that which attaches to the vagina, the paracolpium.

The parametria are made up of the cardinal (transverse cervical) and uterosacral ligaments, which are two different condensations of a single mass of tissue. Opposite the external cervical os, the sheet of tissue that attaches the genital tract to the pelvic wall arbitrarily changes name from the parametrium to the paracolpium. These supportive tissues contain prominent blood vessels, nerves, and fibrous connective tissue that can be thought of as mesenteries that supply the genital tract bilaterally.

The paracolpium attaches to the upper two thirds of vagina and it consists of two portions. The upper portion (level I) consists of a relatively long sheet of tissue that suspends the vagina by attaching it to the pelvic wall. In the midportion of the vagina, the paracolpium attaches the vagina laterally and more directly to the pelvic walls (level II). This attachment stretches the vagina transversely between the bladder and rectum and has functional significance. The structural layer that supports the bladder is pubocervical fascia and is composed of dense fascia from the cervix to the pelvic wall. The suburethral endopelvic fascia is better developed than that higher in the area of bladder, thereby providing better support for the vesical neck. This layer attaches laterally to the arcus tendineus fascia pelvis and also to the medial border of levator ani muscles. Loss of this normal support at the vesical neck is one of the factors responsible for stress urinary incontinence. The posterior vaginal wall and endopelvic fascia (rectovaginal fascia) form the restraining layer that prevents the rectum from protruding forward. In the distal vagina (level III), the vaginal wall is directly attached to surrounding structures without any intervening paracolpium.[9]

Damage to the upper suspensory fibres of the paracolpium (level I) causes different type of prolapse from that caused by damage to the midlevel supports of the vagina (level II). Defects in the support provided by level II vaginal supports (pubocervical and rectovaginal fasciae) result in cystocele and rectocele, and loss of the upper suspensory fibers of the paracolpium, and parametrium (level I) is responsible for the development of vaginal vault and uterine prolapse.

Levator Ani Muscles

The levator ani consists of two portions: the pubovisceral muscle and the iliococcygeus muscle.[10,11] The pubovisceral muscle is a thick U-shaped muscle whose ends arise from the pubic bones on either side of the midline and pass behind the rectum, forming a sling-like arrangement. It has several components. The pubococcygeus is the most cephalic portion of the levator and passes from the pubic bones to insert on the inner surface of the coccyx. This portion does not contribute substantially to supporting the pelvic organs. The puborectalis portion of the pubovisceralis passes beside the vagina, and lateral vaginal walls are attached to it. The muscle then continues dorsally where some fibres penetrate the rectum between internal and external sphincter, while others pass behind the anorectal junction. Laterally, the iliococcygeus arises from the fibrous band on the pelvic wall (arcus tendineus levator ani) and forms a relatively horizontal sheet that spans the opening within the pelvis and forms a shelf on which the organs may rest.

The opening in the levator ani muscle, through which urethra and vagina pass (and through which prolapse occurs) is the urogenital hiatus. The normal baseline activity of the levator ani muscle keeps the hiatus closed and thereby the lumen of vagina, urethra and rectum. This eliminates any opening in the pelvic floor through which prolapse could occur and forms a shelf on which the pelvic organs are supported.

The interaction between pelvic floor muscles and supportive ligaments is critical to the support of pelvic organs. As long as the levator ani muscles function normally, the pelvic floor is closed and the ligaments and fascia are under no tension. The fasciae stabilize the organs in their position above the levator ani muscles. When the pelvic floor muscles relax or are damaged, the pelvic floor opens and the vagina lies between the high abdominal pressure and low atmospheric pressure. Although the ligaments can sustain the organs in place for short periods of time, if the pelvic floor muscles do not close the urogenital hiatus, then the connective tissue will become stretched or damaged and eventually fail to hold the vagina in place. This situation is likened to a ship in its berth on the water, attached by rope on either side to a dock—where the water supports ship's weight and the moorings simply keep the ship from straying away.[12]

SECONDARY ANATOMICAL CHANGES

Uterus gets retroverted before prolapsing through the vagina. The prolapse leads to further kinking of its blood supply, especially the venous drainage and results in congestion. The chronic congestion of the cervix will be responsible for the bulky cervices seen in menopausal women with prolapse.

The venous congestion over a period of time leads to decreased oxygenated blood in the most dependent portions of the cervix. Decubitus ulceration is the result of such tissue hypoxia. It is a trophic ulceration and heals on reposition of the uterus into the vagina, which restores venous drainage and improves availability of oxygenated blood.

In a patient with prolapse the exposed vaginal skin shows areas of keratinization and pigmentation due to exposure and friction. It looses rugosities from lack of estrogen.

Childbirth injury usually affects pelvic floor and traction from below by the weight of the uterus or any strain imposes pull of parametrium (cardinal and uterosacral ligaments) to keep the cervix and uterus in position. This results in stretching and elongation of softened, congested supravaginal portion of cervix.

Anterior vaginal wall prolapse and the resultant descent of posterior bladder wall near trigone cause stretching of the ureteric openings. It may also result in cystoureteric reflux of urine. The effect of these is hydroureter and hydronephrosis in a case of long-standing prolapse of severe degree.

SYMPTOMS

The degree of prolapse bears little relationship to the presenting symptoms. Someone with a severe prolapse, say procidentia, may have a few symptoms, whereas others with a small anterior wall descent may complain of more symptoms.

Symptomatic prolapse may manifest in several different ways. Majority of the patients referred to hospital with genital prolapse complain of 'something coming down'. There may be only a feeling of pressure or insecurity 'inside'.

Low backache may be one of the symptoms due to strain on the periosteal attachment of uterosacral ligaments caused by downward pull of uterine descent. The patient is unable to pinpoint the site of pain. It is felt more at the end of a day's work and is relieved after taking rest by lying down.

Anterior vaginal wall prolapse leads to urethral hypermobility, loss of urethrovesical angulation and descent of proximal urethra below the pelvic floor. This results in the failure of direct transmission of increased abdominal pressure to urethra whilst it is transmitted to the bladder, which often (but not necessarily) results in stress urinary incontinence. A larger prolapse, prolapsing posterior bladder wall through anterior vaginal wall coming out below the urethra, can produce symptoms of voiding difficulty. Such patients may have the sensation of incomplete voiding and require digital pressure on the prolapsed vaginal wall for completion of the act. They may also have frequency and urgency of micturition due to cystitis.

Protrusion of the posterior vaginal wall by rectum can cause symptoms of inefficient rectal emptying, often described by the patient as constipation, necessitating splinting of the posterior vagina to reduce the pocket of trapped stool.

A sexually active woman may complain of dyspareunia or obstruction to the penetration because of tissues protruding outside the introitus. Lax vagina and introitus could be the reason for decreasing sexual pleasure or there may be diminished frequency of sexual intercourse because of anxiety on the part of her partner.

Congested and hypertrophied cervix by itself or the secondary infection may be the cause for discharge per vagina. The patient with decubitus ulcer on cervix will present with blood-stained discharge.

CLINICAL EVALUATION[13]

Since pelvic support defects are frequently associated with specific alteration in bowel, bladder or sexual function, both the evaluation and management of poor support and abnormal visceral function are important in developing a treatment plan and assessing therapeutic outcome.

There are no universally agreed definitions for normal pelvic support or for pelvic support defects.

The patient is examined in the dorsal lithotomy position with moderate amount of urine in the bladder to help evaluate stress incontinence. Pelvic support is assessed when the patient is straining maximally as each individual site is identified. The defects are based on an imaginary line in the midvaginal axis extending from the midportion of the hymen to the hollow of the sacrum. During maximal strain in women with normal support, the urethra, bladder, cul-de-sac, and rectum will not cross the midvaginal axis. Support defects may occur at any or all of these sites.

Using any of the classification of grading the descensus (*vide supra*), the urethra, bladder, cervix or vaginal cuff, cul-de-sac, and rectum are described as grade 0 to 3 (or 4). If the patient is not straining effectively, the prolapse may not be apparent. If one is unable to make prolapse protrude when the patient is in lithotomy position, repeat examination may be necessitated while she is standing and straining.

Urethra

Urethral support defects are associated generally with paraurethral loss of support. As the patient with urethral hypermobility strains, the urethra rotates posteriorly, and its junction with the bladder straightens. The meatus rotates anteriorly. The paraurethral support defect can be confirmed by using an open curved ring forceps in a position lateral to the urethra to provide support paraurethrally as the patient bears down. As lateral support is applied, one should look to see if there is any correction in the rotational descent. The cotton swab (Q-tip) test objectively quantifies the degree of mobility. When an individual is straining, the urethra usually does not rotate more than 30° from the horizontal plane, but some continent multiparas may have loss of urethral support with no stress incontinence.

Bladder

Support defects involving the anterior vaginal wall may occur in the midline, laterally or paravaginally, superiorly, or in any combination of these sites. Defects can be identified clinically by evaluating each individual area. Using the sponge forceps with the curve pointing posteriorly toward the ischial spines, the lateral aspects of the anterior vagina and pubocervical fascia can be returned to their normal point of attachment along the arcus tendineus fasciae pelvis. The forceps then is placed laterally, and the patient is asked to strain maximally; if there are no evident anterior defects, she has lateral or paravaginal loss of support. If, when she strains, there is some improvement in anterior support, but she continues to have a midline bulge through the open arms of the forceps, she also has a midline defect in pubocervical fascia. The forceps may be closed and used to support the base of the bladder centrally. When the patient strains and she has no midline descent, the support defect is central or midline.

Superior loss of support is characterized by several clinical clues. When the patient strains, if the anterior vaginal epithelium appears thin and, with loss of rugae from the vaginal cuff along the base of the bladder, and the anterior vaginal wall is longer than the posterior vagina, the patient is likely to have superior loss of support of her pubocervical fascia. Superior defects are usually associated with midline defects.

Cervix/vaginal Cuff

Descent of the cervix or that of cuff as made out by dimples seen at 3- and 9-o' clock areas from the level of ischial spines signify inadequate cardinal uterosacral ligament (level I) supports.

An attempt should be made to evaluate the length of the cervix.

Cul-de-sac

With the loss of support in the cul-de-sac, the epithelium overlying it generally becomes thin, shiny and distended by intestines. Placing a speculum over protruding posterior vaginal wall and asking the patient strain will result in cul-de-sac gliding over it confirming the enterocele.

Rectum

Defects in the perirectal fascia occur most commonly in the midline but may occur laterally or transversely near the perineum or the vaginal cuff. The curved ring forceps may be placed posteriorly and laterally in an effort to reduce the posterior defect. If there continues to be a bulge between the open arms of the forceps, the defect is midline. The forceps may be closed and used to support the midline. If there is no loss of support when the patient strains, the defect is in the midline.

Perineum

The distance between the anal orifice and posterior fourchette should be noted. With a finger in the rectum and the thumb pressing against the perineum, the thickness of the perineum can be felt.

Loss of support at cul-de-sac and at perineal body is best identified intraoperatively. A full general and abdominal examination is necessary. It is necessary to exclude chronic chest problems, gross obesity and abdominal masses. Bimanual vagino-abdominal palpation should always be carried out to exclude pelvic masses such as ovarian cysts or fibroids.

DIFFERENTIAL DIAGNOSIS

Diagnosis of prolapse is not difficult, but the correct identification of site-specific defect in the pelvic floor may pose a problem.

Descent of anterior vaginal wall along with portions of bladder or hypermobile urethra may at times have to be differentiated from vulval cyst/ tumor, Gartner's duct cyst, or urethral diverticuli.

Congenital elongation of cervix needs to be considered while diagnosing uterine descent or vault prolapse. Cervical fibroid polyps or chronic inversion of uterus are rare conditions that may be reported as a uterine descent and need to be recognized.

Rarely, the patient complains of vaginal prolapse, but in fact she will be suffering from true rectal prolapse.

TREATMENT OF PELVIC ORGAN PROLAPSE

The modalities of treatment include conservative follow-up, surgical repair, or use of a vaginal pessary.

Expectant Management

Prolapse may be discovered during a routine gynecological examination. Such patients may or may not have symptoms due to pelvic support defect. One should keep in mind the axiom of medicine that "the asymptomatic patient cannot be made to feel better by medical or surgical therapy". The patient should be informed of the physical examination finding and the problems that could make the condition worse over time. The importance of buttock squeezing exercises in improving perineal muscle tone should be emphasized,[5] and in some vaginal cones of increasing weight[14] are prescribed for use in vagina for the same purpose. It is to be remembered that pelvic muscle exercises are virtually never harmful, but they are not likely to correct the problem if there is neuromuscular damage as the underlying pathology. In postmenopausal women use of estrogens as replacement therapy may help strengthen the supports and alleviate trivial symptoms. Periodic examinations while on follow-up will provide comparisons regarding the status of pelvic support defect, changes in patient's physical condition or symptoms.

Surgical Management

Traditionally, prolapse has been treated by surgery, the nature of which depends on degree and type of prolapse, patient's general health status and the need for preservation of menstrual, reproductive or coital function. The goal of surgery should be to relieve the patient of her symptoms by repairing each aspect of abnormal pelvic support in a durable and long-lasting manner. A detailed description of the various operations for managing pelvic support defects is beyond the scope of this chapter, however, a few general remarks are in order.

Removal of the uterus is not the surgery for prolapse. It is the repair of support tissues of uterus and vagina, which is the corrective surgery for prolapse. The surgical approach for each patient needs to be tailored to the specific symptoms, objective physical findings, and tests of visceral function. Most patients with prolapse have defects in more than one location, so attention should be paid to correcting all defects during the same operation. Operations for prolapse are generally, but not always, carried out through the vaginal rather than through the abdominal surgical route. Some conditions, such as stress urinary incontinence, are most reliably handled by an abdominal operation.

Repair of Anterior Vaginal Wall Defects

Patients with a central defect are best treated by anterior colporrhaphy, which reapproximates the pubocervical fascia in the midline under the bladder neck. Lateral defects require a different approach in which the vaginal attachments to the pelvic sidewall are reconstituted. These defects are commonly corrected either with a paravaginal repair via the abdominal or vaginal approach where endopelvic fascia is reattached to the arcus tendineus fasciae pelvis,[15] or with a 4-corner bladder neck suspension.[16]

Operations for Uterovaginal Prolapse

Vaginal hysterectomy and repair: Uterine prolapse is generally treated with vaginal hysterectomy and repair, which may be accomplished by several different techniques. It is preferred in a woman who has desired number of children and is not particular about preserving menstrual function. The advantage of vaginal hysterectomy is that it allows other vaginal surgery (viz., anterior and posterior colporrhaphy or enterocele repair) to be performed at the same time, without the need for a separate incision or for repositioning the patient. At the time of hysterectomy for prolapse, special attention should be paid to closing the cul-de-sac using a McCall culdoplasty and to reattaching the endopelvic fascia and the uterosacral ligaments to the vaginal cuff to provide additional support.[17]

Manchester/Fothergill repair: An alternative to hysterectomy for patients with uterine prolapse who wish to retain the uterus is the Manchester operation. In this operation, the bladder is dissected off the cervix and cervix is amputated. The cardinal ligaments are sewn to the anterior of cervical stump. Anterior colporrhaphy and colpoperineorrhaphy form the essential components of the repair.

Shirodkar's modification of Manchester repair: In a patient desirous of retaining childbearing function where amputation of cervix could compromise fertility, Shirodkar's modified Manchester repair may be a better option. In this operation, uterosacral ligaments are divided close to their attachment to cervix; the stumps are brought in front of the cervix, crossed and stitched to the cervix. High closure of the peritoneum of the pouch of Douglas is carried out. The cervix is not amputated. The rest of the operation is similar to Manchester repair.

Utero/cervicopexy and sling operations: Occasionally, marked uterine prolapse may develop in a young nulliparous patient due to inherent weakness in suspensory supports. The basic principle behind these operations is to fortify the supporting ligamentary structures. Abdominal round ligament (Gilliam) uterine suspension with uterosacral plication and culdoplasty may be helpful.[18] There have been efforts to use ribbons of rectus sheath brought out retroperitoneally between leaves of broad ligaments to be attached to isthmus of uterus. As a modification, some surgeons have used mersilene/nylon tapes instead, to be attached between uterus and external oblique aponeurosis.[19] A fascial strap or mersilene/nylon tape can also be interposed between the cervix and the sacrum.[20] Another attempt is to fix the mersilene tape to isthmus posteriorly and bringing the free ends out retroperitoneally to emerge laterally through anterior oblique abdominis for anchoring to anterior superior iliac spines on either side.[21] There is anecdotal evidence of success in such patients using sacrospinous ligament fixation or retroperitoneal abdominal uterosacropexy, suturing mesh or fascia to the uterosacral ligaments and then to the anterior longitudinal ligament of the sacrum. There is little information available regarding long-term follow-up of such patients.

LeFort repair: This is reserved for the very elderly menopausal women who are poor medical risks. It is not suitable for a sexually active woman. In this operation, rectangular flaps of the vagina from anterior and posterior walls are excised, the raw areas apposed with absorbable sutures. The repair converts vagina into a double barrel where uterus sits atop the midline adhesions.

Operations for Vault Prolapse

Among the most challenging cases are those involving complete eversion of the vagina in patients who have had a previous hysterectomy. Vault prolapse requires surgical correction because of the large size of the prolapse, its propensity to increase over time because of increase in intra-abdominal pressure, and the possibility of vaginal evisceration if it is not treated.

a. *Colpectomy and Colpocleisis:* For some patients, particularly elderly women who are not sexually active and who lead a sedentary lifestyle, surgically removing the vagina and closing off the space is a suitable option.

b. *Colpopexy:* An alternate procedure is required for younger women and women who wish to retain sexual function. For these women, the condition can be managed transvaginally or transabdominally. With the transvaginal approach, vaginal eversion is corrected by suturing one side of the vaginal apex (usually the right side) to the sacrospinous ligament with one or two sutures—a transvaginal sacrospinous colpopexy.[22] In the transabdominal approach, the vaginal apex is suspended from the anterior longitudinal ligament along the sacrum using a graft of fascia or artificial mesh that is sutured to the vagina and to the sacrum in a retroperitoneal position—a transabdominal sacral colpopexy.[23] Both the operations are highly successful in resuspending the vaginal apex.

Repair of Posterior Vaginal Wall Defect

Repair of posterior vaginal prolapse for rectocele and enterocele is performed vaginally using posterior colporrhaphy. In a rectocele repair, the posterior vagina is opened, the rectum is dissected away from the pararectal fascia, and the levator ani muscles are plicated over the rectum in the midline, after which the vaginal epithelium is closed. It is important to note that a rectocele is a defect of the vaginal supporting tissue and not a defect of the rectum. An enterocele is a peritoneal hernia over the rectum, often seen as a second bump higher up in the vaginal canal on examination. The peritoneal sac should be carefully identified, opened, and closed with several purse-string sutures of permanent material; the sac should be excised, and the vagina should be closed once more over the defect. If the perineal body is noted to be deficient and the patient has a gaping introitus, this deficit may be repaired by a perineorrhaphy or a perineoplasty, in which the vaginal fourchette is opened and the base of the levator ani muscle is pulled together in the midline, providing renewed support for the lateral vagina at its outlet. The latter step (perineorrhaphy) is better avoided in the sexually active woman for the fear of causing dyspareunia, unless gaping introitus and related sexual dissatisfaction are the symptoms.

Conservative Management

Conservative management of prolapse usually involves fitting the patient with a pessary. It should be emphasized that pessary will not cure prolapse but relieves the symptoms by stretching the urogenital hiatus. The patient who is using a pessary should have a well-estrogenized vagina. For women who are post-menopause, it is preferable to use intravaginal estrogen cream 4-6 weeks before the pessary is inserted, because this makes the pessary more comfortable to wear and dramatically increases compliance and promotes long-term use. Pessaries are advised not only to test as to whether the low backache or urinary stress incontinence is due to prolapse condition, but also as an interim therapy to avoid and/or postpone surgery in early pregnancy, puerperium, patients unfit for surgery with limited life expectancy, or while awaiting surgery. Postmenopausal women should use intravaginal estrogen cream on a regular basis if they are not on hormone replacement therapy.

SUMMARY

Pelvic organ prolapse is not due to single etiology. Normal support of the pelvic organs depends on a combination of fascial and muscular support. The specific type of prolapse that exists in an individual corresponds with specific defects in the anatomic structures responsible for normal support. Hence, surgical management needs to be individualized.

REFERENCES

1. Thompson JD. Surgical correction of defects in pelvic support. In Rock JA, Thompson JD (Eds): Te Linde's Operative Gynecology. 8th edn, Philadelphia. New York: Lippincott-Raven 1997;963.
2. Cramer DW. Epidemiology for the Gynecologist. In Berek JS, Adashi EY, Hillard PA (Eds): Novak's Gynecology. 12th edn, Williams and Wilkins 1996;63.
3. Baden W, Walker T. Surgical repair of vaginal defects. Philadelphia: JB Lippincott, 1993; 9-24.
4. Bump RC, Mattiasson A, Bø K, Brubaker LP, DeLancey JOL, Klarskov P, Shull BL, Smith ARB. The standardization of terminology of female organ prolapse and pelvic floor dysfunction. Am J Obstet Gynecol 1996;175:10-17.
5. Milton PJD. Utero-vaginal prolapse. Progress in Obstetrics and Gynecology 1989;7: 319-30.
6. Smith ARB, Hosker GL, Warrel DW. The role of partial denervation of the pelvic floor in the aetiology of genito-urinary prolapse and stress incontinence: A neurophysiological study. Br J Obstet Gynecol 1989; 96: 24-28.
7. Allen RE, Hosker GL, Smith ARB, Warrell DW. Pelvic floor damage and childbirth: A neurophysiological study. Br J Obstet Gynecol 1990; 97: 770-79.
8. Norton PA. Pelvic floor disorders: The role of fascia and ligaments. Clin Obstet Gynecol 1993; 36: 926-938.
9. DeLancey JOL. Anatomy and biomechanics of genital prolapse. Clin Obstet Gynecol 1993; 36: 897-909.
10. Lawson JON. Pelvic anatomy, I: Pelvic floor muscles. Ann R Coll Surg Engl 1974; 54: 244-52.
11. Lawson JON. Pelvic anatomy, I: Anal canal and associated sphincters. Ann R Coll Surg Engl 1974; 54: 288-300.
12. Paramore RH. The uterus as a floating organ. In the statistics of the female pelvic viscera. London: HK Lewis and Co; 1918; 1: 12-15.
13. Shull BL. Clinical evaluation of women with pelvic support defects. Clin Obstet Gynecol 1993; 36: 939-951.
14. Plevnik S. New methods for testing and strengthening the pelvic floor muscles. In Proceedings of the 15th Annual Meeting of the International Continence Society, London, 1985: 267.

15. Shull BL, Benn SJ, Kuehl TJ. Surgical management of prolapse of the anterior vaginal segment: An analysis of support defects of morbidity and anatomic outcome. Am J Obstet Gynecol 1994; 171: 1421-39.

16. Raz S, Klutke CG, Golomb J. Four-corner bladder and urethral suspension for moderate cystocele. J Urol 1989; 142: 712-15.

17. McCall M. Posterior culdoplasty: Surgical correction of enterocele during vaginal hysterectomy: A preliminary report. Obstet Gynecol 1957; 10:595-602.

18. Gilliam DT. Round-ligament ventrosuspension of the uterus: A new method. Am J Obstet 1900; 41: 299.

19. Purandare VN, Patel K, Aryan R. Operative treatment for genital prolapse in young woman. J Obst Gynae India 1966; 16: 53-56.

20. Shirodkar VN. The problem of prolapse. In: Contribution to obstetrics and gynecology. London: Churchill Livingstone, 1960;16.

21. Khanna SD. A new sling operation for nulliparous prolapse. Procedings 19th All India Obst Gynae Congress, New Delhi, 1972.

22. Morley GW, DeLancey JOL. Sacrospinous ligament fixation for eversion of the vagina. Am J Obstet Gynecol 1988; 158: 872-81.

23. Addison WA, Livengood CH, Sutton GP, Parker RT. Abdominal sacral colpopexy with Mersilene mesh in the retroperitoneal position in the management of posthysterectomy vaginal vault prolapse and enterocele. Am J Obstet Gynecol 1985; 153: 140-46.

VP Paily

19.
Urinary and Fecal Incontinence (Including Fistulae)

INTRODUCTION

The ability to store urine and feces and void them at socially acceptable times and places is a characteristic that distinguishes the adult human from animals.

Unfortunately, there are many situations when this ability is disrupted to varying degrees and these can be grouped together under the term of incontinence. Since urine and feces are produced continuously, and are to be voided only periodically, there has to be a storage mechanism. The bladder and the rectum act as the storehouses and the concerned sphincters provide the voluntary control. Integrity of the pelvic floor is essential for their normal function. In this chapter, the normal mechanism of micturition and defecation and the pathogenesis and management of incontinence will be discussed.

For convenience, urinary and fecal incontinence are considered separately, even though there is overlap in etiological factors and management strategies.

URINARY INCONTINENCE

Definition

The International Continence Society defines incontinence of urine as "an involuntary loss of urine which is objectively demonstrable and a social or hygienic problem."

Knowledge of the normal mechanism of storage and voiding of urine is essential to understand the etiology, pathology, and management of incontinence.

Normal Filling and Voiding

Bladder can store about 200-300 ml of urine without rise in the intravesical pressure because of the compliance of the detrusor. When the volume rises still more, the intravesical pressure slowly rises and the person becomes aware of the fullness of the bladder. If conditions are not favorable for voiding, micturition can be voluntarily delayed, but there will be a gradual rise in intravesical pressure until it becomes distressing. Beyond this, voluntary tightening of pelvic floor muscles will be required to prevent escape of urine.

When conditions are favorable for voiding, the first step is voluntary relaxation of the pelvic floor muscles. This allows descent and coning down of the bladder neck and escape of urine into the proximal urethra. Contractions of the detrusor muscle raise intravesical pressure further and result in complete emptying of the bladder. The cycle of bladder filling and emptying is then repeated.

Neuronal Control of Micturition

Knowledge of the nerve supply to the bladder and pelvic floor is essential to understand the neuronal control of micturition.

Bladder and proximal urethra are supplied by the autonomous nervous system—both parasympathetic and sympathetic. The parasympathetic cholinergic fibers are stimulatory to the detrusor. The sympathetic fibers have both alpha and beta nerve endings. The beta nerve endings supply predominantly the detrusor and are inhibitory. The alpha nerve endings supply the bladder neck and proximal urethra and their stimulation increases outflow resistance. Abnormalities of function of both parasympathetic and sympathetic supply can result in voiding dysfunction.

Parasympathetic stimulation or drugs that have cholinergic activity increase detrusor contractions and can lead to overactive bladder; as a corollary, anticholinergic drugs inhibit such contractions and even lead to urinary retention. On the other hand, sympathetic stimulation inhibits detrusor contractions and increases urethral resistance thus leading to retention. Alpha sympatholytic drugs may help to reduce urethral resistance and favor micturition. When urethral resistance is the cause of retention, alpha sympatholytic drugs help to overcome it.

Mechanism of Continence

Continence is possible only when the pressure inside the bladder is less than the pressure in the urethra. When the intravesical pressure overtakes the urethral pressure, urine will flow out. The proximal part of urethra being an intra-abdominal organ, the intra-abdominal pressure acts here also. In addition, there is contraction of the urethral sphincter and the resistance offered by the spongy lining of the urethra. If this lining gets thinner as happens after menopause, the urethral closure pressure will be reduced. This can lead to incontinence. Normally, at rest, the intravesical pressure is less than the pressure in the urethra.

Classification

A practically useful classification of urinary incontinence is to divide it as urethral and extra urethral (Table 19.1).

Table 19.1: Classification of urinary incontinence (Adapted from Stanton)[1]

Urethral	Extra urethral
Genuine stress incontinence	Congenital e.g ectopic ureter
Detrusor instability	Fistula
Retention with overflow	Ureteric
Congenital e.g. epispadias	Vesical
Miscellaneous	Urethral

Genuine Stress Incontinence (GSI)

Definition

GSI is the involuntary loss of urine with activities that raise intra-abdominal pressure such as coughing and sneezing. There are many terms used to describe this condition. The International Continence Society has recommended the term genuine stress incontinence. The other terms commonly used are urethral sphincter incontinence, stress urinary incontinence and anatomic stress incontinence.

Clinical Features

Genuine stress incontinence is much more common in the female than in the male. The quantity lost may vary from a few drops to substantial amounts that can make the clothes wet and become a social embarrassment. In its severe form the constantly wet underclothes may cause changes on the skin and can lead to sodden skin, dermatitis, etc. The patient may be conscious of the smell of urine emanating from the clothes. She may withdraw from social functions and this can have psychological impact.

Incidence

The prevalence of genuine stress incontinence varies widely depending on sex, age, parity, race (Bump and Norton).[2] A rough estimate is that about 23.5% of women will leak urine. The major type of incontinence among them will be GSI.

Pathogenesis

The exact pathogenesis of GSI is still unclear. Excess mobility of the bladder neck is believed to be the leading cause. When the bladder neck is in its normal position, any rise in intra-abdominal pressure will be transmitted equally to the bladder and the urethra and the pressure differential will be maintained, thereby preventing urinary leakage. On the other hand, when the bladder neck is below this pressure transmission zone, urine leaks.

Urethral pressure profile studies show that when the bladder neck is restored to its retropubic position, improvement or cure occurs for the stress incontinence. The other reason for incontinence could be weakness of the urethral sphincter. Rigidity of walls of the urethra, as can happen with scarring following surgery, also can interfere with the mechanism of urethral closure.

Diagnosis

Stress urinary incontinence is a symptom as well as a diagnosis. Demonstration of leakage of urine on coughing with a full bladder, therefore, helps to make the diagnosis. But, occasionally, there could be overlap with urge incontinence, as a detrusor contraction may be elicited by cough. Hence, ideally urodynamic studies are required to make a correct diagnosis of GSI. Urodynamics will also help to throw light on the type of surgery that will be best suited for the particular patient. For example, if it is a hypermobile bladder neck, a retropubic fixation of the bladder neck may be the ideal treatment. On the other hand, if it is a case of urethral sphincter weakness, a sling or injection of bulking agents periurethrally may be the better method.

A Q-tip test gives an idea about the mobility of the bladder neck. In this, a lubricated Q-tip is introduced up to the bladder neck and the patient is asked to cough. The movement of the Q-tip projecting outside the urethra will indicate how mobile the bladder neck is—usually, it makes an arc less than 30 degree. If the arc created by its movement is more, then the bladder neck is proportionately more mobile.

Treatment

The need for treatment will depend on how much the patient is bothered by her symptoms. There are different approaches to treatment—conservative or surgical.

Conservative treatment: It is generally agreed that conservative treatment should be tried first. Attempts to increase the strength of the pelvic floor muscles come under this category. Various methods of systematic exercise to increase the strength of the pelvic floor are suggested. One such method is to give gradually increasing weights, shaped like cones, to be kept in the vagina while the patient is standing. She is instructed to prevent the cone from falling by contracting the muscles of the pelvic floor. Unfortunately, a lot of motivation is required to persevere with this type of treatment. Majority of studies suggest that the beneficial effects slowly disappear once regular exercise is stopped.

There have been many studies using electrical stimulation as treatment for stress and urge incontinence, but consistent benefit has not been reported.

Surgery for genuine stress incontinence (GSI): Many surgical procedures are described to treat GSI. The choice of operation should take into account the age, general health of the patient, mobility of urethra and supports and associated pathology like descent of uterus or vaginal walls. Ideally, urodynamic studies should be done prior to the choice of operation. Some of the commonly done procedures and the factors that influence the choice are given in Table 19.2.

    i. *Anterior colporrhaphy*: Most parous women will have some degree of prolapse of anterior vaginal wall. Anterior colporrhaphy will help in correcting that. Identifying and using the pubocervical fascia to support the bladder is the essential part of the procedure. If there is GSI, special care is taken to imbricate the paraurethral fascia under the bladder neck and elevate it. This may, however, lead to post-

Table 19.2: Various surgical procedures for urinary incontinence and factors influencing their choice

Route	Procedure	Factors influencing the choice	Remarks
Vaginal	Ant.colporrhaphy Periurethral injection	Presence of ant.vaginal wall descent (cystocele) Physically frail patients. Can be done under local anesthesia.	High failure rate on long-term follow-up Long-term follow-up lacking
Vaginal and retropubic	Needle suspension (Endoscopically)	Can be done under local or regional anesthesia	High failure rate on long term follow up.
	Sling procedures	Can be done as primary and secondary procedures	Voiding difficulties more common. *De novo* detrusor instability more common
	Tension-free vaginal tape (TVT)	Can be done under local anesthesia and sedation.	Voiding difficulties less. No long-term follow-up available.
Suprapubic	MMK. Burch colposuspension	Carries good results Can be combined with hysterectomy	MMK-osteitis pubis as a complication. Is considered the gold standard.
	Artificial sphincter	Often chosen as the last resort	Patient has to be conscious and alert to use it.

MMK—Marshall-Marchetti–Krantz operation

operative urinary retention in a large number of patients. Training the patient on clean intermittent self-catheterization (CISC) before surgery will help to overcome this problem. The medium and long-term results are poor for anterior colporrhaphy as treatment for GSI. However, it is an essential step, if coexisting anterior vaginal wall prolapse is present.

ii. *Periurethral injection of bulking agents:* Periurethral injection of bulking agents at the location corresponding to the intrinsic urethral sphincter has been suggested as treatment for patients with sphincter deficiency. A variety of materials have been tried, but the ones currently popular are glutaraldehyde cross-linked collagen (GAX collagen, BARD, Crawley, UK) and Macroplastique (Uroplasty, Reading, UK).
The exact mechanism of action of this method is not clearly understood. The material is placed periurethrally by transurethral injection under cystoscopic control. Alternatively, the needle can be inserted by the side of the external urinary meatus and advanced to the correct location. The bulking agent may bring about cooption of the mucosa. As a response to the collagen injected, fibrosis and new collagen tissue formation may occur. This is believed to be the mechanism of action.
The special attraction of this procedure is that it is simple to perform and can be done under local anesthesia. The procedure can be repeated. In patients who have not completed the family this method has particular relevance as future pregnancy and vaginal delivery are not affected by this.

iii. *Needle suspensions* (Fig. 19.1): Armand Pereyra[3] in 1959 described the use of a long needle to take sutures from the vaginal end to the suprapubic region, to pull up the bladder neck and suspend it from the anterior abdominal wall. He continually modified the procedure and in 1982 proposed the use of prolene.

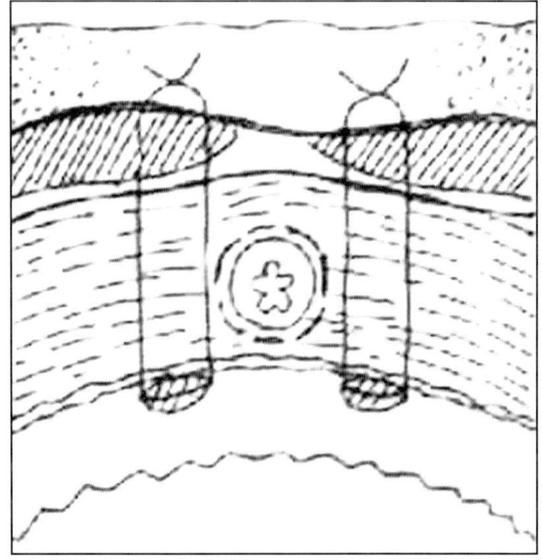

Figure 19.1: Needle suspension procedure for stress incontinence

Stamey[4] developed special needles for the purpose and used nylon sutures. Dacron buffers were used to prevent the suture cutting through the vaginal tissues.

Raz[5] advocated lateral dissection of vaginal epithelium and taking helical stitches through paravaginal tissues. There were many further modifications of these techniques. Gittes and Loughlin[6] suggested that dissection of vaginal epithelium was unnecessary and they recommended taking the helical stitches through the full thickness of vaginal tissues including the epithelium. His argument was that the vaginal epithelium would grow over the suture and cover it.

Use of cystoscope is recommended in all types of needle suspensions to verify if the suture has gone into the bladder cavity.

The short-term results of needle suspensions are very good giving nearly 90% cure rate. However, the long-term results are poor, coming down to as low as 18% at 5 years, O'Sullivan et al.[7] Still the simplicity and lower rate of complications make it an attractive procedure in the elderly.

Needle suspensions can be combined with anterior colporrhaphy in cases with anterior vaginal wall prolapse.

Bone anchors have been introduced to simplify the procedure further. In this, the abdominal end of the suture is anchored into the pubic bone. Commercial kits are available to anchor the suture to the pubic bone. The short-term results are good and comparable to needle suspension procedures. Long-term results and complications are still to be evaluated.

iv. *Sling procedures*: Use of a strip of material passed under the urethra or bladder neck and anchored to anterior abdominal wall structures to give support to urethra is an attractive proposition. There were many procedures described, but the one reported by Aldridge[8] in 1942 is the prototype of modern sling procedures. Various materials are used for preparing the sling—strip of rectus fascia, fascia lata, porcine dermis and a variety of synthetic materials like silastic, prolene mesh, mersilene and Goretex. One problem common to all synthetic materials is its erosion into bladder or urethra. Persistent infection may also necessitate early removal of the foreign body. *De novo* detrusor instability and retention can develop following sling procedures.

In most centers, sling procedures are reserved for those in whom other simple methods have failed. In spite of this, overall subjective cure rates of about 82% are reported. If employed as the primary procedure, the results could be even better.

v. *Tension-free vaginal tape (TVT)* (Figure 19.2): This procedure is similar in a broad sense to sling procedures described above but has many differences when we look at the details. The support is provided at the mid-urethra based on the principle that urethral pressure profilometry shows maximum closing pressure at the mid-urethra and not at the bladder neck. The TVT procedure does not aim to elevate the bladder neck, but rather provides a platform for the urethra to rest when there is downward movement caused by raised intra-abdominal pressure. Based on this principle, the tape is left below the urethra without trying to elevate it much. Prolene mesh is used and fibrous tissue will grow into the mesh giving it strength.

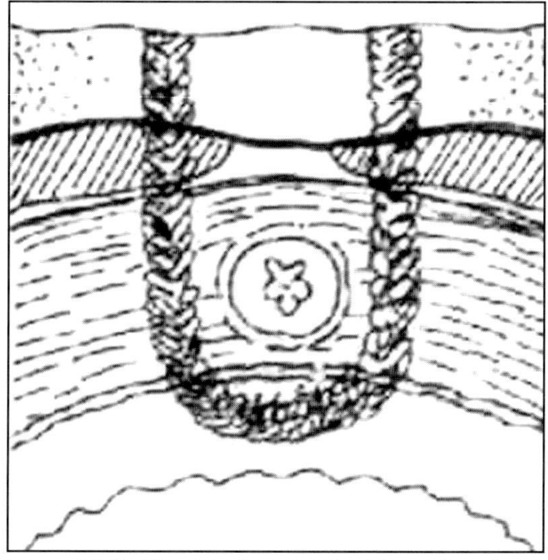

Figure 19.2: Tension-free vaginal tape for stress incontinence

The vaginal wall below the urethra is dissected laterally and the suburethral space is developed. From this space, the tape is taken retropubically to the anterior abdominal wall using the curved needle provided. The abdominal ends of the tape are pulled up and the patient is asked to cough. It is left at that position which is just enough to prevent leakage of urine; but at the same time, not too much as to kink the urethra. The polythene cover of the tape is slit off leaving the mesh to rest on the tissue by its friction. It is not sutured to any structure on the abdominal wall.

Ulmsten et al[9] have reported 86% objective cure rate after 3-year follow-up.

Recently, reports of tape erosion have started to appear in the literature. The final status of this procedure is yet to evolve; but at present, its low morbidity, technical simplicity and attractive immediate cure rate make it one of the preferred options for the elderly high-risk patients.

vi. *Retropubic procedures:* Marshall, Marchetti and Krantz[10] in 1949 described the retropubic technique for elevation of the bladder neck. Even though they initially described it for use in male patients who had urinary incontinence following prostatectomy, it soon became more popular for treating stress incontinence in the female. In this technique, the paraurethral tissues are attached to the periosteum of the pubic bone. It had good cure rate (about 90%), but went into disrepute because of the complication of osteitis pubis which may occur in 5 to 7%. In many centers the MMK procedure has been replaced by Burch colposuspension

Burch[11] described modifications to MMK procedure in 1961(Fig. 19.3). Instead of anchoring tissues to the periosteum of the pubic bone, Burch suggested use of Cooper's ligament as the anchoring site. In addition, he suggested elevation of bladder neck by taking stitches through the paravaginal tissue lateral to the bladder neck. Suture materials with delayed absorption like polyglactin (vicryl) and polydioxanone (PDS) are used. Two or three sutures may be taken on either side. These sutures are used to pull up the paravaginal tissues.

Incidentally, this will correct some degree of cystocele as well, but may increase the risk of development of posterior wall defects like enterocele and rectocele.

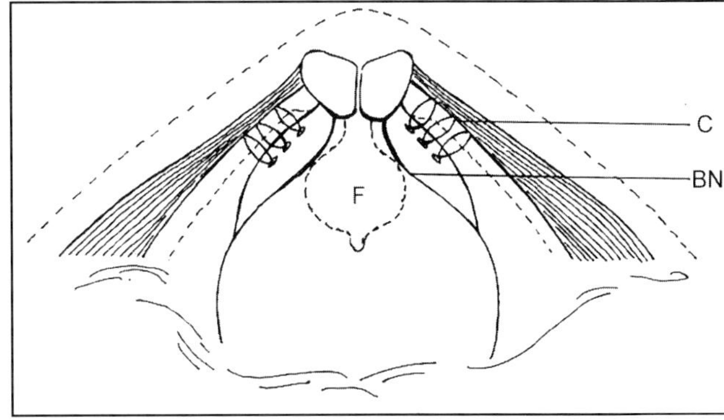

Figure 19.3: Burch colposuspension for stress urinary incontinence. F—Bulb of Foley's catheter, BN—Bladder neck, C—Reflected part of Cooper's ligament

Voiding difficulties are not uncommon following Burch colposuspension. However, as time goes by, the situation improves. In a study by Smith and Cardozo,[12] the initial voiding difficulties of 21% reduced to 2% after 6 months. *De novo* detrusor instability occurs in about 12-18.5% of cases.

Even now, Burch colposuspension remains the gold standard for surgical management of stress urinary incontinence. Success rates of 80-100% are claimed. Herbertsson[13] reported a 90.3% continence rate after 10-year follow-up. Burch colposuspension can be employed as the procedure for cases where previous attempts at surgical correction have failed.

A survey from Norway and Finland published in 1998 (Lose et al)[14] showed that more than 90% of Obstetrics and Gynecology departments still practised Burch colposuspension as the treatment for GSI.

Burch colposuspension can be done laparoscopically. Many modifications to the conventional procedure have been suggested. Synthetic mesh or direct suturing can be used to pull up the paravaginal tissues to Cooper's ligament. The short-term results are good but long-term results are yet to be assessed.

vii. *Artificial urinary sphincter*: In cases of intractable stress incontinence, where all other methods have failed, implantation of an artificial sphincter may be considered. After a lot of trial and error, the one model manufactured by American Medical Systems (AMS 800) has found clinical acceptance. The main components of this are a cuff that will go round the bladder neck, a pressure regulating balloon and a control pump inserted in the labium majus. The cuff could be deflated at will and the urethra opened to let the urine flow. This can be used in GSI where other surgical methods fail or in refractory cases of neurogenic bladder dysfunction. Long-term complications like erosion of the cuff, pump failure, etc. can occur and the need for repeated operations is not rare.

Detrusor Instability

Definition

The International Continence Society defines unstable bladder as "one that is shown objectively to contract spontaneously or on provocation during the filling phase while the patient is attempting to inhibit micturition." This is known by other terms like overactive bladder, detrusor reflex instability, etc. The term detrusor hyper-reflexia is reserved for abnormal detrusor activity secondary to a neuropathy (e.g. spinal cord injury) wherein the central inhibitory effect is gone and detrusor overactivity results.

Detrusor instability is not synonymous with urge incontinence, even though irresistible urge to pass urine is, probably, the most common symptom of unstable bladder.

Incidence

It is the second commonest cause of urinary incontinence (first being genuine stress incontinence). Detrusor instability is estimated to occur in about 6% of adult women.

Etiology

The exact etiology of detrusor instability is not known. Some associations noted are neurotic personality, bladder neck surgery and outflow obstruction. The basic problem could be at the level of neuromuscular junction or even in the detrusor muscle itself. This uncertainty in etiology is a hindrance to the development of effective medical management.

Symptomatology

Symptoms of detrusor instability vary a lot. The most common features are urgency (a strong and sudden desire to void) and frequency. When urine escapes because the contractions cannot be inhibited, it is called urge incontinence. Urgency and frequency can be the result of various other causes like urinary tract infection, bladder pathology, pressure due to pregnant uterus or other pelvic masses, medical disorders like diabetes, diuretic therapy or psychological factors.

Some women may have a detrusor contraction triggered by physical activity like sexual contact or cough. This makes it difficult to differentiate between genuine stress incontinence and detrusor instability purely on clinical grounds.

Diagnosis

To make a definitive diagnosis, urodynamic studies are required. However, a frequency volume chart may give a clue to the possibility. This will show the frequent voiding of small quantities of urine and the leakage. A cystometrogram will show the uninhibited contraction during the filling phase and the consequent leakage. Ambulatory urodynamic studies may show detrusor contractions, which were missed in the conventional urodynamic studies.

Treatment

The main treatment options available are behavioral modifications, drugs, electrical stimulation and surgery.

Explanation regarding the pathogenesis of the condition and reassurance about absence of serious problems like cancer may help to get the cooperation of the patient. Lifestyle changes like avoiding drinking too much tea, coffee or water may be all that will be required for some women.

Behavioral therapy: This aims to encourage the woman to go for voluntary bladder retraining (bladder drill). Best results are obtained when the patient is admitted to hospital. She is encouraged to gradually increase the interval between voiding and when she succeeds, it is acknowledged and encouraged. Very good results, up to 90% success, are reported even though high relapse rate, up to 40%, may occur on stopping the treatment.

Biofeedback, electric stimulation and acupuncture are other methods that may improve the situation.

Medical treatment: Since parasympathetic stimulation causes bladder contraction, inhibition of these contractions achieved with anticholinergic drugs is treatment for detrusor instability. Propantheline acts this way, but its side effects are unacceptably high. Oxybutinin is the currently used effective drug for detrusor instability, but its side effects on other organs (e.g. dry mouth due to effect on salivary glands) limits its widespread use. Daily intake up to 5 mg three times daily is recommended even though many may find a lower dose adequate. Tolterodine is a new antimuscarinic agent with more specific effect on the bladder and less effect on the salivary glands.

Tricyclic antidepressants like imipramine (50 to 150 mg at night) and amitryptiline (25 to 75 mg at night) may help particularly in nocturia

Surgical treatment: Surgery is usually reserved as the last resort. Since the basic problem is increased contractility of the detrusor, one technique or other for denervation forms the basis of surgical treatment. Transection and resuturing of the bladder, transvesical phenol injection of the bladder base, or deliberate prolonged cystodistension under spinal blockade, are some of the techniques available but not widely practised.

The clam augmentation cystoplasty is the most widely used surgical method for detrusor instability. In this, a segment of ileum with intact blood supply is attached to the bisected bladder thereby increasing its capacity and providing an inert segment on its wall. However, there are worries of future development of malignancy in the ileal segment so used.

Other Causes of Incontinence

The other causes of incontinence include retention with overflow, epispadias and miscellaneous causes.

Retention with Overflow

There are many gynecological causes for retention with overflow, but patients with even nongynecological causes may present to the gynecologist.

In situations where retention is anticipated, as in pelvic floor surgery, a prophylactic catheterization should be advised. Otherwise, unrecognized retention may lead to overstretching of the bladder wall. This can lead to chronic retention. If repeated catheterization is required to keep bladder empty, a suprapubic rather than transurethral catheter will be a better option. This helps to know when the patient has regained proper voiding without removal of the catheter.

It is also important to teach the patients clean intermittent self-catheterization (CISC) before surgery or after the retention has been diagnosed.

Epispadias

This is usually diagnosed in childhood, but occasionally may present for the first time in adult life. Reconstructive surgery will be required.

Miscellaneous Causes

Urethral diverticulum presents with incontinence, but the history is peculiar. Typically they complain of dribbling after voiding. Depending on the size of diverticulum, it may or may not be palpable. Treatment of this condition is surgical correction.

Urinary infection with frequency sometimes can be so severe as to present with incontinence. This occurs more commonly in the elderly.

Disorders of the bladder can restrict its ability to expand (e.g. tuberculosis or schistosomiasis) to such an extent that the patient may present with extreme frequency bordering on to incontinence. Treatment of the primary condition along with procedures to increase bladder volume (e.g. clam cystoplasty) is indicated.

Urinary Fistulae

Introduction

Urinary fistula resulting from obstructed labor was a major cause of suffering for women all over the world. After obstetric services improved, the picture totally changed in the industrialized nations. However, this scourge continues to cause suffering and social isolation for many women in the developing countries, especially in Africa. They are isolated from the mainstream of society, often as social outcasts. The magnitude of the problem is not clearly known as many of them live outside the reach of modern medical facilities.

Definition

A fistula is defined as an abnormal communication between two or more epithelial surfaces. It can be between two or more viscera or between one viscus and the exterior. On the urinary side, it can involve the ureter, bladder or urethra.

Etiology

The etiology of urinary fistula has changed over the last 150 years. For the developing world, the main etiological factor remains obstetrical injuries; whereas in the developed countries, injuries during obstetric or gynecological operations top the list. Other etiological factors include malignancies, radiation and infections.

In my own practice, the prevalence and types of fistulae have changed over the last 30 years. Earlier, it used to be predominantly obstructed labor leading to large vesicovaginal fistulae. At present, obstetric fistulae are seldom seen. The types of fistulae seen now are the result of accidental injuries to ureter, or bladder during hysterectomy and cesarean section. Cesarean section done late in labor or after a trial of forceps or ventouse is particularly liable to lead to injury to urinary tract.

Rarely, the fistulae, especially ureteric fistulae, could be congenital. The ureter could open into the vagina or even to the exterior.

Diagnosis

Diagnosis often is confirmed on clinical examination. Tiny fistulous communications, especially congenital ones, can pose a diagnostic challenge. If it is congenital in origin, an intravenous urogram may be needed.

Large fistulous openings on bladder wall can often be located with a metal catheter. Sometimes, excess amount of vaginal discharge or urine leaking from external urinary meatus can confuse the issue. Passage of transurethral catheter and instillation of methylene blue will help in locating the fistula.

Before repair is planned, the number and site of the fistulae and if it is at the bladder base, its proximity to the ureteric opening should be ascertained.

The fistula is usually described indicating the viscera between which it runs, e.g. vesicovaginal, uretero-vaginal, vesicocervical, etc.

Management

When there is reason to anticipate the development of a fistula, prophylactic measures can be taken. In cases of prolonged labor with impacted head, continuous bladder drainage for about 2 weeks may prevent stretching and sloughing of the bladder wall and development of a fistulous track. If injury to the bladder is identified, proper anatomical closure of the defect followed by continuous bladder drainage for about 10 days will help proper healing.

If an injury is missed during primary surgery and leakage of urine is noted within a day or two, immediate attempts should be made to take care of such injuries. Once a fistula is established, the general recommendation is to delay surgical correction for at least 10-12 weeks allowing time for the inflammation to settle.

The route of repair will depend upon the location of the fistula and the surgeon's personal preference. Gynecologists usually approach vesicovaginal fistula transvaginally, whereas the urologists usually repair them transabdominally.

For repair of vesicovaginal fistula, there are mainly two surgical techniques—saucerization and repair in layers.

Saucerization is possible only when the defect is relatively small. In this, the defect is closed in a single layer, after the edges are freshened. In layered closure, the bladder wall is separated from the vaginal wall and the edges are approximated in layers with water-tight closure. Proper mobilization to allow closure without tension is essential.

Where there is much scarring and devitalization, as occurs in radiation fistulae, interposition of healthy tissues to increase blood supply to the wound is advisable. Fat, muscle or omentum can be mobilized for this purpose. Meticulous postoperative care is essential for success of the repair. Continuous drainage of urine to keep the bladder empty should be ensured.

In cases of ureteric fistulae with scarring, implantation of proximal ureter to bladder (bladder neocystostomy) may be better than attempting to repair the defect.

FECAL INCONTINENCE

Definition

Fecal incontinence is defined as the involuntary loss of stool at any time of life after toilet training.

The above definition does not include incontinence of gas, which may be equally embarrassing and bothersome. Hence, some authorities recommend that the correct term should be anal or anorectal incontinence rather than fecal incontinence.

Anatomy of the Anorectum

The anal canal extends from the level of puborectalis sling to the anal verge. Its length is 2 to 6 cm. The internal anal sphincter, which is a continuation of the circular smooth muscle of the rectum, forms its wall. Outer to it is the external anal sphincter which has three components-subcutaneous, superficial and deep. Fibers of the puborectalis muscle interdigitate between the

external and the internal sphincters (Fig. 19.4).The rectum acts as a reservoir for feces and can distend to accommodate the stool. The anal canal joins the rectum at about 90 degrees as the junction between the two is pulled anteriorly by the puborectalis.

The hemorrhoidal (inferior rectal) branches of the pudendal nerve supply the external anal sphincter. The internal sphincter is supplied by the parasympathetic fibers from first, second, and third sacral nerve roots and sympathetic fibers from L5 carried via the hypogastric nerve.

Mechanism of Fecal Continence

The anal canal normally remains closed due to the tone of the internal and external anal sphincters. Further, the entry of fecal matter into anal canal is prevented by the acute angulation brought about by the contraction of the puborectalis. Fecal matter is emptied into the rectum by the sigmoid. Rectum acts as a reservoir and accommodates the stool without a rise in its intraluminal pressure.

When the contents increase in bulk, stretch reflexes on rectal wall get stimulated and by reflex the puborectalis relaxes allowing small amounts to escape into the proximal anal canal. This fecal matter is sampled by the very sensitive anal mucosa. If conditions are favorable for defecation, relaxation of the anal sphincter occurs and the rectal wall increases its contractions pushing the feces to the exterior. On the other hand, if conditions are not suitable for defecation the contents which escaped into the anal canal are pushed back into the rectum and the voluntary contractions of the sphincter will be maintained. The ability to discriminate between rectal contents and decide on defecation depends on an intact nerve supply and anal sensation.

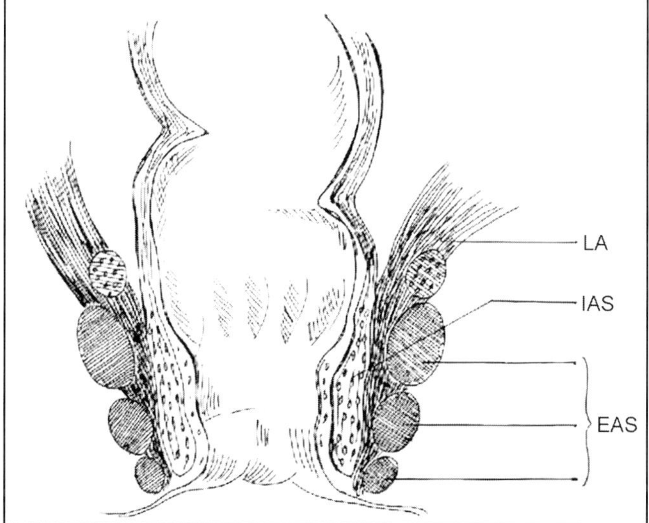

Figure 19.4: Arrangement of puborectalis in relation to external and internal anal sphincter. LA—Levator ani muscle, IAS—Internal anal sphincter, EAS—External anal sphincter

Causes of Fecal Incontinence

Fecal incontinence can result from very many different causes. Most cases presenting to a gynecologist are the consequence of injuries or diseases affecting the anorectum or vagina. A brief list of such conditions is given in Table 19.3.

Table 19.3: Causes of fecal incontinence

Etiology	Examples
Congenital malformations	Anorectal malformations e.g Vestibular anus
Obstetric injuries	Third or fourth degree lacerations Episiotomy breakdown Pudendal nerve injury during vaginal delivery
Injury during pelvic surgeries	Posterior colpoperineorrhaphy Hysterectomy, Colpotomy
Trauma	Impalement, Criminal abortions Coital injuries
Inflammatory conditions	Crohn's disease, Perirectal abscess Tuberculosis
Malignancies	Carcinoma of cervix Carcinoma of vagina Carcinoma of rectum

Of the many causes, the obstetric injuries to the posterior vaginal wall and anorectum is the most common. This can present as a complete perineal tear or as a rectovaginal or anovaginal fistula.

Prevalence of the Problem

The exact prevalence of fecal incontinence is difficult to assess due to various factors. These include the absence of a generally accepted definition, the reluctance of patients to give the information and the variations in the clinical presentations. A prevalence as high as 2.2% in the general population is reported. Sultan and colleagues[14] reported that 13% of women had fecal incontinence or urgency following their first vaginal delivery.

Diagnosis

A proper history and examination will reveal the diagnosis in many of the cases. A rectal examination will indicate the tone of the sphincters. Sometimes there may be tiny fistulous communications which may require examination under anesthesia, passing a probe or injection of dye to locate its openings and tract.

Anal endosonography has evolved as a big boon to diagnose the structural integrity of the sphincter. Nerve conduction studies like pudendal nerve terminal motor latencies (PNTMLs) help to diagnose the integrity of the nerve function.

Management

The main mode of treatment for anal incontinence is surgical. However, dietary manipulation to reduce flatus and liquid stools and pelvic floor exercises to strengthen the external sphincter may help in some cases. The surgical management depends on the defect present. The most common cause being complete perineal tear, its correction will be described in some detail.

Preoperatively, for about three days, the patient should be on liquid diet. The evening before surgery, give enema to clean the rectal contents. There are different surgical techniques to repair a complete perineal tear. The most popular is the layered method of repair. Make a transverse incision at the junction of the posterior vaginal wall and anterior rectal mucosa. The two layers are separated. A vertical midline incision on the posterior vaginal wall will help in dissection. The dissection is continued laterally to identify the retracted ends of the external anal sphincter.

The scar tissues on the margins of the rectal mucosa is excised and rectoanal mucosal edges are closed with 3 '0' delayed absorbable continuous sutures. A second layer approximating the muscular wall (internal sphincter) is taken with 2 '0' delayed absorbable material. The cut ends of the external anal sphincter are then sutured together on top of the previous layer using 2 '0' or 1 '0' delayed absorbable sutures. This layer of stitches may be extended cephalad to approximate the puborectalis muscles. The vaginal mucosa is then trimmed and closed with a continuous suture of 2 '0' or 3 '0' delayed absorbable material. The perineal body is then reconstituted and the skin is closed with subcuticular sutures.

Postoperatively, she is given liquid diet for 3 days and low-residue diet for a few days thereafter. Stool softeners are added from day 4 onwards.

Fecal Fistulae

Fecal fistulae most commonly occur between the rectum and vagina. It may be the result of incompletely healed complete perineal tear or due to the various causes mentioned in Table 19.3.

When the fistula is within 3 cm of the anal verge, it is called anovaginal fistula and the higher ones as rectovaginal.

The treatment of the fistula is almost always surgical. If it is big and the result of an incompletely healed third or fourth degree laceration, the bridge of tissue between the fistula and the anal verge may be cut converting it into a fourth degree perineal laceration. Repair procedure, described earlier for fourth degree tear, may then be followed.

Smaller fistulae may be closed transvaginally or transperineally. Gynecologists generally prefer the transvaginal approach. In this, the vaginal and rectal mucosa around the fistula are separated laterally by careful dissection. The anal mucosa is closed with one or two purse-string stitches using 3 '0'delayed absorbable material. The vaginal mucosa is then closed on top of the previous stitches.

In the transperineal approach, a transverse incision is made on the perineum. Dissection is carried forward anterior to the anal sphincter, and the vaginal and rectal mucosa are separated sufficiently from the margins of the fistula. The openings on both sides are then closed separately, and muscle tissue interposed. The perineal body is then reconstituted and the perineal skin is closed.

If the fistulous communication is very large and surrounding tissues unhealthy, as can happen in fistulae following malignancy or radiation, it is better to divert fecal matter using colostomy. Other principles followed in large urinary fistulae like use of pedicle graft to increase blood supply to the repair site may be employed.

CONCLUSION

Urinary and fecal incontinence are distressing conditions for the patient and the caregivers. A careful evaluation and correct diagnosis are essential pre-requisites for offering the best possible treatment. Fortunately, recent advances in diagnostic procedures and newer approaches to treatment have brightened the prospects for a cure or at least symptomatic relief for the victims of incontinence.

REFERENCES

1. Stanton SL. Classification of urogynecological disorders. In Shaw RW, Soutter WP and Stanton SL (Eds): Gynecology, 2nd edn, Edinburgh: Churchill Livingstone, 1997;693-96.
2. Bump RC, Norton PA. Epidemiology and natural history of pelvic floor dysfunction. Obstetrics and Gynecology Clinics of North America 1998;25: 723-46.
3. Pereyra AJ. A simplified surgical procedure for the correction of stress incontinence in women. Western Journal of Surgery 1959;67: 223-56.
4. Stamey TA. Endoscopic suspension of vesical neck for urinary incontinence in females. Annals of Surgery 1980; 192: 465-71.
5. Raz S. Modified bladder neck suspension for female stress incontinence. Urology 1981;17: 82-85.
6. Gittes RF, Loughlin KR. No-incision pubovaginal suspension for stress incontinence. Journal of Urology 1987; 138:568-70.
7. O'Sullivan DC, Chilton CP, Munson KW. Should Stamey colposuspension be our primary surgery for stress incontinence? British Journal of Urology 1995;75: 457-60.
8. Aldridge AH. Transplantation of fascia for relief of urinary incontinence. American Journal of Obstetrics and Gynecology 1942;44: 398-411.
9. Ulmsten U, Johnson P, Rezapour M. A three year follow up of TVT for surgical treatment of female stress incontinence. British Journal of Obstetrics and Gynecology 1999;106: 345-50.
10. Marshall VF, Marchetti AA, Krantz KE. The correction of stress incontinence by simple vesicourethral suspension. Surgery Gynecology and Obstetrics 1949;88:509-18.
11. Burch JC. Urethrovaginal fixation to Cooper's ligament for correction of stress incontinence, cystocele and prolapse. American Journal of Obstetrics and Gynecology 1961;81: 281-90.
12. Smith RN, Cardozo LD. Early voiding difficulties after colposuspension. British Journal of Urology 1997;160: 911-14.
13. Herbertson G, Iosif CS. Surgical results and urodynamic studies 10 years after retropubic colpocysto urethropexy. Acta Obstetricia et Gynecologica Scandinavica 1993;72: 298-301.
14. Lose G, Kulseng-Hanssen S, Nilsson CG. Aspects of the actual practice of surgical management of urinary incontinence in Norway and Finland. Acta Obstetricia et Gynecologica Scandinavica 1998; Supplement 168(77): 25-28.
15. Sultan AH, Kamm MA, Hudson CH, Tomas JM, Bartram CI. Anal sphincter disruption during vaginal delivery. New England Journal of Medicine 1993;329: 1905-11.

20. Breast and the Gynecologist

Behram S Anklesaria
Meenu S Handa

INTRODUCTION

The breast is a dynamic organ throughout a woman's life. As a primary health care provider for women, a gynecologist should thoroughly understand the preventive aspects and management of all common female breast problems.

Until the advent of modern specialization in the field of breast surgery, all aspects of breast pathology were dealt with by gynecologists. All her life she has confided her reproductive health problems to her gynecologist including her breast problems.

Being the most common cancer in women, across all socioeconomic strata, there is a quest for breast cancer prevention and early diagnosis. The gynecologist, or any primary health care provider, should be responsible for breast assessment and detection of breast cancer.

MASTALGIA

Mastalgia is the most common breast complaint in women and is often a concern for the patient because of the fear of cancer. In a study conducted in the US.[1] Sixty-nine percent of women reported regular premenstrual discomfort and 36% consulted health care providers about the symptoms. Mastalgia was moderate to severe in 11%. In patients with breast related primary complaint, pain was the most commonly reported symptom in every age group over 34 years. Breast pain is either cyclic or noncyclic. Cyclic mastalgia is more common. About 50-80% of women experience pain and swelling in breasts before menstruation.[2] Cyclic breast pain peaks premenstrually, lasts for a mean period of 5 days and resolves with the onset of menses. The pain is usually moderate to severe in intensity may be unilateral or bilateral. It is common in women receiving cyclic estrogen. In most of women there is spontaneous cessation of pain or in some, cessation of pain is associated with hormonal changes, e.g. pregnancy or menopause (Table 20.1).

Noncyclic breast pain has three subtypes:

1. *Idiopathic*: This breast pain may be intermittent, continuous or irregular, bilateral or unilateral. It could be sharp, burning or stabbing in nature and subsides spontaneously.
2. *Breast pain along with benign breast lesions* (e.g. macrocysts, duct ectasia, fibroadenoma) is caused by tension on other breast structures.
3. *Referred pain*: This pain arises from musculoskeletal structures of chest, e.g. costochondritis, pectoral muscle spasm.

Table 20.1: Mastalgia classification

Feature	Cyclic	Noncyclic
Age of presentation	30s	40s
Site	Bilateral	Unilateral
Localization	Diffuse	Well localized
Type of pain	Dull, aching	Sharp, stabbing
Association with menopause	Rare	12%
Efficacy of hormonal treatment	80%	40%

Causes

Two major theories about causes of mastalgia:

1. *Role of diet*: Intake of methylxanthine causes breast pain. However, several randomized clinical trials of dietary caffeine reduction have shown minimal changes in pain.
2. *Role of hormones*: It seems logical that breast pain in phase with the menstrual cycle has a hormonal origin. The pain usually is relieved by a disruption of the hormonal milieu including drugs, menopause and surgery. Yet, a few consistent abnormalities have been identified. Circulating hormone levels are normal in cyclic mastalgia patients. With normal levels of circulating hormones, attention has been turned towards theory of altered receptors sensitivity. The histopathological findings of patients with mastalgia do not appear significantly different from that of controls.

Treatment

Treatment consists of symptomatic measures:

1. Support brassieres
2. Local application of heat or cold

Dietary recommendation includes elimination of methylxanthenes and taking vitamins E, A, and B complex which have a placebo effect. Decreasing fat intake also may prove beneficial to improve breast swelling, tenderness and nodularity.

Drug Therapy

Danazol: 200 mg/day produced an improvement in 70% of cases of cyclical and 30% of cases of noncyclical mastalgia.

Bromocriptine: Less effective than danazol but may decrease mastalgia. Most effective for cyclical mastalgia.

Dose should be 1.25 mg nightly for one week and then 2.5 mg nightly for 2 months.

Evening Primrose Oil: It is used as an initial attempt to control cyclic breast pain because of its low incidence of side effects. It may be most useful in younger women who need long-term treatment as well as those who wish to avoid hormonal manipulation.

Tamoxifen in dose of 20 mg/day improves 70% cases but is not licensed for this indication.

The response to treatment is assessed by Cardiff breast score (Table 20.2).

Table 20.2: The Cardiff Breast Score (CBS) for response to treatment of patients with mastalgia

Score	Definition
CBS I	Excellent response leaving no residual pain
CBS II	Leaving some residual pain but bearable
CBS III	Poor response leaving substantial residual pain
CBS IV	No response

NIPPLE DISCHARGE

The secretion of fluid from the nipple of a newborn baby or any mature woman is not unusual nor is it a sign of underlying breast disease. Nipple discharge is more commonly associated with benign rather than malignant lesions.[3] A bilateral nipple discharge usually has a systemic cause, rather than a local one, however, a unilateral nipple discharge may be due to individual breast responsiveness to systemic causes.

There are seven types of nipple discharge:

1. Milky
2. Multicolored and sticky
3. Purulent
4. Clear or watery
5. Yellow or serous
6. Pink or serosanguineous
7. Bloody or sanguineous

The first three types are usually managed by medical treatment. Although the cause of the last four types is usually of a benign nature, they can be due to cancer or precancerous conditions and, therefore, require surgery to obtain tissue for histological examination.

Discharge can also be classified as:

1. *Physiologic discharge*: It is serous, unilateral or bilateral and comes from multiple ducts. This discharge occurs from two neurogenic reflexes from the breast, one to the anterior pituitary that inhibits dopamine and stimulates prolactin and one to the postpituitary that stimulates oxytocin.

2. *Pathologic discharge*: It occurs in benign lesions such as intraductal papilloma and duct ectasia as well as carcinoma Nipple discharge that is nonlactational, spontaneous, unilateral, serous or bloody and single duct in origin is more likely to have pathologic significance. The incidence of malignancy in patients with nipple discharge increases with age and with presence of breast mass.

A bilateral, spontaneous, multiple duct, milky type of discharge that is usually seen in patients of child-bearing age is referred to as galactorrhea (Table 20.3). It is due to increased production of prolactin. The condition is most commonly observed after pregnancy and can last for one to two years or longer. The patient should be tested by obtaining a serum prolactin. A thin layer chromatography test for lactose also should be performed to verify that the discharge is actually milk. The treatment of a pathologic nipple discharge is surgical excision of the involved duct. Preoperatively, mammography ductogram, in which contrast medium is injected into the cannulated duct, will identify the affected duct.

BREAST LUMPS

Dominant lumps are clinically benign breast lesions that are persistent. Their diagnosis is important to distinguish them from carcinomas. The commonest benign lumps are macrocysts, galactoceles and fibroadenoma. They can be diagnosed by fine-needle aspiration, but definitive diagnosis requires histological proof of the nature of tumor.[4]

Macrocysts

They are the commonest lump, manifested between 35 and 50 years. Usually, these cysts disappear after menopause. Clinically, these cysts can be silent or painful and may cause palpable lumps or be seen on ultrasonography. Aspiration is both diagnostic and therapeutic. A few patients will develop multiple cysts that can cause anxiety and discomfort. These cysts can be usually managed by periodic aspirations and menopause brings relief.

Galactocele

This cyst is formed by overdistension of lactiferous duct. It is simply milk-filled cyst. It presents as a firm non-tender mass in the breast. Diagnostic aspiration is often curative.

Fibroadenoma

Those are most common benign solid tumors of female breast and represent most common tumor in women younger than 25 years. These are hormone responsive tumors and may increase in size toward the end of each menstrual cycle. Clinically, these are painless, well-circumscribed freely movable tumors also known as breast-mouse. These tumors do not regress spontaneously so simple gross excision is the treatment of choice.

BREAST CANCER

Investments in basic science and breast cancer research reveal numerous opportunities for our ability to prevent and treat breast cancer. The incidence of breast cancer is on the increase.

Table 20.3: Breast discharge

	Color	Age of presentation	Type of presentation	Special features
Galactorrhea	Milky	Childbearing	Bilateral, multiple ducts	Fat globules
Benign breast diseases	Any (green, yellow, brown)	40-60 yr	Unilateral, few ducts	Leukocyte suggest infection
Malignancy	Any	> 50 yr	Unilateral, few ducts	Heme positive

Risk Factors (Table 20.4)

The most remarkable risk factors are increased age, family history in a first degree relative and geographical location of birthplace.[5] First pregnancy and delivery at an earlier age appear to decrease breast cancer risk. Nulliparity, early age at menarche, older age at menopause increase the risk of breast cancer. Oophorectomy at an early age is considered protective, reducing the risk of cancer by 70%. The fact that the total duration of ovarian activity is related to the risk of breast cancer implicates natural ovarian hormones in the initiation or further progress of the disease. The risk increases in women taking oral contraceptives for 5 years or more. Mutations in gene BRCA-1 (located on chromosone 17 having tumor suppressor capabilities) produce susceptibility to both breast and ovarian cancer.

Table 20.4: Risk factors for breast cancer

- Age
- For any group of 9 women, one will develop breast cancer at some time during their life and 8 will not
- In 30's: Risk 1/250
- In 40's: Risk 1/77
- Never gets to be over 1/34 in any decade
- Prior history of breast cancer
- Nulliparity
- Age of completion of first pregnancy > 30 years
- Oral contraceptive pills for more than 5 years
- Early menarche or late menopause
- Ionizing radiation during menopausal years.
- Ovarian or endometrial cancer
- Carcinoma present clinically as ill-defined, firm mass without pain or cyclic variation
- History of benign proliferative lesion

It is associated with inflammation or dimpling of skin and palpable axillary lymph nodes.

It is staged initially on a clinical basis which includes physical examination, radiological evaluation and laboratory workout.

It includes physical examination, a complete blood count, mammography liver function tests and chest radiograph.

The staging system used is the TNM classification. This system more accurately assess prognosis which is related to extent of axillary disease.

Treatment consists of total mastectomy or breast conserving therapy.

Breast conserving treatment is recommended as the preferred treatment for stage I and II invasive breast cancer. This includes lumpectomy, axillary node dissection and postoperative radiation therapy. Modified radial mastectomy involves removing the breast totally, dissecting the axilla and preserving both pectoral muscles. The patients with large tumors and another associated unfavorable prognostic factors should be given adjuvant chemotherapy.

The most common regimes are:

1. Cyclophosphamide, methotrexate and 5-fluorouracil (CMP)
2. 5-fluorouracil, adriamycin and cyclophosphamide (FAC)

Pregnancy and Breast Lumps

Two percent of breast carcinomas are diagnosed during pregnancy, but pregnancy does not change the outcome of cancer (Fig. 20.1). It has, however, been shown to delay diagnosis. Any breast lesion should be evaluated as it would be in the nonpregnant patient to prevent diagnostic delay and early management. Screening mammography can be postponed to limit fetal exposure. If cancer is suspected, however, shielding will protect the fetus and diagnostic mammography can be performed (Table 20.5).

If breast cancer is diagnosed, treatment options depend on the period of gestation. In general, management remains same as for the nonpregnant women during the first and second trimesters, mastectomy and axillary node dissection may be done. Radiation is contraindicated because of fetal risks. If diagnosed in third trimester, the patient may elect to be observed until delivery when prompt treatment is initiated. Most tumors recur within 2 years of treatment, so patients are advised to avoid pregnancy during this time.

American Cancer Society Guidelines for Preventive Breast Care

- Breast self-examination:
  Monthly for women > 20 yr of age.
- Clinical breast examination:
  Every 3 years for women 20-40 years of age. Every year for women over 40 years of age.

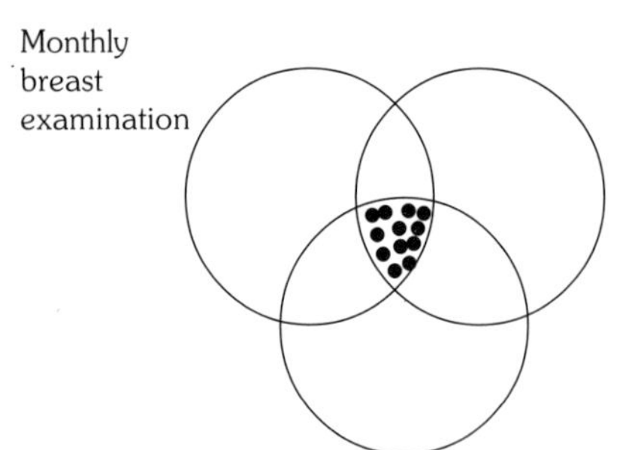

Figure 20.1: The diagnostic triad

Dotted area represents the co-relation of the three diagnostic modalities In cases of suspicion, these three modalities together help to diagnose the breast cancer in patients

Table 20.5: Diagnosis of breast lumps

Method	Positive aspects	Negative aspects
Clinical examination	Easy to perform	Low sensitivity in women aged < 50
Mammography	Useful for screening women aged > 50	Requires dedicated equipment and experienced personnel Low sensitivity in women aged < 50 Unpleasant (discomfort)
Ultrasonography	Same sensitivity in all ages Useful in assessing impalpable lesions Painless	Operator dependent Less sensitive & less specific than mammography
Fine-needle Aspiration cytology	Cheap High sensitivity Provides definitive diagnosis in most instances Low incidence of false positives	Operator dependent Needs experienced Cytopathologist Painful

- Screening mammography:
  Baseline between 35-40 years
  Every 1-2 years for women 40-49 years of age.
  Every year for women 50 years of age or older.

Role of Obstetrician and Gynecologist

The Obstetrician-Gynecologist should know about breast diseases both benign and malignant. When a breast disorder is diagnosed requiring patient's referral, the following must be done:

- Explain the patient about the disease.
- Explain that she needs further care.

- Provide her the names of qualified oncologist from whom she can receive care. Women with breast cancer require multidisciplinary team effort. The gynecologist must be an informant in their care.

Hormone Replacement Therapy and the Breast

The traditional belief that HRT is an absolute contra-indication in breast cancer survivors is now challanged and has led to a reassessment of its role in breast cancer etiology (Table 20.6). Postmenopausal HRT acts on women who otherwise would be subject to little if any endogenous hormonal stimulation. As the late natural menopause increases the risk of breast cancer, there is concern about the use of HRT in women. But the reason for its use is the decreased sensitivity of mammary tissue to hormones with age. The body weight affects the relationship between HRT and breast cancer risk. The risk of having breast cancer increases with increasing duration of its use. The effect disappears about 5 years after stopping HRT use. Family history of breast cancer is of significance in concern about the safety of HRT.[6] Combined HRT with progesterone carries more risk than unopposed (estrogen only) HRT. Whether HRT is to be given after breast cancer is controversial. Some studies say that HRT is contraindicated for a woman who has had breast cancer as estrogen may stimulate proliferation of residual cancer cells. Others suggested that some women may be troubled by symptoms of estrogen withdrawal. So the decision whether to start HRT or not should be individualized.

Table 20.6: HRT and breast cancer

- Risk is higher in HRT users with a family history of breast cancer.
- The route of HRT does not affect the risk in any way.
- Adding a progestogen does not reduce the risk; on the contrary, may cause interference with mammographic evaluation due to diffuse hyperplasia of fibroglandular tissue.

Tissue Specific HRT Agents

Hormone replacement with estrogens has many beneficial effects in the body, but has some disadvantages, since it affects all estrogen sensitive tissues, e.g. estrogens stimulate receptors in a breast tissue which can induce breast tenderness. More over, long-term use is potentially associated with a slight, albeit, small, increased risk of breast cancer. That is why, various tissue specific agents are developed (Table 20.7) so that long-term HRT can be safely given.

Table 20.7: Types of tissue specificity[7]

Biochemical	Receptor based	Phytestrogens e.g. Tibolone
	Selective estrogen receptor modulators (e.g. SERMS - Raloxifene)	

Phytestrogens: These are naturally occurring plant sterols which have an action similar to estrogen. Diet rich in soy foods that has phytestrogens increases LH levels and reduces estrogen levels through various mechanisms. They modify the hormone production and hormone metabolism thus limiting the cancer growth. Phytestrogens relieve postmenopausal symptoms without stimulating breast tissue. These are known to inhibit the growth of breast cancer cell lines.

Raloxifene: This new agent is a SERM. It reduces breast pain significantly as compared to HRT. It has antiestrogenic action in breast tissue and reduces the incidence of invasive breast cancer by 76% and estrogen receptor positive tumors by 90%. However, raloxifene is not approved for this indication in the United States.

Tibolone: Tibolone has important effects on the breast that are different from those of estrogens. Unlike conventional HRT, women using Tibolone rarely complain of breast tenderness. Preclinical studies show no evidence of carcinogenicity of Tibolone. Tibolone and its metabolites are potent inhibitors of the stimulation of breast tumors.[8]

BENEFITS OF LACTATION

From embryo to puberty, the breasts of the human male and female are the same, both histologically and functionally. The increase of estrogen and progesterone beginning at puberty is responsible for ductal growth and lobuloalveolar development. Changes during pregnancy, both hormonal and structural, prepare the breast for lactation.

A contraceptive effect accompanies lactation. This effect is temporary and is less reliable. The effectiveness of lactation as a contraceptive depends on the level of nutrition of the mother, the intensity of suckling and the extent to which supplemental food is added to the infant diet (Table 20.8). Women who wish to breastfeed but avoid pregnancy should use a mechanical method of contraception beginning 4-5 weeks postpartum.

When breastfeeding is used exclusively and menstrual bleeding has not occurred, ovulation does not occur before the end of the 10th postpartum week.

Table 20.8: Mechanism of amenorrhea and anovulation in lactating mothers

Repeated suckling stimulus of breastfeeding increases prolactin concentration	
FSH concentration in normal range	LH values below normal
Ovaries show less follicular growth	No LH surge
Hypoestrogenic state	Anovulation
Amenorrhea	

Enhancement/Suppression of Lactation

To improve adequate milk yield, the following steps should be taken:

1. To guide the mother about nursing the baby, mention the advantages of breastfeeding.
2. Nipple care and preparation include advising the patient how to express out the colostrum and to take care of the crust formed on the nipples.
3. Advice the mother to feed the baby every 4-6 hours.
4. To prevent engorgement, manual expression should be taught.

Suppression of Lactation

This is required when the baby is born dead or dies in infancy or in conditions where nursing is contraindicated like women with cytomegalovirus, chronic hepatitis B and human immunodeficiency virus infection. The hormones suppress lactation only if started soon after delivery. These suppress lactation through inhibition of pituitary hormone. Drugs include:

- Combination of testosterone and estrogen (Mixogen) 2 ampoules intramuscularly.
- Pyridoxine 100 mg 2 tabs three times a day for 2 days and then 1 tab three times a day for 3 days.

- Tight compression bandage of breast for 3-4 days.
- Analgesics to relieve pain
- Application of cold packs.
- Bromocriptine, a dopamine agonist stimulates the production of prolactin inhibitory factor which in turn causes a fall in plasma prolactin and the suppression of lactation.
- Carbogoline

Breast Problems during Lactation

Breast Engorgement

This develops after 2-3 days of starting lactation. The breasts become distended, firm and nodular. This condition is also known as caked breasts. It produces considerable pain and may be accompanied by a transient elevation of temperature. Puerperal fever from breast engorgement is common. It ranges from 37.8 to 39°C. The incidence and severity of fever associated with it were lower if treatment was given for lactation suppression. Treatment consists of supporting the breasts with a binder applying an ice bag and an analgesic. Manual expression of milk may be required.

Mastitis

It is occasionally observed during the puerperium and lactation. Suppurative mastitis usually develops before the end of the first week postpartum. It is invariably unilateral and engorgement of breast precedes the inflammation, the first sign of which is chills followed by fever and tachycardia. Most commonly offending organism is *Staphylococcus aureus*, others are group B *Streptococcus* and *Streptococci viridans*. Source of organisms is usually infant's nose and throat. Staphylococcal infections are caused by organisms sensitive to pencillin or cephalosporins. Erythromycin is recommended to penicillin sensitive women.

Abscess

Abscess development is due to failure of early treatment of mastitis and it develops within 48 to 72 hr of a palpable mass.

Surgical drainage under general anesthesia is required. The incision should be made corresponding to skin lines for good cosmetic results.

Galactocele

It is produced by clogging of a duct by milk secretion, milk may accumulate in one or more lobes of the breast. Excess accumulation may form a fluctuant mass that may give rise to pressure symptoms. Mostly, they resolve spontaneously or require aspiration.

Nipple Abnormalities

Retracted nipples: The lactiferous ducts open directly into a depression at the center of the areola. When the depression is superficial, milk can be expressed with use of a breast pump.

Cracked nipples: The fissures on the nipple almost invariably render nursing painful. Such lesions provide a convenient portal of entry for pyogenic bacteria. To promote healing and to protect them from further injury, a nipple shield and topical medication are used.

Abnormalities of secretion: There are individual variations in the amount of milk secreted, which are dependent upon the development of the glandular portions of the breasts. Very rarely, there is complete lack of mammary secretion (agalactia). Occasionally, the milk secretion is excessive (polygalactia).

SUMMARY

As a primary health care provider, a gynecologist plays a vital role in the preventive and management aspects of breast problems. The most common breast problems faced by a woman are mastalgia, nipple discharge and breast lumps. Patients with breast problems should be thoroughly investigated for underlying breast pathologies. As breast carcinomas constitute the second most common cancers in women, women above age of 35 years should undergo screening for breast cancer regularly as per guidelines. Tissue specific HRT agents like SERMS can be given safely to women without increased risk of breast cancer. Naturally occurring phytestrogens play a major role in prevention of breast cancer globally in the near future by dietary means.

REFERENCES

1. Ader DN, Browne MW. Prevalence and impact of cyclic mastalgia in a United States clinic-based sample. Am J Obstet Gynecol 1997;177:126-32.

2. Goodwin PJ, Miller A, Richie K. Breast health and associated premenstrual symptoms in women with severe cyclic mastopathy. Am J Obstet Gynecol 1997;176:998-1005.

3. Leis HP Jr. Management of nipple discharge. World J Surg 1989;13: 736.

4. Henderson IC. Risk factors for breast cancer development. Cancer 1993;71: 2127-40.

5. Colditz GA, Egan KM, Stampfer MJ. Hormone replacement therapy and risk of breast cancer: Results from epidemiologic studies. Am J Obstet Gynecol 1993;168: 1473-1480.

6. Leis HP Jr. Concepts regarding breast biopsies. Breast Disease An international Journal, 1991;4:223.

7. Anklesaria BS. The New Science of Tissue Specificity. FOGSI FOCUS, 2000; 5-6.

8. Anklesaria BS. The New Science of Tissue Specificity. FOGSI FOCUS, 2000; 7-8.

21.

AP Manjunath
Jayaraman Nambiar

Gynecological Operations

ABDOMINAL HYSTERECTOMY

Abdominal hysterectomy is a common operation performed in gynecology. Abdominal hysterectomy is performed three times more common than vaginal hysterectomy. Abdominal hysterectomy carries an increased morbidity compared with vaginal hysterectomy but has an advantage of adequate exposure especially in patients with malignancy and other intra-abdominal disease.

Types of Abdominal Hysterectomy

Subtotal Hysterectomy

Here the body of uterus is removed and the cervix is left behind. This is generally done in cases of emergency like postpartum hemorrhage and in cases where approach to lower part of uterus is difficult as in cases of adhesions.

Total Abdominal Hysterectomy

In total abdominal hysterectomy the uterus and cervix is removed. This is usually done in cases of benign uterine pathology when the patient's age is less than 40 years.

Total Abdominal Hysterectomy with Bilateral Salpingo-oophorectomy

Here the uterus and cervix is removed along with the adenexa. It is also known as pan abdominal hysterectomy. It is generally done for patients above the age of 50 years and in some centers above the age of 40 years.

Radical Hysterectomy (Wertheim's Hysterectomy)

This is a special surgery done in cases of cervical malignancy. Here the uterus, cervix, parametrium, adnexa and upper third of vagina are removed. The removal of ovaries is optional depending on the age of women. Grossly normal ovaries are generally preserved if the woman is less than 40 years of age.

The draining pelvic lymph nodes are also removed in addition to the removal of above structures for complete treatment of cervical cancer.

Indications for Abdominal Hysterectomy

Common indications for hysterectomy include fibroid uterus, dysfunctional uterine bleeding (DUB) and endometriosis. Other indications include pelvic inflammatory disease and malignancies of genital tract. Hysterectomy may also be performed for cases of severe intra-epithelial neoplasia (CIN III) of the cervix if the patient is not willing for ablative therapies. Hysterectomy may be performed as an emergency procedure to control atonic postpartum bleeding.

Preoperative Preparations for Hysterectomy

Prior to surgery a detailed history and physical examination should be undertaken. Apart from detailed gynecological history, careful urological and gastrointestinal history should be taken. These organs lie close to the uterus and previous surgery in thee systems may make gynecological operations difficult. Details regarding previous gynecological operations should be carefully asked as these procedures may make the surgery difficult. Thorough gynecological examination should be done. Apart from this assessment of cardiovascular system and other systems should be undertaken which may make anesthesia difficult. Investigations preoperatively include a full blood count, platelet count, fasting blood sugar, renal function tests, liver function tests, chest X-ray and ECG. Patients should be subjected to routine HIV and HBsAg screening. Adequate amount of blood should be arranged before surgery depending on the blood loss expected during the procedure.

Choice of Incision

Incisions for abdominal hysterectomy may be a sub-umbilical midline incision or a suprapubic transverse incision. A midline incision is used when there is a large uterus to be removed or there is malignancy. Transverse incisions do not provide adequate exposure and are generally reserved for benign uterine pathology and when the uterine size is not big. A transverse incision produces a more cosmetic and stronger scar.

Prophylactic-oophorectomy at the Time of Hysterectomy

Ovaries are generally left behind if they are grossly normal and if the patient is below 40 years. After the age of 40 ovaries are removed with the consent of the woman to prevent the occurrence of ovarian carcinoma at a later date.

Steps of Abdominal Hysterectomy

The operation begins with placement of clamps by the side of the uterus. This clamp apart from lifting the uterus, tubes and ovaries out of the pelvis also helps in dissection and homeostasis (Fig. 21.1). The round ligaments are clamped, cut and ligated (Fig. 21.2). The incision on the anterior leaf of broad ligament is now extended anteriorly to the midline of uterus. Next the bladder is separated from the lower uterine segment by sharp dissection (Fig. 21.3). If tubes and ovaries have to be conserved tubes and ovarian ligament are clamped, cut and ligated close to uterus after making a window in the posterior leaf of broad ligament (Fig. 21.4). If ovaries have to be removed, the infundibulo pelvic ligament is clamped cut and ligated. Next structure that is clamped is uterine vessels. One should

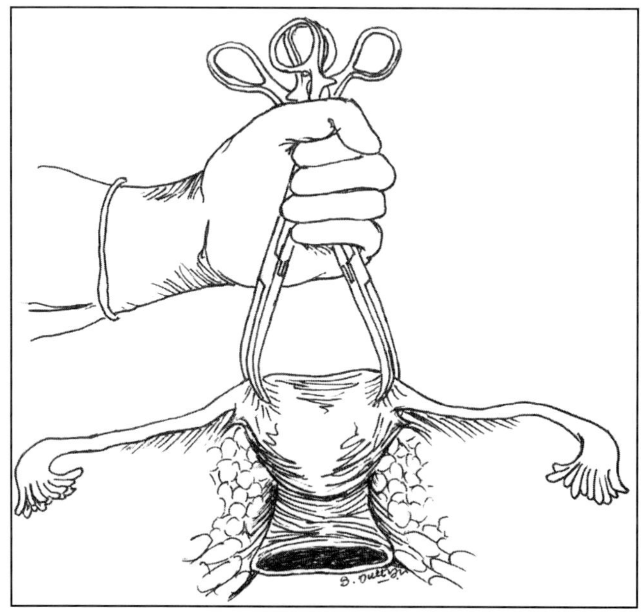

Figure 21.1: Clamps applied at the cornual structure

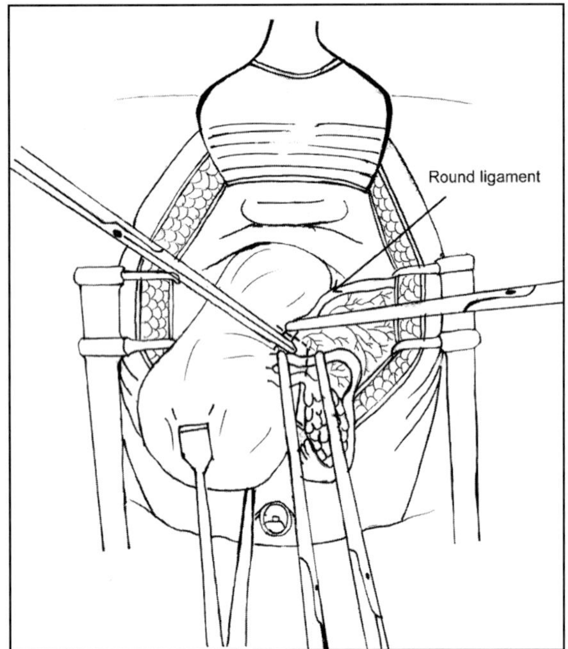

Figure 21.2: Round ligament clamping

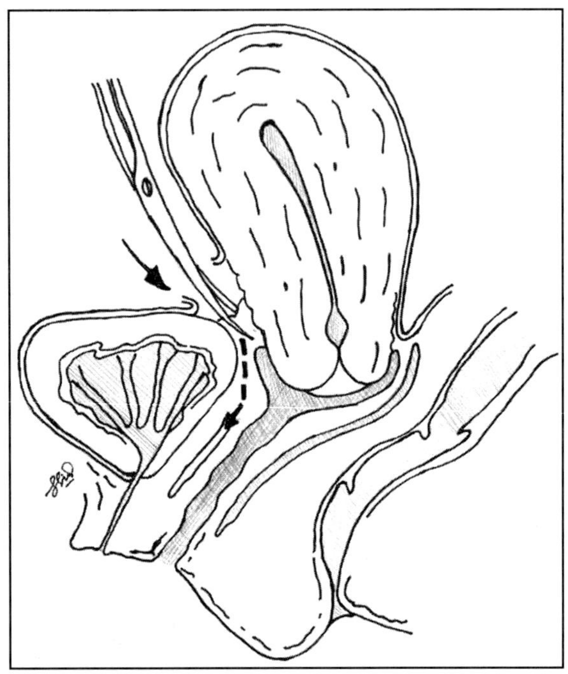

Figure 21.3: Bladder separated from lower uterine segment

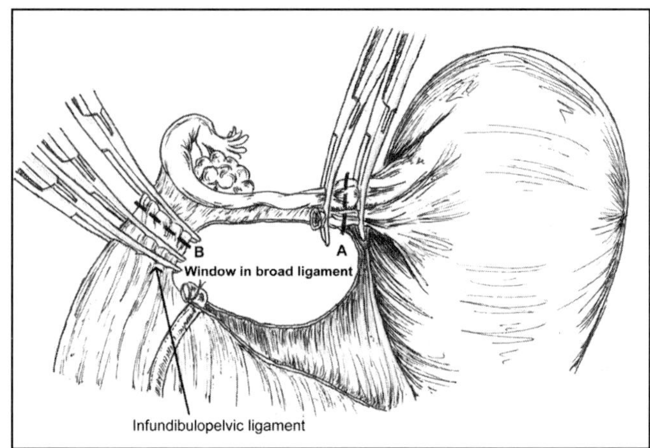

Figure 21.4: Window in broad ligament

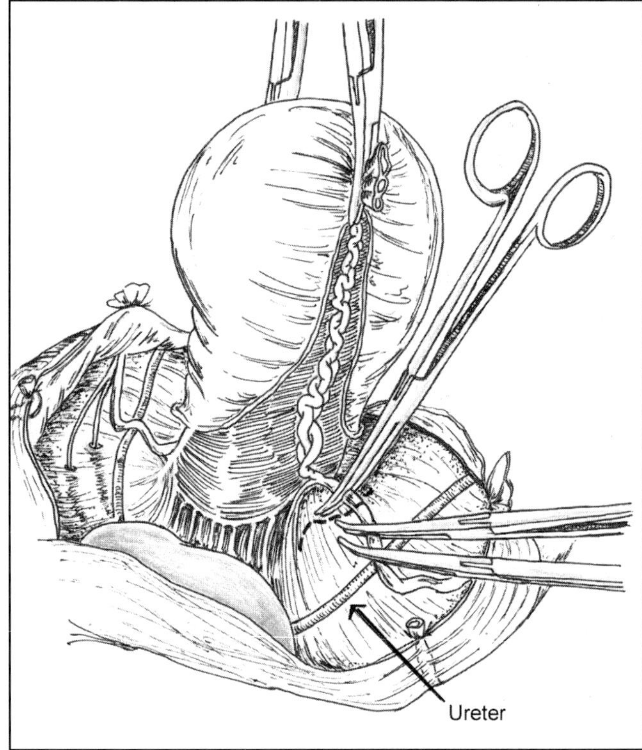

Figure 21.5: Clamping of uterine vessels

remember three cardinal rules in clamping uterine vessels.

1. The clamp is placed at the level of internal cervical os

2. It is placed at right angle to the lower uterine segment

3. The lowest clamp is placed initially

If these principles are followed the injury to the ureter is avoided. Ureters lie close to the cervix as they travel through the pelvis. One should carefully palpate and identify the ureter during its course through pelvis. By gentle upward uterine traction and downward

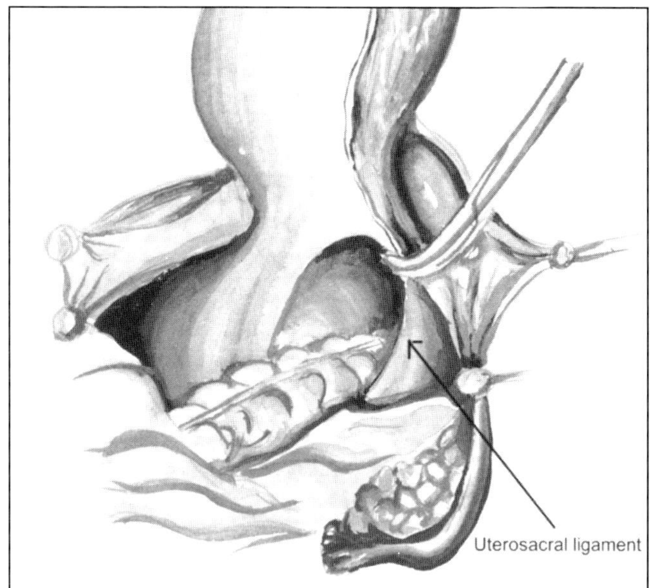

Figure 21.6: Clamping uterosacral and cardinal ligament complex

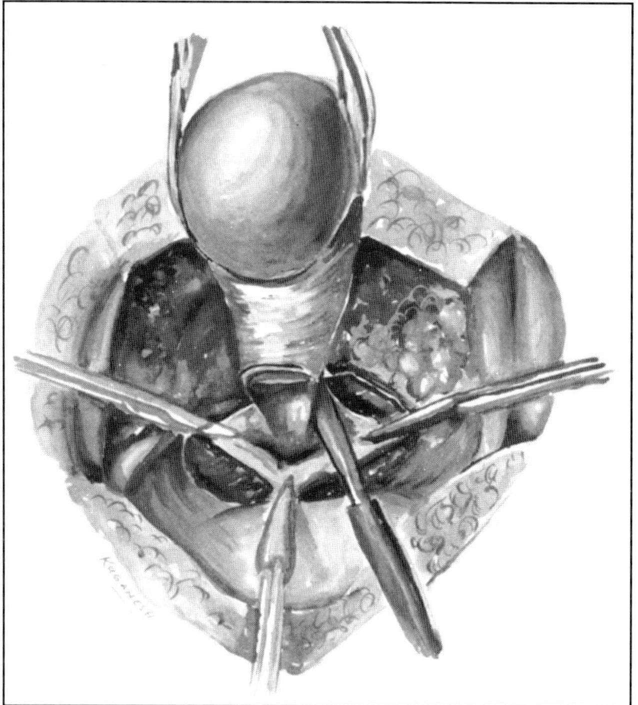

Figure 21.7: Uterus and cervix removed

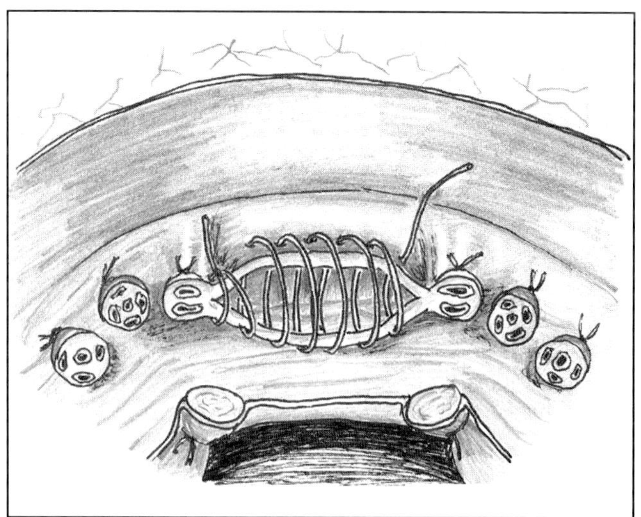

Figure 21.8: Closure of vaginal vault

mobilization of bladder, the ureters that usually lie 2 cm and lateral to the cervix are further displaced from the uterine vessels (Fig. 21.5). The uterosacral ligaments and cardinal ligaments are clamped cut and ligated (Fig. 21.6). Next the anterior vaginal fornix is opened and the incision is extended circumferentially close to the cervix to maintain the length of the vagina. Straight clamps are placed on lateral vaginal angles and the uterus and cervix are removed and angles sutured (Fig. 21.7). Vaginal angles are supported with uterosacral and cardinal ligaments to prevent vault prolapse in later life. Vaginal vault is closed with interrupted 0 chromic catgut sutures (Fig. 21.8). Prior to closing the abdomen all the stumps should be inspected for hemostasis.

Postoperative Care after Hysterectomy

Patient is kept in the postoperative ward closely to monitor vital signs and urine output in the postoperative period. Patient is kept nil by mouth for the first 24 hours after surgery. Intravenous fluids are administered in this period to maintain fluid and electrolyte balance. In case the operation has involved handling of the bowel, patient may be kept nil by mouth for a longer time till peristalsis returns. Postoperative pain relief is achieved with pethedine intramuscularly every 8 hourly. When the surgery has been done under epidural anesthesia the same may be continued for postoperative pain relief. Urinary retention is common after pelvic surgeries and continuous bladder drainage is usually kept for first 24 hours. If there has been bladder injury during the surgery a catheter should be kept for a longer time for about 14 days. Early ambulation is encouraged and patients are advised to move out of the bed after first 24 hours of surgery. Early ambulation prevents deep hastens recovery. Patient after hysterectomy can resume their household work in 3 to 4 weeks. However, heavy activities like lifting weight should be delayed for 6 weeks after hysterectomy. Coitus should be delayed for 6 weeks after hysterectomy. Patient is called for postoperative check up 6 week after hysterectomy to assess the healing and complete recovery.

Postoperative Complications

Hemorrhage

One of the most dangerous complications of hysterectomy is the bleeding that occurs in the immediate postoperative period usually with in the first 24 hours following hysterectomy. This is manifested in the postoperative period by hypotension, tachycardia and altered sensorium. This needs exploration and suturing of the bleeding points in the vault under anesthesia. If bleeding is intraperitoneal, it may need relaparotomy and suturing of bleeding points. Bleeding which occurs late after hysterectomy is called secondary hemorrhage. It usually occurs between 8 and 14 days following hysterectomy and is usually due to infection and separation of the slough at the vault. Bleeding is usually small in amount and it needs to be treated with systemic antibiotics. Suturing is generally not recommended for secondary bleeding as bleeding is generalized and not limited to a particular point. If bleeding is of concern, vaginal packing under anesthesia is recommended.

Postoperative Fever

Slight rise of temperature is very common following a hysterectomy with in the first 48 hour after hysterectomy. This is usually due to absorption of products of tissue damage and absorption blood in the pelvis. This usually subsides as blood and other tissue damage is absorbed. If the surgery was done under general anesthetic, pulmonary atelectasis can be the cause of the rise in temperature in the first 48 hours. More serious rise in temperature accompanied by systemic and localizing signs need investigation. Most common causes of temperature elevations include urinary tract infection, infection of abdominal wound or pelvic peritonitis, which needs to be treated.

Urinary Tract Injuries

Injuries to urinary tract occur in about 0.5%-1% cases of abdominal hysterectomy. Injuries to bladder occur when entering the abdominal cavity and when bladder is dissected from the lower uterine segment especially when there are adhesions between the bladder and lower uterine segment due to previous lower segment Cesarean section. Injuries to bladder should be repaired with 2-0 or 3-0 interrupted or continuous sutures. The first layer should include the bladder mucosa and second layer include the muscularis. The course of ureter is such that it is liable to get damaged during hysterectomy. Ureters are liable to get injured during situations where there is a large uterus, large pelvic mass and in cases of extensive adhesions as seen in pelvic inflammatory disease or endometriosis. In such cases where ureteric injury is expected a preoperative intravenous pyelogram (IVP) may be undertaken. One should be careful in applying haemostatic clamps blindly in the presence of bleeding. Ureteric injuries should be repaired with the help of an urologist.

Wound Dehiscence and Infection

Factors that can predispose to wound dehiscence and wound infection include improper haemostasis at the time of surgery, anemia, hypoproteinaemia, malignancy, obesity, poorly controlled diabetes mellitus, vitamin C deficiency and old age. If abdominal wall dehiscence occurs it needs immediate resuturing in a single layer with tension sutures. Superficial wound break down and infection is treated with daily cleaning, dressing and antibiotics. It may require resuturing of the wound.

Bowel Injuries

Injury to the bowel is uncommon during hysterectomy. It commonly occurs in patients with previous surgeries when there are adhesions. One should be very careful when opening the peritoneum and if possible the peritoneum should be opened away from the previous incision taking care to avoid the bowel. Intra-abdominal bowel adhesions if present should be carefully dissected with sharp dissection with the help of a general surgeon.

If bowel injuries are recognized during surgery it should be closed with 3-0 absorbable sutures in 2 layers. Larger lacerations on bowel need to be closed transversely to prevent narrowing of the bowel lumen.

Deep Venous Thrombosis

Postoperative venous thrombosis is more common in western races than in the Afro-Asian races. General incidence of postoperative venous thrombosis is said to be around 3-5%. Factors that can predispose to venous thrombosis include age more than 45 years, obesity, immobilization after surgery, dehydration, anemia, malignancy, injury to vein walls by pressure or hypoxia. There is a familial predisposition to deep vein thrombosis. Deep vein thrombosis generally occurs 7-14 days after the operation and symptoms include calf pain and stiffness in the legs, which is often dismissed by the patient as a muscle ache. Within 2-3 days after the pain the limb edema develops which begins in the foot and ankle and may involve the whole lower limb. Local signs include edema, pain and Homan's sign. Methods for prevention of deep vein thrombosis include correction of anemia, prevention of pressure on popliteal fossa and calf during surgery and use of pneumatic calf pumps during surgery. Patient should be encouraged early postoperative ambulation to prevent postoperative venous thrombosis. Patients who are confined to bed should avoid venous stasis in their legs by wearing elastic stockings. Prophylactic anticoagulants may be prescribed for patients who are at high risk for venous thrombosis. Usual recommended prophylactic dose of low molecular weight heparin (e.g. Fragmin) is 5000 IU subcutaneously on a daily basis postoperatively for five to seven days. Low molecular weight heparin, which can be used as a once daily dose with little need for monitoring, is becoming popular.

Remote Complications

Remote complications that can follow a hysterectomy include vault prolapse, incisional hernia and menopausal symptoms if ovaries have been removed at the time of hysterectomy. Vault prolapse can be prevented by giving proper attention to vault suspension at the time of hysterectomy and obliterating an enterocele with culdoplasty sutures. The symptoms of surgical menopause are more severe than a natural menopause.

Vaginal Operations

There are various operative interventions available for vaginal prolapse. These operations are aimed at the restoration of normal anatomy. Preoperative evaluation includes fitness for major surgery, any problem to control micturation or defecation, and the surgeon should be fully aware of the sexual activity of the patient and desire to preserve fertility. These evaluations will enable the surgeon to choose the particular operation and modify the techniques to suit the individual patient. Various operations are listed below:

1. Anterior colporrhaphy
2. Colpoperineorrhaphy
3. Manchester operation (Fothergill's operation)
4. Extended Manchester operation (Shirodkar's vaginal repair)
5. Vaginal hysterectomy with pelvic floor repair
6. Le Fort's operation
7. Shirodkar's sling operation
8. Abdominal cervicopexy (Purandare)

- *Anterior colporrhaphy or operations for cystocele*
  It is done in almost all cases of prolapse. It may be combined with other operative treatment of prolapse.
  Objectives
  1. To mobilize bladder
  2. To return bladder to normal anatomical position
  3. To prevent the recurrence of bladder decent
  Surgical technique has been explained under vaginal hysterectomy with pelvic floor repair.
- *Posterior colpoperineorrhaphy*
  Objectives
  1. Reduction of gaping of introitus
  2. Reconstruction of the perineal body
  3. Reinforcement of pelvic diaphragm by approximation of levator ani muscle
  4. Correction of rectocele
  Surgical technique has been explained under vaginal hysterectomy with pelvic floor repair

- *Manchester operation (Fothergill's operation)*
  Objectives:
  1. Amputation of vaginal portion of cervix
  2. Approximation of cardinal ligament in front of the cervical stump. This shortens the ligaments and elevates and displaces the cervix posteriorly. This backward displacement encourage anteversion and helps prevent prolapse of the uterus.
  3. This operation is always combined with anterior repair. Posterior repair is common but not obligatory
- *Extended Manchester operation (Shirodkar's vaginal repair)*
  Shirodkar modified the Manchester operation, where the cervix is not amputated. The uterosacral ligaments were dissected from posterolateral aspect of the uterus and brought forward and stitched in front of the uterus. Here pouch of Douglas is routinely opened to get the greater length of uterosacral ligaments and also to correct the enterocele if present. Because the cervix is not amputated, the pregnancy complications are minimized.
- *Vaginal hysterectomy with pelvic floor repair*
  This procedure is done on women who have completed their family, who also suffer from other pathologies like DUB, fibroids, cervical dysplasia or who have complete procedentia and in postmenopausal women. It must be emphasized that removal of uterus in itself does not cure prolapse. Uterus is not at fault. The main objective is to repair and reinforce the weakened tissues of pelvic floor. Hysterectomy is incidental as it is technically easier to do pelvic floor repair if uterus is removed and the ligaments are available to reinforce the repair.

Principles

There are three pedicles, which are clamped cut and ligated from below up wards:
1. The cardinal and uterosacral ligament complex
2. Uterine vessels
3. Tub ovarian and round ligament bundle

The two peritoneal pouches, the anterior uterovesical pouch and posterior cul de sac pouch need to be opened to facilitate the procedure.

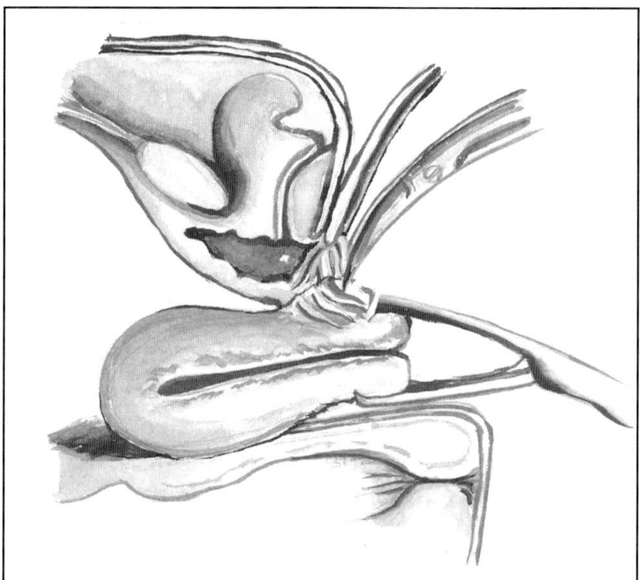

Figure 21.9: Bladder separation in vesicocervical plane

Surgical Technique

Vaginal Hysterectomy

With the patient in dorsolithotomy position appropriate preparation and draping of the surgical field is accomplished. Circular incision is made around cervix. Blunt and sharp dissection is carried out between ant cervix and posterior bladder wall (Vesico cervical plane) to separate bladder from the cervix (Fig. 21.9). Dissection is continued till anterior peritoneum (utero vesical) is reached and opened. Then posterior cervical fascia is dissected. Similar dissection is carried out separating posterior vaginal wall from cervix till pouch of Douglas is reached and opened (Fig. 21.10). Next step is to clamp cut and ligate the uterosacral cardinal ligament complex close to the cervix on both sides (Fig. 21.11). This stump of uterosacral cardinal ligament complex is held long with the stitches to carry out prophylactic cooptation to prevent future enterocele and vault prolapse.

Then uterine vessels are doubly clamped and doubly ligated (Fig. 21.12). Now the uterus is attached only with round ligament, ovarian ligament and infundibulopelvic ligament. The fundus of the uterus is eventrated and brought out side the introitus. Now clamps are applied close to the body of uterus to ligate cornual structures, i.e. round ligament, ovarian ligament, and fallopian tube (Fig. 21.13).

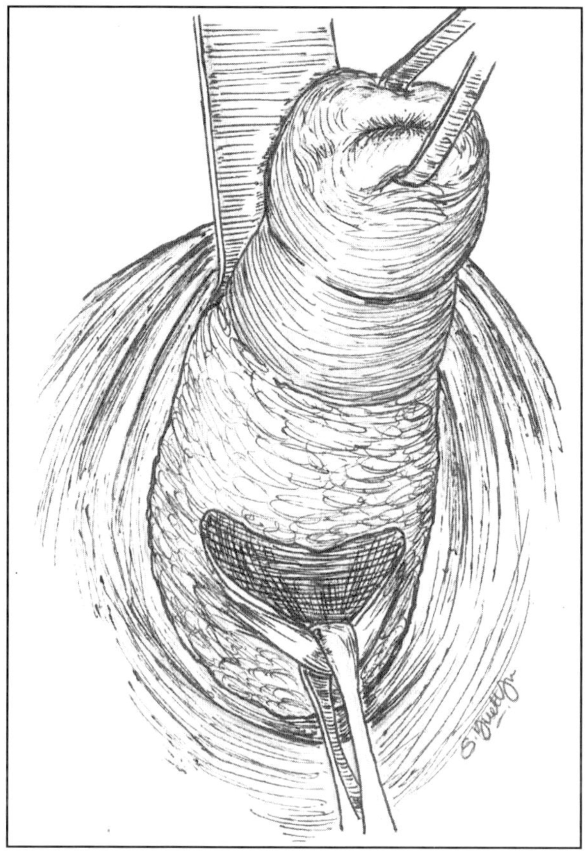

Figure 21.10: Pouch of Douglas is opened

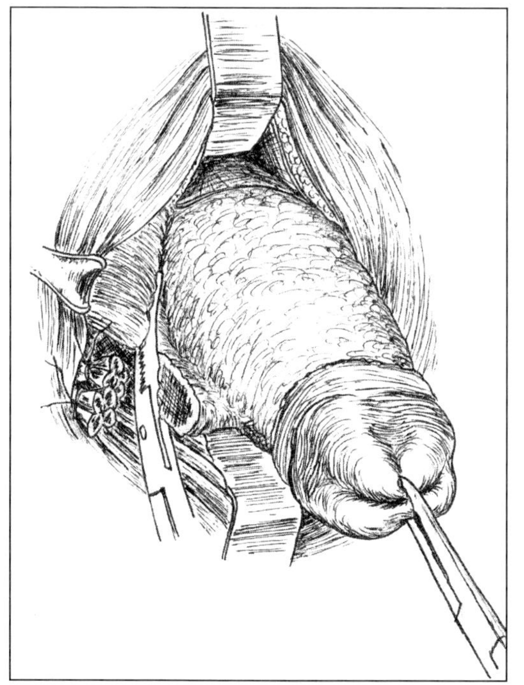

Figure 21.11: Clamping uterosacral cardinal ligament complex

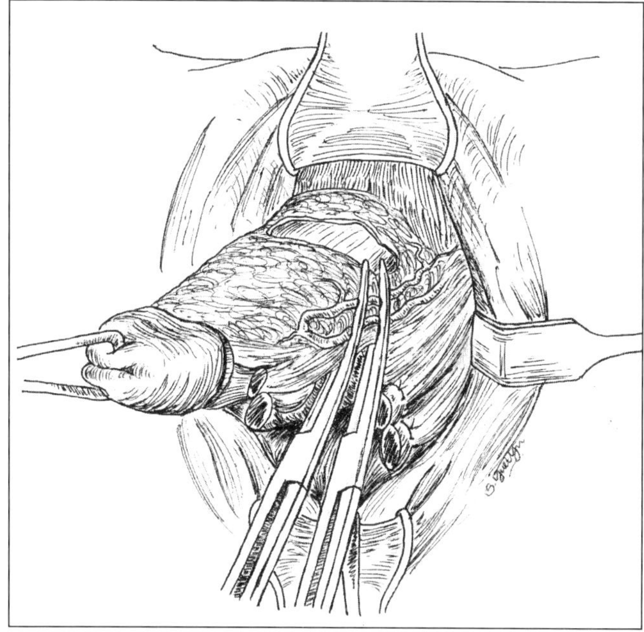

Figure 21.12: Uterine vessel ligation

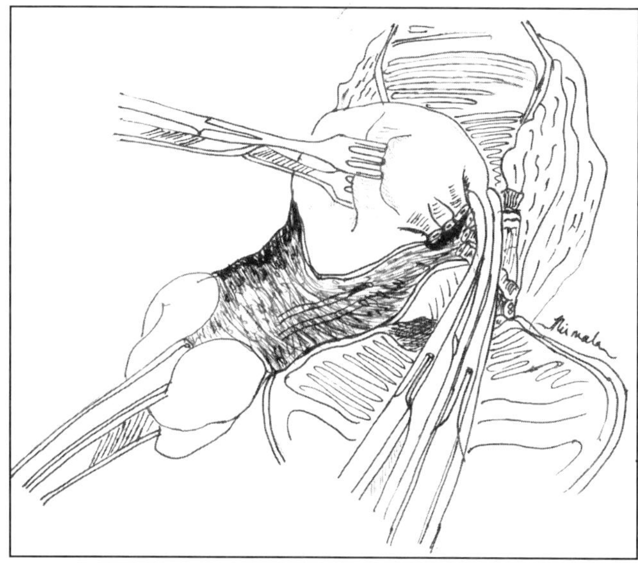

Figure 21.13: Clamping cornual structures

After completing, three pedicels (stumps) are observed on each side. Anteriorly cornual structures, in the middle uterine vessels and posteriorly cardinal uterosacral ligament complex. Complete hemostasis is achieved. All pedicles are extraperitonised by applying perstring stitches on the peritoneum (Fig. 21.14). If there is presence of enterocele it should he repaired after removal of uterus. The redundant peritoneum is excised and high peritonisation is done.

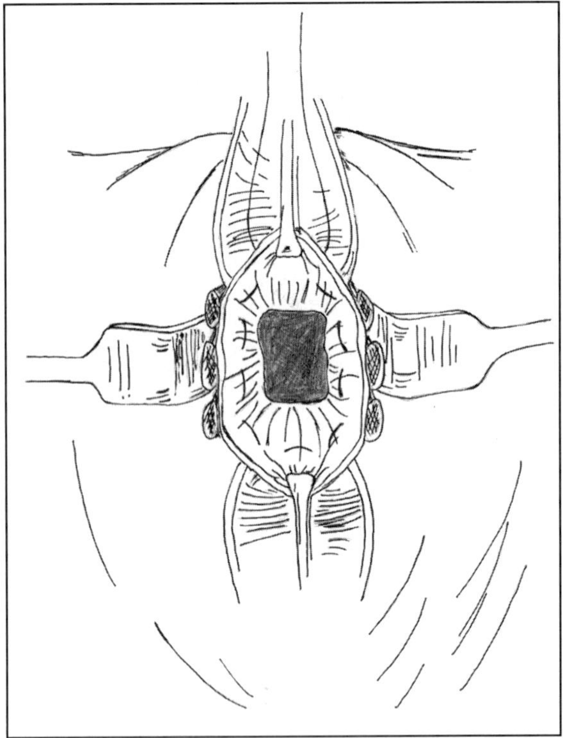

Figure 21.14: Three pedicles seen at vaginal vault

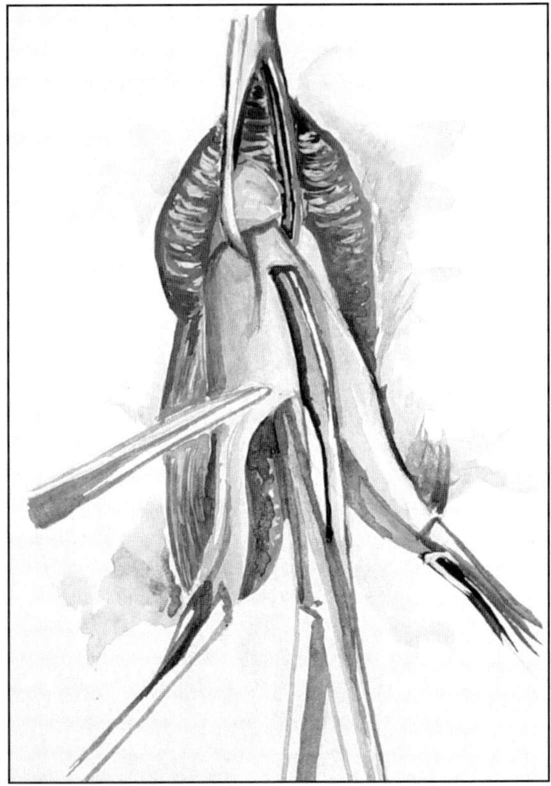

Figure 21.15: Cystocele repair

Anterior Repair/Anterior Colporrhaphy

Cystocele repair immediately follows vaginal hysterectomy. Two Allis forceps are applied to the lower edge of cystocele (free cut edge of vagina where ultimately the vaginal cuff will be closed) and one at the sub urethral sulcus (Fig. 21.15). Now bladder is separated from the vagina in the midline with blunt as well as sharp dissection, till the point corresponding to the urethrovesical junction is reached. Bladder is pushed gently upwards and medially with a gauze in the vesico vaginal plane bilaterally. Interrupted bladder buttressing stitches are applied with 2-0, absorbable material (Fig. 21.16). The bladder-buttressing stitches are tied so that the cystocele is reduced. Redundant vaginal skin is trimmed and then incision is closed with continuous 3-0 sutures. Plication of cardinal uterosacral ligament complex pedicle in to the vaginal wall is accomplished to prevent subsequent development of vault prolapse. The vaginal cuff is closed.

Posterior Repair/Posterior Colpoperineorrhaphy

Two Allis tissue forceps are placed at the lateral aspect

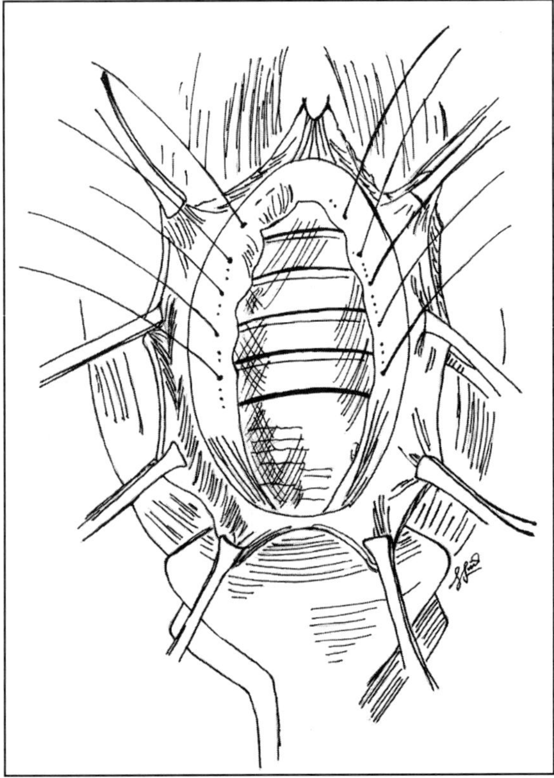

Figure 21.16: Bladder buttressing stitches

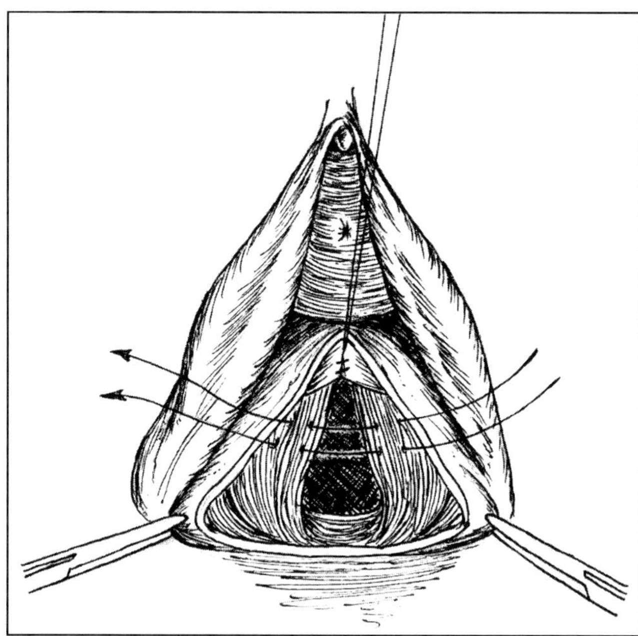

Figure 21.17: Levator ani plication

of mucocutaneous junction and one at the point above the rectocele. An incision along the mucocutaneous junction is made. Rectovaginal space is opened by sharp as well as blunt dissection. Full thickness of posterior vaginal wall is transected along the midline. The rectovaginal space is opened bilaterally by sharp and blunt dissection to expose the perirectal facial tissue. Care is taken to avoid inadvertent damage of the rectum. Lateral margin of the lower vaginal cut edge is separated shapely from the underlying levator ani (pubococcygeus) muscle bilaterally. The perirectal fascia is plicated in the mid line over the rectum throughout its entire length. Excessive posterior vaginal skin is excised. Levator ani is plicated in the midline with one or two interrupted stitches (Fig. 21.17). Posterior vaginal skin is closed with running suture. Perineal skin incision is closed.

Vaginal packing is done with roller gauze soaked with glycerin acriflavine. Foley's catheter is inserted for continuous bladder drainage for 24 to 48 hours.

Postoperative Care

The principles of postoperative care are
- Monitoring of vital signs:
  - Temperature, pulse, blood pressure and urine out put
  - Pulse and BP are measured every 15 minutes till the patient is stable. This is essential to recognize the reactionary hemorrhage.
- Fluid and electrolyte management
- Pain management
- Antibiotic prophylaxis
- Thromboembolism prophylaxis
- Physiotherapy-
  - Chest and leg exercises to prevent postoperative chest infections and thromboembolism respectively.
- Nutrition-
  - Patient is kept fasting till the bowel sounds are heard (approximately 12-24 hr) Then slowly starts with sips of clear fluid, soft diet and regular diet.
- Bladder care—catheter care and remove catheter after 24 to 48 hr later

Vaginal packing removed after 12 to 24 hours of surgery.

Complications

Hemorrhage is a very important complication of vaginal hysterectomy.

Primary hemorrhage: Here the bleeding is due to technical difficulty at the time of surgery. It is often possible to control bleeding by one or two suture ligature above and below the bleeding point.

Reactionary hemorrhage: It is a delayed primary hemorrhage from a vessel which has not been secured of secured adequately as a result of return of normal blood pressure. It occurs with in 24 hours of surgery. Most often it is vaginal bleeding that can be recognized easily. Internal hemorrhage is more insidious and is a dangerous condition because the patient would have suffered considerable blood loss before the diagnosis and active intervention. Exploration under anesthesia is needed to identify the bleeding point and secure hemostasis. If the major vessel pedicle responsible for internal hemorrhage has retracted upwards, there is no choice but to open the abdominal cavity to identify the responsible pedicle and secure it.

Secondary hemorrhage. Here the bleeding is due to secondary infection. It is manifested on seventh to tenth postoperative days. If the bleeding is minimal only change of antibiotics and observations may be sufficient. If there is severe bleeding, exploration under anesthesia is required after arranging for blood. Tight vaginal packing will be sufficient in most of the cases. Rarely internal iliac artery ligation is required to control the hemorrhage

Postoperative complications are listed as follows:

1. Hemorrhage
2. Postoperative fever
3. Urinary tract injury
4. Gastrointestinal injury
5. Psychological response to surgery
6. Complications of general anesthesia
7. Risks from blood transfusions

- *Le Fort's operation (Colpocleisis)*

    It is an excellent operation for the treatment of uterine prolapse for patients who are medically unfit, elderly and sexually not active.

    Objectives and principle

    - Cervix should be healthy and Pap smear should be normal
    - It is performed using local, epidural or spinal anesthesia
    - There is no need for general anesthesia
    - Approximates the anterior and poster vaginal wall
    - Small tunnel on either side for drainage of discharge
    - Takes 45 minutes to perform
    - Minimal pain or complications
    - 90-95% cure rate
    - It is not a suitable operation for a woman who is sexually active.

- *Shirodkar's abdominal sling operation*

    This operation is for nulliparous prolapse or congenital prolapse where supporting ligaments of pelvis are congenitally very weak. This is technically a difficult operation. One should have a sound anatomical knowledge to perform this surgery.

    Objective

    An 18-inch mersilene tape is attached to the posterior surface of supravaginal portion of the cervix

and the free ends of the tape are brought extra-peritoneally on either side of pelvis towards the sacral promontory. On right side the tape is carried extraperitoneally along the brim of the true pelvis. On left side the sigmoid colon prevents the direct extraperitoneal passage of tape. It may interfere with blood supply by kinking the sigmoid colon. It can be over come by creating a psoas loop. By traction on free ends of the tape the uterus can be pulled up to its correct location in the pelvis. The free ends of tapes are stitched to the anterior sacral ligaments and periosteum of sacral promontory.

- *Purandare cervicopexy (Abdominal cervicopexy)*

    Objective

    Abdomen is opened by low transverse incision and two strips of anterior rectus sheet are prepared and brought down in to the pelvis extraperitoneally and stitched to the front of the uterus. Whenever intra abdominal pressure raises, the strips pull the cervix anteriorly towards symphysis pubis and prevents its prolapse.

LAPAROSCOPY

Definition

The word laparoscopy simply means visual examination of the abdomen by means of a laparoscope (A small telescope). It is also called as "belly button surgery", endoscopy, or keyhole surgery. It is a surgical technique involving small incisions in the abdomen that allows direct visualization and remote handling of pelvic organs.

Laparoscopy was described several decades ago. It was used as a diagnostic and simple operative procedure. Recent advances in optics electronics and physics have allowed the development of excellent visualization system, which provide brilliant views of entire pelvis and abdominal cavity. These new system provide close up and magnified views far superior to those obtained at conventional open surgery. Video laparoscopy offers superb visualization technique and with the accessories like laser, bipolar cautery and harmonic scalpel, it is possible to perform almost every type of surgery laparoscopically, which were traditionally performed by laparotomy.

Laparoscopy has several clear advantages over laparotomy, which is highlighted in Table 21.1.

Table 21.1: Advantages of laparoscopy over laparotomy

- Avoidance of large painful skin incision
- Less intraoperative blood loss
- More precise surgery because of superior view
- Less tissue handling and trauma
- Shorter hospital stay
- Less infective morbidity
- Avoid use of retractors and packs
- Less post operative pain and less analgesic requirement
- Quicker mobilization
- More rapid return to full activities.
- More rapid convalescence
- Reduced postoperative adhesion formation
- Cosmetic
- Reduced cost

Currently laparoscopy accounts for large proportion of all gynecological procedures.

This keyhole surgery will be an added advantage in women's health care if the principles are followed regarding the selection of cases keeping in mind the contraindications and prerequisites.

General Guidelines

Basic prerequisites for laparoscopic surgery:
1. Adequate surgical skills
2. Appropriate equipments
3. Proper indications based on the risk and benefits

Laparoscopy is generally performed under general anesthesia. However, laparoscopic tubal ligation and other minor diagnostic tests can be performed under sedation and local anesthesia.

Indications for Laparoscopy

Diagnostic Laparoscopy

- Evaluation of acute abdomen
  Laparoscopy is a valuable tool for diagnosis of acute abdomen or acute pelvic pain, in which the differential diagnosis includes ectopic pregnancy, pelvic inflammatory disease, adnexal torsion, and appendicitis.
- Elective diagnostic laparoscopy
  The most common indications for this category are pelvic pain and infertility. In infertile patients it permits evaluation of tubal and peritoneal factors. A thorough evaluation of severity of pelvic adhesions and extent of endometriosis which allows selection of appropriate treatment. Table 21.2 gives the overview of various indications.

Table 21.2: Indications for laparoscopy

Diagnostic laparoscopy	Operative laparoscopy
Infertility • Chromotubation for tubal patency Pelvic pain • Endometriosis • Pelvis inflammatory disease • Ectopic pregnancy • Unexplained pain Assessment of pelvic masses • Ovarian cysts • Fibroids • Pelvic adhesions Fertility problems • Location of misplaced IUCD • Prior to reversal of sterilization • Primary amenorrhoea • Congenital anomalies of genital tract Second look procedures • After cancer treatment • After Infertility surgery	• Tubal sterilization • General adhesiolysis • Ovariolysis and salpingolysis • Fimbrioplasty and salpingostomy • Salpingostomy or linear salpingotomy • Ovarian cystectomy and oopherectomy • Ovarian drilling for PCOD • Adnexectomy • Ovarian biopsy Advanced operative laparoscopy • Laparoscopic assisted vaginal hysterectomy (LAVH) • Myomectomy • Burch procedure • Pelvic and para aortic lymphadenectomy • Laparoscopic Radical Hysterectomy

IUCD—Intrauterine contraceptive device
PCOD—Polycystic ovarian disease

Operative Laparoscopy

In recent years the spectrum of gynecological indications for operative laparoscopy has expanded dramatically. The definite indications are Ectopic pregnancy, pelvic adhesions, endometriosis, benign ovarian masses, and tubal sterilization. Other controversial indications are laparoscopic assisted vaginal hysterectomy (LAVH), myomectomy, Burch Procedure, Pelvic and aortic node dissection and even laparoscopic radical hysterectomy.

Contraindications

Contraindications to laparoscopy include bowel obstruction, ileus, peritonitis, intraperitoneal hemorrhage, diaphragmatic hernias and severe cardiorespiratory disease.

Other relative contraindications are massive obesity, inflammatory bowel disease, large intra-abdominal masses and advanced intrauterine pregnancy (Table 21.3).

Table 21.3: Contraindications for laparoscopy

Absolute	Relative
• Generalized peritonitis	• Large pelvic or abdominal masses of >26 weeks size
• Class IV cardiac disease	• Intrauterine pregnancy of > 16 Weeks
	• Hypo volemic shock
	• Intestinal obstruction
	• Chronic pulmonary disease
	• Previous laparotomy

Techniques of Laparoscopy

1. "Closed" laparoscopy—employing a Veress needle to create pneumoperitonuem followed by blind insertion of the first trocar.
2. "Open" technique where the fascia and the peritoneum are surgically opened and the trocar inserted under direct visualization.

The various instruments required for laparoscopy are shown in Table 21.4.

- *Veress needle and primary trocar insertion (Close laparoscopy)*

  The patient is placed in dorso lithotomy position. The patient must be in the complete horizontal position (not Trendelenburg). The site of abdominal entry is

Table 21.4: Equipments for laparoscopy

Basic equipments	Ancillary instruments	Hemostatic instruments
Laparoscope	Probes	Electro coagulation
Veress needle	Forceps	Laser
Trocars	Scissors and scalpels	Suture
Gas insufflators	Aspirators and irrigators	Clips and staples
Light source	Morcellators	Chemical substances
Cameras	Harmonic scalpel	

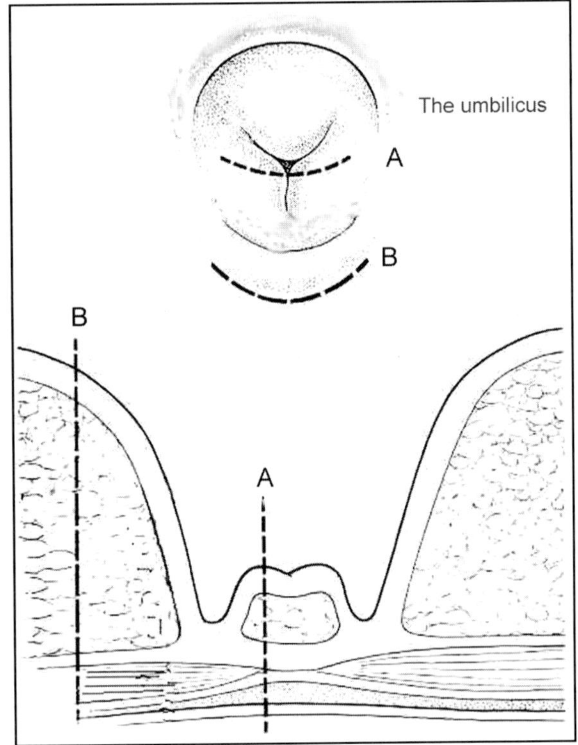

Figure 21.18: Site of abdominal entry. Cross-section view of the umbilical area. A—At the umbilicus the rectus sheath and peritoneum is underneath. B—just below the umbilicus there is subcutaneous fat, anterior rectus sheath, rectus muscle, posterior rectus sheath and peritoneum

intraumbilical or subumbilical, since it is a natural location for scar concealment and also this point offers the advantage of attenuation of the layers of abdominal wall and least vascularity (Fig. 21.18).

First step of laparoscopy is to achieve pneumoperitoneum with carbon dioxide gas using Veress needle. Veress needle is a relatively small gauge instrument with a spring-loaded tip and is used for initiation of pneumoperitoneum (Fig. 21.19).

This device consists of sharp needle containing within its lumen a spring-loaded gas-carrying

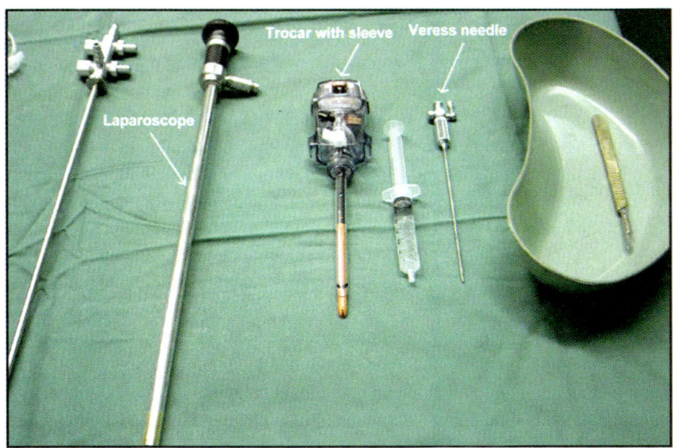

Figure 21.19: Basic instruments for laparoscopy

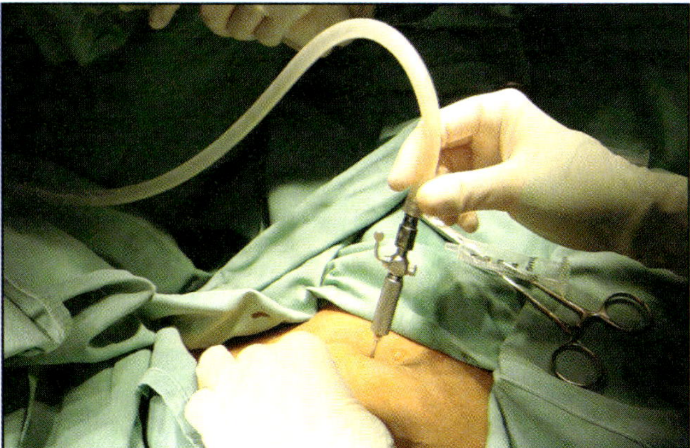

Figure 21.21: Carbon dioxide insufflation

channel. When the needle is inserted through the skin the blunt ended gas channel is forced against its spring and in to the central channel of the needle exposing the cutting edge of the needle. This sharp edge easily penetrates the all layers of abdominal wall. When the tip enters the abdominal cavity, the gas channel with its perforations is released and protrudes beyond the sharp bevelled needle tip to permit the free flow of gas. A small subumbilical incision is made. The Veress needle is placed by the controlled entry. The lower anterior abdominal wall is elevated by manually grasping the skin and subcutaneous tissue to maximize the distance between the umbilicus and the retroperitoneal vessels. The Veress needle is inserted toward the hollow of the sacrum at a correct angle of 45° aimed towards the uterine fundus (Fig. 21.20). When the

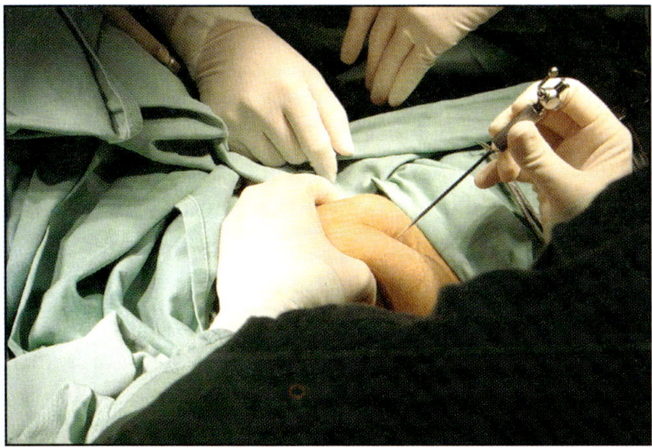

Figure 21.20: Insertion of veress needle

Veress needle is placed through the umbilicus into the peritoneal cavity, avoidance of both the retroperitoneal vessels and the intestinal tract is of paramount importance.

Correct placement of the Veress needle may be confirmed by a number of methods, such as the hanging drop test, injection and aspiration of fluid through the Veress needle, or measurement of intra-abdominal pressure with carbon dioxide insufflation and the hissing sound caused by air rushing through the Veress needle. Once the Veress needle is in place carbon dioxide gas is insufflated (Fig. 21.21). Tympani percussed over the liver is a clinical sign of proper intraabdominal insufflation.

- *Umbilical trocar insertion*

  After a pneumoperitoneum has been achieved with a Veress needle, the primary trocar with sleeve is placed at a similar angle to the Veress needle (Fig. 21.22). Intra-abdominal trocar placement is accomplished by hearing a rush of gas through the trocar sheet. Then laparoscope is inserted through the trocar sheet to visualize and confirm intra peritoneal access (Fig. 21.23).

  Secondary trocar sites are chosen for manipulatory and operative instruments. Care should be taken to avoid injury to the inferior epigastric vessels. Operative laparoscopy with two secondary trocars is shown in Figure 21.24.

  The complications of laparoscopy are summarized in Table 21.5.

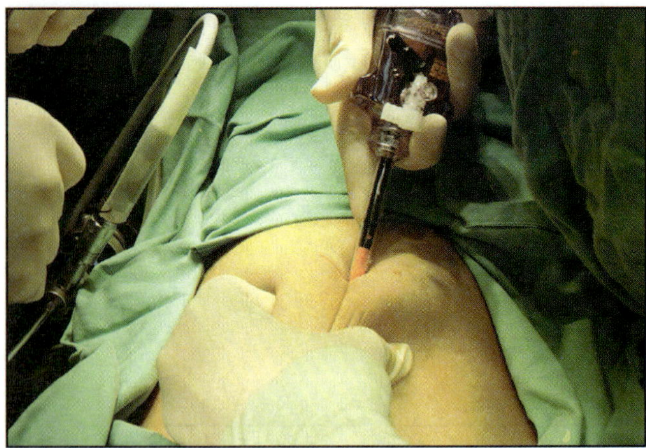

Figure 21.22: Umbilial trocal insertion

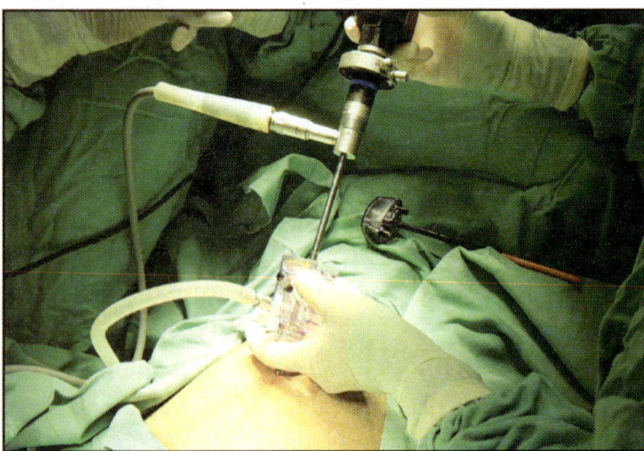

Figure 21.23: Insertion of laparoscope through trocar

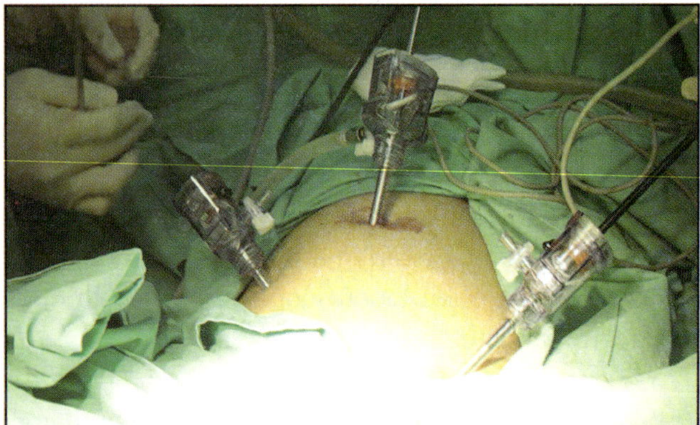

Figure 21.24: Operative laparoscopy with two secondary trocars

The evolving role of laparoscopy in the field of operative gynecology has a dramatic effect on clinical practice. Laparoscopic surgery is an important technique in the armamentarium of gynecologic surgeon. It is safe, cost-effective, and patient-friendly.

Table 21.5: Complications of laparoscopy

- Major vessel trauma
- Ileum and/or colon perforation
- Bladder perforation
- Inferior epigastric vessel damage
- Incisional hernia
- Hematomas
- Surgical emphysema
- Venous gas embolism
- Ureteric damage
- Pulmonary embolism
- Anesthetic problem

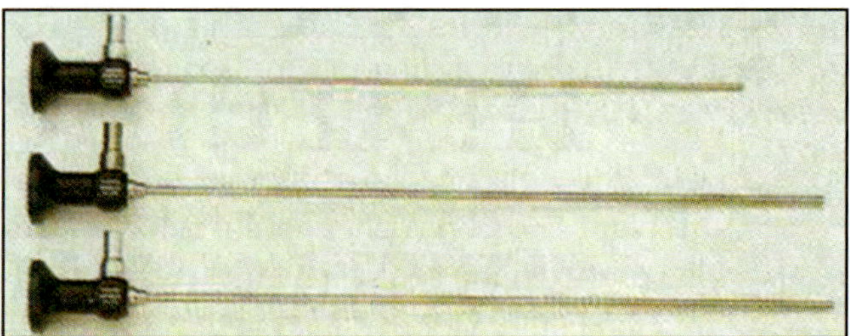

Figure 21.25: Hysteroscopes

HYSTEROSCOPY

Hysteroscopy involves passage of a rigid or flexible instrument into the uterine cavity and visualization of uterine cavity. Various diagnostic and therapeutic procedures can be performed through the hysteroscope (Fig. 21.25).

Procedure for Hysteroscopy

The basic procedure of hysteroscopy involves insertion of hysteroscope via the cervix, if needed after cervical dilatation, distension of the uterine cavity and visualization of uterine cavity. Diagnostic hysteroscopy can be done under paracervical block. Operative hysteroscopy is generally performed under regional or general anesthesia. Most hysteroscopic procedures need cervical dilatation and this may be achieved with insertion of a laminaria tent 3-8 hours prior to the procedure and/or by using Hagar's dilators at the time of surgery. The various distension media that are used to distend the uterine cavity include carbon dioxide, normal saline, Dextran70 and low viscosity fluids such as 1.5% glycine and 3% sorbitol. Carbon dioxide cannot be used in the presence of bleeding and can cause gas embolism if intrauterine pressure exceeds

100 mm Hg. Dextran 70 is a hyperosmolar solution and if it gets into the circulation it may draw water into the systemic circulation and cause fluid overload and circulatory failure. It can also induce an allergic response and coagulopathy. Not more than 300 ml of Dextran 70 should be infused at a time during hysteroscopy. Normal saline is a safe medium and can be used safely even in large volumes if needed as it does not generally cause electrolyte imbalances. But normal saline cannot be used in cases that require eletrosurgical procedures. Low viscosity fluids like glycine and sorbitol can sometimes cause electrolyte imbalances, but they are compatible with electro surgical procedures.

Indications for Hysteroscopy

Hysteroscopy has diagnostic and therapeutic uses. Common diagnostic indications include evaluation of abnormal uterine bleeding, infertility evaluation and recurrent pregnancy losses. Hysteroscopy is indicated in abnormal uterine bleeding especially if a diagnosis cannot be established by curettage. Hysteroscopy allows directed biopsy in cases of endometrial hyperplasia. In patients with infertility when hystero salpingography suggests intrauterine abnormalities, this can be confirmed with hysteroscopy as this allows better visualization of endometrial cavity. Intrauterine pathology like Asherman's syndrome and septum can be resected hysteroscopically at the same time. Many therapeutic procedures can be performed with hysteroscopy. Intra uterine contraceptive device if embedded in the uterine cavity may be removed with hysteroscope. Congenital septum in the uterus can be divided with resectoscope, which is a much simpler procedure than abdominal metroplasty. Small sub mucus fibroids may be resected with a loop electrode. Intrauterine synechiae as seen in Asherman's Syndrome may be divided under hysteroscopic vision. Endometrial ablation in patients with abnormal uterine bleeding can be achieved with electrosurgical resection or with laser. But the relief of menorrhagia with endometrial ablation is not as promising as it was originally thought to be.

Complications of Hysteroscopy

Complications of hysteroscopy include perforation, bleeding, thermal trauma and complications related to distension media. Perforation during hysteroscopy warrants termination of the procedure and laparotomy in case there is damage to other intra-abdominal structures like bowel or urinary tract. Bleeding during hysteroscopy generally is due to damage to the myometrial vessels during resection. This needs either electrocogulation of the bleeding vessel or balloon tamponade of uterine cavity with Foley catheter. Injection of dilute vassopressin has also been tried locally to control bleeding from the myometrial vessels. Thermal injuries can occur during electro surgical procedures of endometrium. If there is thermal injury to surrounding structures this may need laparotomy and repair of the defect. Complications related to distension media has been already described above.

Krishnendu Mukherjee

22.
General Surgical Problems in Gynecology

INTRODUCTION

The overlap of general surgery in the practice of Obstetrics and Gynecology is appreciated by all clinicians. Acute abdominal pain in pregnancy, symptomatic diseases of the breast and urinary or fecal incontinence often present first to the gynecologist. These topics have been dealt with elsewhere in this textbook. The present chapter shall focus on other areas where knowledge and understanding of general surgical principles is essential to the good practice of obstetrics and gynecology.

CATEGORIES OF GENERAL SURGICAL PROBLEMS IN GYNECOLOGY

General surgical disorders may co-exist with gynecological diseases or may masquerade as one. During the course of pregnancy or treatment for a gynecological condition, surgical problems may be precipitated.

Three broad categories can be identified, which encompass these areas:

a. Diagnostic dilemmas in females presenting with lower abdominal pain.
b. Extra-abdominal general surgical problems in pregnancy.
c. Operative surgical considerations with relevance to iatrogenic injuries of planned surgery on non-reproductive organs or structures during the course of pelvic surgery in females.

Diagnostic Considerations in Lower Abdominal Pain

Lower abdominal pain in females often poses diagnostic dilemma. The gynecological clinicians would most often consider the following differential diagnosis.

- Acute or recurrent appendicitis
- Ureteric colic, urinary tract infections
- Irritable bowel syndrome.
- Inflammatory bowel disease (IBD), i.e. Crohn's disease, ulcerative colitis, indeterminate colitis
- Infective enteritis; tuberculosis

While a typical presentation of acute appendicitis is a straightforward diagnosis, not all cases will present with the usual features. History of "shifting pain" should be carefully sought in all cases as it is highly suggestive of acute appendicitis. In the absence of signs of peritoneal inflammation the diagnosis becomes more difficult. It is rational to perform full blood count and urinalysis. However, one should bear in mind that polymorpho-nuclear leucocytosis is neither specific for, nor invariable in appendicitis. Microscopic hematuria or pyuria also does not negate or refute a diagnosis of appendicitis. High resolution ultrasonography performed by an experienced sonologist may be able to demonstrate an inflamed appendix directly (luminal gas shadow) and it should be used in the evaluation of lower abdominal or right iliac fossa (RIF) pain. Though an invasive investigation, laparoscopy is useful in distinguishing acute appendicitis from other pathologies.

Low grade, persistent (chronic) RIF pain is not a feature of recurrent appendicitis. The pain in this condition is typically recurrent in fashion and localised in the RIF and adjoining areas. Only if, repeated clinical assessment and other investigations fail to resolve the problem and provided acute abdominal signs are absent, a barium study may be performed. Barium enema is preferable to barium follow through. Though non-filling of the appendix is suggestive, but not diagnostic of appendicits, a completely filled appendicular lumen rule out the diagnosis. Reproduction of the crampy abdominal pain during performance of a double contrast barium enema is highly suggestive of irritable bowel syndrome. Laparoscopy may not help in diagnosing recurrent appendicitis but visualisation of the pelvis and distal small bowel may be helpful in the final assessment.

Irritable bowel syndrome is a common condition. These patients often complain of pellet-like stools, tenesmus and a myriad of non-specific abdominal symptoms in addition to pain. Though a psychosomatic component is common, these patients do not usually have any recognisable psychiatric morbidity. Presence of systemic symptoms. (e.g. low grade fever), extra-abdominal manifestations (e.g. oral apthous ulcers), mucous diarrhea with rectal bleeding should raise the possibility of inflammatory bowel disease. Even in the absence of these features, irritable bowel syndrome should not be diagnosed without full evaluation and it is customary to perform colonoscopy and small bowel barium enema (which is preferable to barium follow through) in these patients.

In the presence of pregnancy, evaluation of lower abdominal pain of non-acute nature poses special difficulties because conventional radiology and laparo-scopy are both contraindicated. Hence, for example, gallstones detected by ultrasonography need to be treated by the conventional cholecystectomy as opposed to the laparoscopic procedure. Symptoms of biliary tract disease can be reduced by adherence to a low fat diet and operation should be advised in the second trimester of pregnancy. Management of asymptomatic gallstones detected in pregnancy evokes controversy. Since pregnancy itself increases the lithogenicity of gallbladder bile, operation is the preferred option in the second trimester or soon after delivery.

Unlike intestinal colic, ureteric colic is not a colicky pain. The pain is usually constant with exacerbations and classically, radiates from loin to groin though the later is by no means invariable. The pain is produced by increasing luminal pressure in the upstream collecting system and is mediated by prostaglandins. Hence, the pain responds well to non-steroidal anti-inflammatory agents. Urinalysis demonstrates hematuria in 85% of cases and a straight X-ray of the KUB (Kidney, Ureter, Bladder) demonstrates calculi in over 80% of patients. Ultrasono-graphy may not demonstrate the stone but usually shows the dilatation of the pelvicalyceal system and the ureter. Combining the three investigations in the said order, a diagnostic accuracy of nearly 100% can be achieved.

Dysuria and hypogastric pains are common manifes-tations of urinary tract infections (UTI), and rarely, may be the first manifestation of a gynecological or bladder malignancy. In post-menopausal women, the frequent co-existence of bladder neck obstruction and vaginal dryness predispose to UTI. However, in recurrent UTI, especially if abacterial pyuria is repeatedly demonstrated, one must consider the possibilities of tuberculous cystitis, interstitial cystitis and carcinoma-in-situ of bladder. Appropriate workup should include culture for acid fast bacillus (AFB) and cystoscopy.

Extra-abdominal General Surgical Problems in Pregnancy

Anorectal Diseases

The actual frequency of proctological diseases in

pregnancy is poorly documented; it is estimated, however, that 85% primi or multiparae with anorectal disorders develop them during or after their first pregnancy.[1]

Proctological diseases provoked or aggravated by pregnancy are:

- Congestion of anal canal and anal varices.
- Changes in stool movements.
- Hemorrhoids and their complications.
- Acute perianal hematoma (thrombotic "piles")
- Anal neuralgias
- Pruritus ani.

Increased tendency to constipation is almost universal in pregnancy. Dietary adjustments are crucial and specific dietary advice is more rewarding than general statements like "increasing fiber intake". Bran and wheat cereals, apricot, dessicated coconut, peas, spinach and lentils are high in fiber. Osmotic laxatives (e.g. Lactulose) can be prescribed in pregnancy.

Topical preparations containing astringents, anti-inflammatory (e.g.corticosteroids) and local anesthetic agents are popularly used to treat ano-rectal problems. Though there is little evidence of their efficacy, temporary symptomatic relief may be achieved. They may, however, aggravate pruritus ani by causing maceration of perianal skin. Most anorectal disorders in pregnancy will respond to adequate bedrest (decrease of perineal congestion), suitable diet and judicious use of laxatives. Hygiene is important. The hypersecretory state of the vagina with modified pH of secretions and extension of vaginal mycosis predisposes to pruritus ani. Secondary bacterial infections are common. Treatment of vaginal mycoses, endoanal application of antifungals, maintaining dry perianal skin, dusting with antiseptic powder will help to alleviate pruritus ani. Local nystatin is useful in thrush; its systemic absorption from the gastrointestinal tract is negligible.

Hemorrhoids present with rectal bleeding which is fresh, painless and usually not mixed with motions. Internal hemorrhoids are not palpable by digital rectal examination and need to be visualized with a protoscope. Hemorrhoids are best treated conservatively except in permanently prolapsed bleeding hemorrhoids, which require hemorrhoidectomy. Since hemorrhoidal bleeding exacerbates the anemia of pregnancy and since early cases can be dealt with by non-operative means, hemorrhoids should be treated energetically in pregnancy. Topical creams have little to offer in hemorrhoids except short-term relief.

Table 22.1: Different degrees of hemorrhoids, signs and treatment

	Signs	*Injection Sclerotherapy (Oily phenol)*
First degree	Internal hemorrhoids	Laser photocoagulation
Second degree	Prolapse, and reduces spontaneously	Rubber band ligation Cryosurgery
Third degree	Prolapse, requiring digital repositioning	
Fourth degree	Permanently prolapsed	Hemorrhoidectomy

Acute Perianal Pain

The common causes of acute perianal pain are listed in Table 22.2.

Table 22.2: Causes of acute perianal pain

- Acute perianal hematoma
- Anal fissure
- Prolapsed thrombosed internal hemorrhoids
- Anal neuralgias
- Anorectal suppuration (abscess)

Pregnancy carries a higher than usual incidence of the first four causes of acute perianal pain.

1. *Acute perianal hematoma* is a common condition often referred to by the misnomer, "external thrombotic pile" because it is not a true hemorrhoid. It presents with a typical globular and exquisitely tender swelling on the perianal margin. The condition is very painful. The 'clot' can be evacuated by a simple incision-drainage under a local anesthetic with dramatic symptomatic relief.

2. *Fissures* are usually posterior splits in the anoderm but anterior fissures are relatively more common in women. Spasm of the external sphincter precludes examination and heightens the pain. Acute anal fissures can be treated by local application of glyceryl trinitrate cream. However, in pregnancy the consequent

hypotension may be detrimental. Hence, it must be used with caution only in hospitalized states with adequate supervision and bedrest. Fissures are best treated by a subcutaneous lateral sphincterotomy of the internal sphincter. Conventional manual anal stretching (Lord's procedure) should be avoided whenever possible; however, a gentle anal stretch may ameliorate the pain of prolapsed thrombosed hemorrhoids which must be distinguished from acute perianal hematoma.[2]

3. *Hemorrhoids* have been discussed above.

4. *Anal neuralgias*, attributed to the stretching of pelvic neural plexuses, usually presents with constant burning pain which, often radiates to the thighs, vagina and sacral region. A psychogenic component may be prominent. Exacerbations occur during impaction of solid feces; such acute periods should be treated with enemas followed by long-term administration of laxatives.

5. *Condyloma accuminatum* may be aggravated during pregnancy. Severe cases need electro-coagulation as podophyllin is contraindicated in pregnancy.

Venous Disorders

Pregnancy is a hypercoagulable state and deep vein thrombosis (DVT) is not uncommon. Recent studies have identified genetic susceptibility to protein C resistance in pregnancy and these women have a higher incidence of DVT.[3] The risk of potentially fatal pulmonary embolism dictates that DVT should be diagnosed and treated urgently. Heparin is safe in pregnancy as it does not cross the placental barrier but Warfarin is best avoided in pregnancy.

Varicose veins are also common in pregnancy. Though distressing symptoms are rare, there may be a slight predisposition to DVT. Venous disorders are best investigated by Duplex Doppler imaging and patency of deep venous flow can be accurately judged in most patients. Varicose veins are best managed conservatively with elastic compression stockings and adequate bed rest with elevation of feet.

Operative Surgical Considerations

In the course of difficult pelvic surgery inadvertent injuries are prone to occur to the ureter, intestine and major blood vessels.

Ureteric Injuries

The pelvic surgeon must have accurate knowledge of the course of the ureters and be proficient in locating the ureter at different sites and steps of pelvic dissection. The ureter is posterior to the ovarian vessels at the origin of the infundibulopelvic ligament. During ligation of the ovarian vessels it can be inadvertently incorporated in the pedicle and it is at this site the ureter is most commonly injured during pelvic surgery.[4] The ureter continues in the base of the broad ligament and courses under the uterine artery and is 0.7 to 1.5 cm lateral to the uterine isthmus. While ligating the uterine vessels at this situation, the ureter is again vulnerable to injury. The ureter traverses the parametrium lateral to the cervix, ultimately entering the bladder trigone at the level of anterior vaginal fornix. This is the third common site of ureteral injury, left side being commoner than the right side.

The common causes of iatrogenic ureteral injury are outlined in Table 22.3.

Table 22.3: Common causes of ureteric injury

- Abdominal hysterectomy
- Vaginal hysterectomy
- Salpingo-oophorectomy
- Laparoscopy (rarely)
- Cystocele repair

Identification of ureteral injury is of paramount importance, because primary repair has the best chance of success. Unrecognized traumas lead to delayed diagnosis usually with the formation of fistulae, infected urinomas or obstructive uropathy, which presents with fever, flank pain and ileus in the postoperative period. Presence of mild hematuria should arouse suspicion of urinary tract injuries. In the postoperative period, these injuries are best investigated by intravenous urography. Partial injuries may be dealt with by stenting the ureter by a double J stent passed over a guide, either from

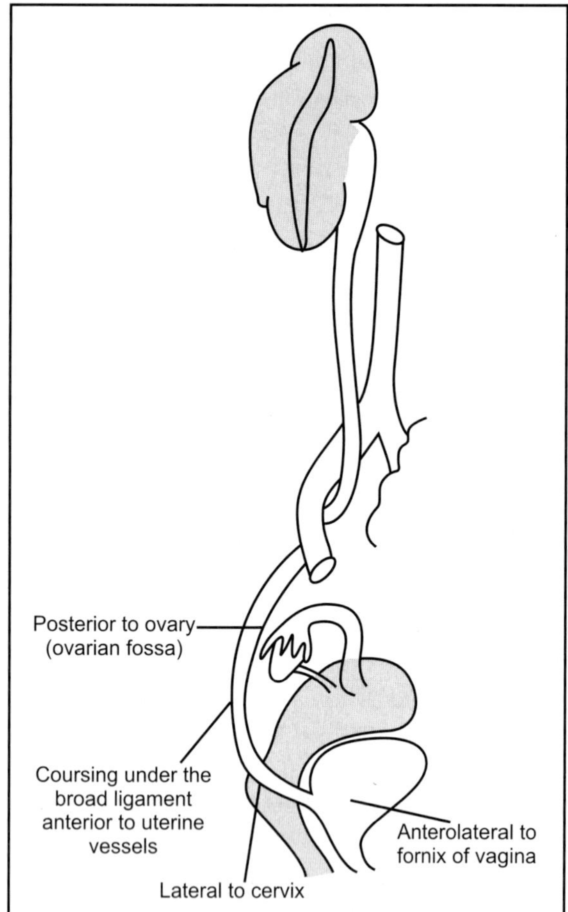

Figure 22.1: Common sites of ureteral injury during pelvic operations

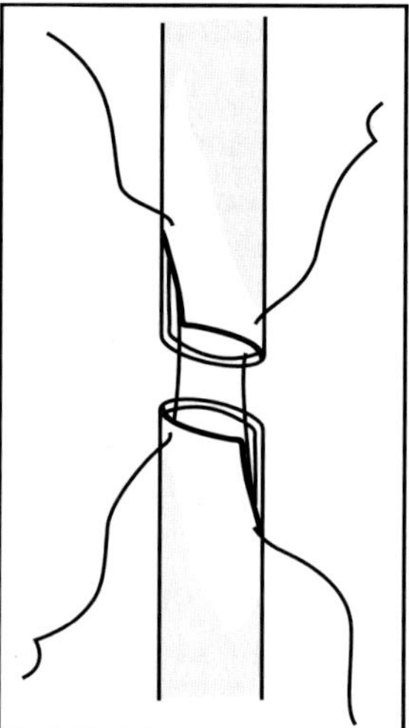

Figure 22.2A: End to end ureteroureterostomy (note the obliquity and spatulated ends)

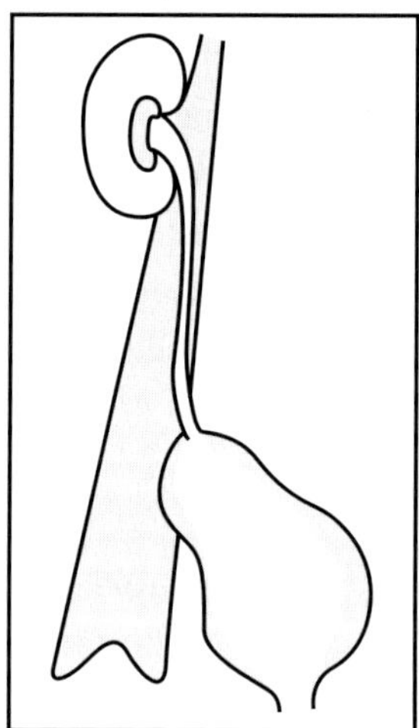

Figure 22.2B: Ureteroneocystostomy with psoas hitch (The dome of bladder is fully mobilised, contralateral superior vesical pedicle may be divided

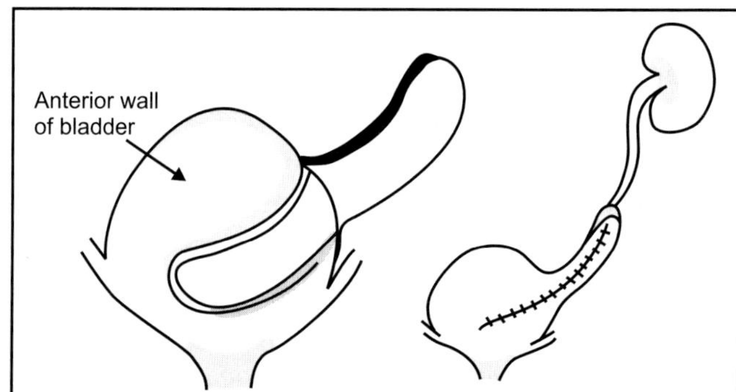

Figure 22.2C: Ureteroneocystostomy with Boari flap (The flap is based posterolaterally on the ipsilateral superior vesical artery. Base of flap: 4 cm in width, tip of flap: 3 cm. in width)

below by cystoscopy or from above through a percutaneous nephrostomy. Ureteric repairs or reimplantations should be performed with interrupted sutures of absorbable variety, e.g. Polyglycolic acid. The repair should be drained extraperitoneally. A double J stent may be used to splint the anastomosis, and it is customary to keep the bladder decompressed with an indwelling catheter for 6 to 7 days. Uretero-neocystostomy (ureteric reimplantation) is generally performed by a tunnelled anti-reflux procedure. Additional length of the bladder may be obtained by mobilization of the dome and suturing the ipsilateral extension to psos major muscle ('the psoas hitch') as per diagram (Figures 22.2A to C). Avoidance of tension is crucial as tension at the site of ureteric anastomoses predisposes to stenosis.[5] Bladder injuries are best-repaired in two layers and decompression is maintained with a catheter for 10 to 14 days.

Table 22.4: Surgical techniques for ureteral reconstruction

Procedure	Ureteral defect
Uretero-ureterostomy	1-3 cm
Uretero-neocystostomy alone	3-5 cm
Uretero-neocystostomy with psoas hitch	5-10 cm
Uretero-neocystostomy with Boari flap	10-15 cm

Bowel Injuries

Intestinal injuries are particularly prone to occur in the presence of adhesions, usually from previous surgical procedures. Endometriosis, multiple surgeries, previous intraperitoneal sepsis and previous irradiation for malignancy increase the density of adhesions. In surgery involving resection for pelvic cancers, particularly ovarian carcinoma, en-bloc resection of loops of small intestine may be necessary if they are involved with tumor.

It is salutory to consider the possibility of adhesions and bowel injuries before the operation. A knowledge of the pathology of the individual patient should alert the discerning clinician of technical difficulties. Resection of a large chocolate cyst in the presence of pelvic endometriosis or resection of a bulky tubo ovarian mass may lead to inadvertent injury of the rectosigmoid, necessitating a proximal colostomy. It is difficult to site a colostomy with perfection in an anesthetized, supine patient. Such a patient may therefore, benefit from a preoperative physical evaluation to select the site of a stoma should the eventuality arise. A stoma should avoid the creases produced by abdominal fat rolls, which can only be assessed by sitting the patient up. Stoma should also be at least 4 cm away from bony prominences (e.g. anterior superior iliac spine), the umbilicus and surgical scars.

Key Points

- It is important to *anticipate* difficult pelvic dissections, adhesions and possible bowel injury.
- *Repair* of intestinal injuries or resections of bowel are contaminated procedures. Appropriate antisepsis protocols should be employed, e.g. change of gloves and wound drapes and use of fresh instruments for wound closure.
- Perioperative *antibiotics* are best administered by the intravenous route at or before induction of anesthesia. A second-generation cephalosporin is usually adequate. Anti-anerobic cover must be added as soon as possible if bowel injuries have occurred. Continuing prophylactic antibiotics beyond the first postoperative day confers no additional benefit.[6]
- *Bowel preparation* should be considered preoperatively, if left colonic or rectal injury is anticipated. Its role in small bowel resections or right colonic repairs remains unclear.
- *Adhesions* are best separated under direct vision with blunt tipped fine dissection scissors. Interloop adhesions of small bowel need not be separated. All adhesions distal to the site of an intestinal repair, however, must be carefully lysed; presence of distal obstruction is the single most important factor contributing to anastomotic leaks. All bands must be divided. Bands originating from the mesentery and crossing the ileum and attached inside the pelvic cavity should be ligated before division as rarely, they harbor blood vessels.[7]
- Whenever possible synthetic absorbable *sutures* (e.g. polyglactin 910 (Vicryl) or polyglycolic acid) should be chosen over chromic catgut.
- Small bowel is usually repaired in two layers. However, a single layer of inverting sutures is equally acceptable. Injuries of the colon or rectum should be repaired with a single layer closure. The repair, especially in unprepared bowel may be protected by a proximal loop colostomy or a loop ileostomy. Such proximal venting does not decrease the incidence of leaks. However, they do reduce the magnitude of septic complications should a leak occur.[10]
- *Diathermy injuries* should be repaired after trimming the edges of the injured gut.
- *Irradiated bowel* must be resected if perforated during dissection. An adequate margin of macroscopically normal bowel must be included in the resection.

- There is no evidence that routine use of *nasogastric tube* alters the outcome after intestinal surgery.[8]
- Most patients can usually tolerate small amounts of *oral fluids* by the second postoperative day and a *diet* can usually be introduced by the fourth day. There is no evidence that withholding oral feeds in the postoperative period lessens the incidence of anastomotic leak.[9]
- *Intraperitoneal drains* may be used in left colonic or rectal repairs. Closed system of drainage employing soft tube drains avoiding direct contact with the suture line is preferable. Following small bowel resections the abdomen need not be drained.
- All mesenteric gaps should be closed.
- Peritoneal wash *(lavage)* is not necessary unless gross macroscopic contamination has occurred. Sterile normal saline is adequate for lavage; strong antiseptic solutions, e.g. Povidone iodine should be avoided.
- It is rational to avoid over infusion of sodium in the early postoperative period, though clear evidence to justify this is unavailable.
- Unexplained tachycardia, persistent distention with adynamic ileus, episodes of hypotension and copious wound discharge are often early signs of an anastomotic leak and may precede enterocutaneous fistulation or gross peritonitis or abscess formation by several days.
- Incidental appendicectomies are sometimes performed during the course of gynecological procedures. Routine incidental appendicectomy is difficult to justify. It must be remembered that appendicectomy is a "major" intestinal operation with a low but appreciable risk of complications particularly intra-abdominal and wound sepsis.[11]

Vascular Injuries

Injury to major pelvic blood vessels, the iliac veins in particular, may give rise to catastrophic intraoperative hemorrhage. As with the bowels or the ureter, care to avoid such injuries during difficult dissections is of paramount importance. Proximal and distal control of the vessel makes repair of injuries easier and safer. A selection of vascular clamps and appropriate suture materials (5-0 or 6-0 Prolene) should be available in the operating room. Panic laden attempts to apply hemostatic forceps to injured vessels causes greater injury and laceration. Bleeding can be usually controlled with localised pressure with a finger or small swab while proximodistal dissection is continued to mobilize the vessel to perform an anastomosis or repair without tension on the vessel.

CONCLUSION

Understanding the principles, which underlie general surgical problems and operative surgery, will significantly help obstetricians and gynecologists in their own field of work.

REFERENCES

1. Marti MC: Pregnancy and Proctological disease, Surgery for ano-rectal diseases 1989: 305-309 Springer-Verlag.
2. Hancock BD: Hemorrhoids and Anal fissures, ABC of colorectal disease, BMJ publishing group; 1998, 24-26.
3. Barbieri RL, Repke JT: Medical disorders during pregnancy, Harrison's Principles of Internal Medicine (15th edn), Mc Graw Hill 2001; 25-30.
4. Montz FJ, Berek JS: Gynecologic Pelvic Procedures, Maingot's Abdominal Operations, (10th edn), Appleton and Lange 1997;2133-49.
5. Franke JJ, Smith JA: Surgery of the ureter, Campbell's Urology, 7th edn, WB Saunders company, 1998; 3069-72.
6. E Patchen Dellinger: Surgical infections, Sabiston Textbook of Surgery, 43, 15th Edn, WB Saunders Company, 1997.
7. Mukherjee K, Fryer L, Stephenson BM: Mesodiverticular bands. British Jour Surg 1997; 84(1): 43.
8. Savassi-Rocha PR, Conceicao SA, Ferreira JT, et al. Evaluation of routine use of nasogastric tube in digestive operations by a prospective controlled study. Surg Gynecol Obstet 1992;174:317-20.
9. Bickel A, Shtamler B, Mizrahi S: Early oral feeding following removal of narogastric tube and gastrointestimal operations. Arch Surg 1992;127:287-89.
10. Fielding LP: Lessons from the Large Bowel Cancer Project 1976-88, Recent Advances in Surgery. Churchill Livingstone 1998; 13, 143-157.
11. Hayes RJ: Incidental appendectomis; current teaching. JAMA, 1977;238: 31.

23.

Vani Ramkumar

Puberty

INTRODUCTION

In many societies throughout history, puberty has been a time of celebration.[1] Puberty has been defined as the state of being functionally capable of procreation.[2] The cascade of events initiated by the release of pulsatile gonadotropin releasing hormone (GnRH) from prepubertal feedback and central negative inhibition results in increased levels of gonadotropins and steroids with appearance of secondary sexual characteristics and eventual adult function (menarche and, later ovulation).[1]

Adolescence is the span of human growth extending from the immaturity of childhood to the physical and psychological maturity of adulthood. This period extends from 10 to 20 years (WHO, 1977). Puberty marks the beginning of adolescence. During puberty, the secondary sexual characteristics appear and mature, the adolescent growth spurt takes place, fertility is attained, and significant physical, psychological, and behavioral changes occur, transforming the child into an adult.

ENDOCRINE CHANGES OF PUBERTY

Maturation of the hypothalamic pituitary complex and the input of the central nervous system (CNS) that integrates a variety of intrinsic and extrinsic stimuli bring about the initiation of puberty. This hypothalamic pituitary complex was named the gonadostat by Grumbach and, as currently understood, develops in two stages: First, the negative feedback mechanism is operative early in childhood, probably from mid to late fetal life. The gonadostat is extremely sensitive to the suppressive effect of small amounts of circulating gonadal steroids. The circulating concentrations of estrogens and gonadotropins are also correspondingly low. With the onset of puberty, the hypothalamic gonadostat becomes progressively less sensitive to the suppressive effect of the gonadal steroids and more gonadotropins are secreted from the pituitary. Grumbach et al showed that the hypothalamic gonadostat in prepubertal children is 6 to 15 times more sensitive to circulating estrogens than after puberty. There is no evidence of episodic luteinising hormone (LH) secretion in children before puberty, but beginning in early puberty intermittent LH secretion is observed only during sleep. This is characterized by widely fluctuating plasma LH concentrations. There is, most probably, a maturation phenomenon related to changes in the CNS that affects pulsatile release of GnRH and possibly participates in the prepubertal increase in pituitary response to GnRH.[3]

The second stage of pubertal development is maturation and activation of the positive feedback effect of estrogens that occurs in girls about mid to late puberty. The progressive maturation of the hypothalamic pituitary gonadal axis and increasing secretion of gonadotropins and gonadal steroids occur simultaneously with the development stages described by Tanner and correlate better with bone age than with chronological age.

The sensing area in the brain is sensitive not only to estrogens but also to adrenal androgens. An increase in adrenal activity takes place in the latter half of childhood prior to the onset of puberty. This phase of development is called adrenarche. Maturation of the hypothalamic pituitary adrenal circuit probably begins with the production of an unidentified hormone by the hypophysis referred to as cortical adrenal stimulating hormone (CASH). This stimulates androgen production by the adrenal reticularis. The earliest evidence for production of such a hormone is the maturation of the androgenic zone of the adrenal cortex at about 8 years in girls. The initial biochemical effect is an increase in the production of dihydro epiandrosterone (DHEA) and dihydro epiandrosterone sulphate (DHEAS) followed by increased levels of androstenedione.[3]

Changes in the hypothalamic pituitary ovarian circuit begin after the development of the androgenic zone of the adrenal cortex. The sensitive gonadostat of the childhood years responsible for maintaining a low output of both gonadotropins and ovarian steroids becomes less sensitive after the age of 8 years. A modest rise of follicle stimulating hormone (FSH) and lutenising hormone (LH) is characteristic of the resulting increase in prepubertal gonadotropin secretion. FSH levels are initially slightly higher than LH levels. Later, nocturnal episodic discharges of LH are produced and by the end of puberty the same higher levels are maintained during daytime hours. Evidence for the decreased sensitivity of the gonadostat to these maturational changes of the hypothalamus and pituitary is demonstrated by an associated increase in ovarian estradiol secretion after the age of 10 years. While the pubertal process begins with this diminished sensitivity to negative feedback at the level of the hypothalamus, maturation is not complete until a more complex positive feedback mechanism is operative.

At adolescence, maturation of the gonads is accompanied by acceleration of somatic growth, development of the secondary sex characteristics, and attainment of reproductive capacity. The growth curve of a child runs steeply in early life, after which it gradually levels off. Around the time of puberty, it suddenly becomes steep again.

PHYSICAL CHANGES OF PUBERTY

A. Breast development (Thelarche)
- Stage 1—Infantile stage
- Stage 2—Breast and papilla elevated in a small mound, diameter of areola increases
- Stage 3—Breast and areola are further enlarged (small adult breast)
- Stage 4—Areola and papilla further enlarge to form a secondary mound
- Stage 5—Secondary mound disappears. Smooth rounded contour

B. Pubic hair development (Pubarche)
- Stage 1—Infantile stage. No hair
- Stage 2—Sparse growth of long slightly pigmented hair on labia majora or mons pubis.
- Stage 3—An increase in the amount of hair spreads sparsely over the mons pubis, it is considerably darker, coarser and more curly than in Stage 2
- Stage 4—Hair is adult in character but covers a smaller area than in most adults
- Stage 5—Hair is distributed in an inverse triangular pattern, with some spread to the medial surface of the thighs, characteristic of an adult female.

C. Axillary hair development
- Stage 1—Infantile stage (no hair)
- Stage 2—Intermediate development
- Stage 3—Full development

One should note that breast and pubic hair development need to be staged separately in each patient because they are not necessarily concordant.

Timing and Sequence of Pubertal Phenotypic Changes

Phenotypic changes of puberty begin with acceleration of growth velocity. This somatic landmark is followed by the first visible change in sexual development, thelarche. The appearance of a breast bud occurs between the ages of 9 and 11. It represents the first clinical sign of ovarian estradiol release. It is the initial test of competency of the hypothalamic pituitary ovarian circuit. Adrenarche as evidenced by the initial growth of pubic hair that occurs shortly after the appearance of the breast bud. In 15% of individuals, these first two events in human sexual development are reversed. In some instances menstruation occurs prior to axillary hair formation. The appearance of pubic hair shows that the hypothalamus pituitary adrenal axis is also intact. Appearance of axillary hair usually follows pubarche by approximately 2 years.

The initial growth acceleration in height of approximately 4 cm per year continues through the early stages of sexual development. An additional increment of 5 cm per year is added to this height velocity during the adolescent growth spurt. This peak height velocity of 9 cm per year, occurring at approximately ages 11 to 12, is caused by the production of ovarian steroids. It is an important developmental landmark of puberty. Generally, the pubertal girl's growth spurt is seen 2 years earlier than that of the boy.[4] Once the maximum speed of adolescent growth has been attained and the adolescent female begins her deceleration of growth velocity, menarche heralds the closing stage of puberty. The first menses occurs between chronologic ages 11 and 15 for American girls, with a mean age of 12.8 years. With the continued production of ovarian steroids, epiphyses continue to close and growth velocity slows further. As a result, it is rare for the adolescent to grow more than 6 cm in height following her first menses.

Menarche is not the final event of puberty. Rather, it marks the beginning of the last stage of pubertal development. The most important aspect of this entire process is the continued stimulation of ovarian follicles, which eventually results in the maturation of a positive feedback system to the hypothalamus and in ovulation.

It takes approximately 20 cycles before this last important function of the ovary begins on a regular basis. The teleological purpose of puberty is to produce an individual capable of reproduction for recapitulation of the species. These events occur at the given chronological ages, which are equal to physiological or bone age (Table 23.1).

Table 23.1: Physical and physiological landmarks of puberty

Features	Age in years
Breast bud, enlargement of labia minora and physiological vaginal discharge	9-11
Pubic hair	11-12
Growth spurt (mean peak velocity of 8 cm per year)	12
Areolar pigmentation; further development of breast and axillary hair	12-13
Menarche	13.5 (9-17)

By plotting one's height velocity against physiological or bone age, normal pubertal landmarks can be properly anticipated. Figure 23.1 summarises the developmental landmarks of puberty in the form of a pubertal developmental chart. Thelarche and adrenarche are shown to appear during the early growth acceleration. Menarche follows the ensuing peak height velocity, and ovulation begins when epiphyses continue to close and growth slows towards a halt. In the female with pubertal aberrations, genetic, environmental or systemic processes violate this normal

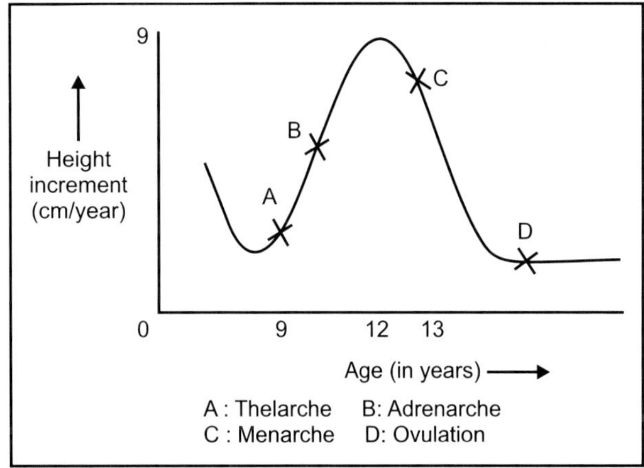

Figure 23.1: Pubertal development chart showing landmarks of the normal pubertal process, superimposed upon growth velocity

temporal relationship of pubertal events. In these patients, bone age (e.g. physiological age) often deviates from chronological age. Pubertal development charts in these individuals often identify these discrepancies. These charts serve as aids for diagnosis and allow therapeutic efforts to be monitored.[3]

Clitoris

In cases of suspected virilization, the clitoral size should be determined by measuring the length and width of the glans. Normal values for a female between 11 and 15 are not more than 3×3 mm, for a girl between 15 and 19 no more than 5×5 mm. A width of 10 mm is significant virilization.

Factors Affecting Menarche

Girls in the higher socioeconomic classes tend to have earlier menarche than do girls in the lower classes. Lifestyle too is very important. Children who are not athletically active have an earlier menarche, as have blind children, who presumably have a more sedentary lifestyle.

The age at menarche in the US is 12.65 years and in UK it is 13 years. A range of 9 to 16 years constitutes the period during which the onset of menses might be regarded as normal. It should be considered abnormal when menses appear before the age of 9 or are delayed beyond age 16. The mean age at onset of menarche precedes the mean age of regular menses by about 14 months. Painful menses are noted at a mean interval of 10 months later.

Frisch hypothesized that weight, or more precisely total body fat, plays a critical role in the onset of menses. Menarche is associated with attainment of an average critical body weight of about 47 Kg.[5] About 17% of body composition as fat are probably needed for menarche to occur and about 22% for onset and maintenance of regular ovulatory cycles. The gene that controls the onset of puberty may be the transforming growth factor a gene. The initiation of this process involves an interaction between percentage body fat and the genetic determinant of the onset of puberty. Some speculation exists as to whether or not leptin will be the coordinating hormone.[6]

In a study, dancers attained menarche later than music students, and were also thinner.[3] It was concluded that energy drain may have a modulator effect on the hypothalamic pituitary set point at puberty, and in combination with low body weight may prolong the prepubertal state. Pubarche was found to occur at a normal age. This is not surprising, since pubarche is related to androgen secretion, and high testosterone levels have been reported in female runners.

The components of physical maturation include statural and ponderal growth, and the development of secondary sexual characteristics and menarche. Various factors including heredity, social class, nutrition and physical or emotional stress influence physical maturation.

In general, menstruation does not occur in girls who are more than 15% below ideal body weight for height. Malnutrition in childhood can cause growth retardation and pubertal delay. Anorexia nervosa is associated with pubertal arrest or delay and is seen in girls from developed nations. Physical illness like diabetes mellitus, inflammatory bowel disease and chronic renal failure can cause pubertal delay.

Excessive exercise delays puberty due to change in endogenous opioid peptides. Other factors which affect onset of pubertal hormonal maturation are hyper or hypothyroid states, growth hormone deficiency and increased sex steroids secretion as occurs in pseudosexual precocity and the congenital adrenal hyperplasias. These effects can be monitored by skeletal age. Onset of puberty in females then occurs when bone age is 10.5 to 11 years, whether or not this coincides with chronologic age. Menarche occurs in the average girl at a bone age of about 13 years.

Precocious puberty refers to the development of any sign of secondary sexual maturation at an age earlier than 2.5 SD less than the expected age of pubertal onset. In North America, these ages are 8 years for girls and 9 years for boys.[4] Those girls who begin menstruating either much earlier or much later than their peers are under extreme stress. Identification with the peer group is important, and girls who are out of step with the group show an increase in anxiety. Precocious puberty can be treated with GnRH analogs.

PSYCHOLOGIC CHANGES OF PUBERTY

The major characteristics of early adolescent period (12- 14 years) include (1) rebellion, (2) preoccupation with one's body and self, (3) the vital importance of peer group, (4) marked increase in emotional and intellectual capacity and (5) experimentation. The years 15, 16 and 17 - middle adolescence—are thought to be a period of settling down. The paradox is that this period is usually one in which the teenager most adamantly rebels against parental values. Substance abuse is common. Late adolescence begins at 17 and lasts through the resolution of adolescent struggles. This is a phase of identity formation.

Erikson suggests that we look at adolescence not as a highly disorganized time of turmoil but as a crisis that is a normal phase. Anna Freud has rightly defined it. It is normal for an adolescent to behave in an inconsistent and unpredictable manner; to deny her impulses and to accept them; to love her parents and to hate them; to be deeply ashamed to acknowledge her mother before others and, unexpectedly, to desire heart to heart talks with her; to thrive on imitation of and identification with others while searching unceasingly for her own identity; to be more idealistic, artistic, generous, and unselfish than she will ever be again, but also the opposite : self-centred, egoistic and calculating. Such fluctuations between extreme opposites would be deemed highly abnormal at any other time of life. At this time, they may signify no more than that an adult structure of personality takes a long time to emerge, that the ego of the individual in question does not cease to experiment and is in no hurry to close down on possibilities.[3]

The adolescent phase of psychological maturation is a crucial and complex step in a process that continues throughout life. If later psychologic maturation is to proceed, the person must successfully resolve and complete the identity versus role confusion that is an issue in adolescence.

Common Problems Associated with Adolescence

1. Delayed sexual maturation
2. Intersex
3. Abnormal uterine bleeding
4. Dysmenorrhea
5. Pelvic pain
6. Androgens in the adolescent—hirsutism, obesity and acne
7. Sexually transmitted diseases
8. Contraception
9. Teenage pregnancy
10. Tumors

* These will be discussed in other chapters.

SUMMARY OF PUBERTAL EVENTS

The onset of puberty is an evolving sequence of maturational steps. The hypothalamic pituitary gonadal system differentiates and functions during fetal life and early infancy. Thereafter, it is suppressed to low activity levels during childhood by a combination of hypersensitivity of the "gonadostat" to estrogen, negative feedback and an intrinsic CNS inhibitor. At the onset of puberty, GnRH secretion is restored.[1]

The five main physical features of puberty include thelarche, adrenarche, growth in height, menarche and ovulation. Menarche corresponds to bone age. Psychologic changes also occur.

1. FSH and then LH levels rise moderately before the age of 10 and are followed by a rise in estradiol. An increase in LH pulses is first seen only in sleep but gradually extends throughout the day.
2. As gonadal estrogen increases (gonadarche), breast development, female fat distribution, and vaginal and uterine growth occur. Skeletal growth rapidly increases.
3. Adrenal androgen (adrenarche) and, to a lesser degree, gonadal androgen secretion, cause pubic and axillary hair growth.
4. At midpuberty, sufficient gonadal estrogen secretion results in proliferation of the endometrium and the first menses (menarche) occurs.
5. Postmenarcheal cycles are initially anovulatory. Sustained, predictable positive LH surge responses to estradiol with ovulation are late pubertal events.
6. The physical events of puberty are as important as the psychological changes.

REFERENCES

1. Speroff L, Glass RH, Kase NG. Clinical Gynecologic Endocrinology and Infertility, 6th edn, Philadelphia: Lippincott Williams and Wilkins, 1999;382.
2. Sheil O, Turner M. Adolescent gynecology. Progress in Obstetrics and Gynaecology 1996; 12: 217.
3. Lavery JP, Sanfilippo JS. Pediatric and Adolescent Obstetrics and Gynecology. New York: Springer Verlag, 1985.
4. Buyalos Jr RP. Puberty and Disorders of Pubertal Development. In Hacker NF and Moore JG (Eds): Essentials of Obstetrics and Gynecology, 3rd edn, Singapore: WB Saunders Company, 1998;572.
5. Rebar RW. Puberty. In Berek JS, Adashi EY, Hillard PA (Eds): Novak's Gynecology, 12th edn, Baltimore: Williams and Wilkins, 1996;772.
6. Edmonds KD (Ed). Dewhurst's Textbook of Obstetrics and Gynecology for Postgraduates, 6th edn, London: Blackwell Science, 1999;14.

24. *Disorders of Ovulation*

Paul Tay Yee Siang

INTRODUCTION

Ovulatory disorder is a very common gynecological problem that presents in a variety of clinical scenarios, including amenorrhea, irregular periods, and hirsutism. Serious consequences of chronic ovulatory dysfunction are infertility and increased risk of developing carcinoma of the breast and endometrium.

Normal ovulation requires the coordination of the menstrual cycle at the central hypothalamus-pituitary axis, the feedback signals and the local response within the ovaries. Any disruption to these factors at each of these levels may result in a dysfunctional state, leading to anovulation and polycystic ovaries.

The basic principles underlying the physiology of menstrual function permit the formation of several compartmental systems on which proper ovulation depends upon. It is useful to segregate the various causes of anovulation into the following compartments:

Disorder of the ovaries

Polycystic ovarian syndrome

Primary Failure

Premature ovarian failure

Resistance ovarian syndrome

Gonadal dysgenesis

Disorder of the anterior pituitary gland

Pituitary tumors (craniopharyngioma, pituitary adenoma, glioma)

Hyperprolactinemia

Disorder of hypothalamus

Hypogonadotrophic hypogonadism

Obesity

DISORDERS OF OVARIES

Polycystic Ovarian Syndrome (PCOS)

In 1935 Stein and Leventhal reported a series of seven women with bilateral polycystic ovaries and thickened ovarian cortex accompanied by amenorrhea, hirsutism, and infertility: a constellation of symptoms now known as polycystic ovary syndrome (PCOS).[1] In general, it is helpful to differentiate polycystic ovaries (PCO) from PCOS. The former specifically describes the ultrasonic appearance of the ovaries, whereas the latter term is appropriate when PCO are found in association with oligomenorrhea with the complications of hyperandrogenism.[2]

Incidence

PCOS is one of the most common endocrine disorders in gynecology and accounts for about 75% of anovulatory infertility. The prevalence of PCOS greatly depends on the criteria used to define it.

Swanson et al were the first to provide an ultrasonographic description of polycystic ovaries (PCO). Using such ultrasonographic description, 22% of unselected women have been reported to have polycystic looking ovaries.[3] However, this marker is relatively nonspecific as 25% of patients with PCO on sonography have regular menstrual cycles.[4] Moreover, not all patients with hyperandrogenic anovulation demonstrate PCO looking ovaries.[5]

Recently, a study by National Institutes of Health/ National Institute of Child Heath and Development (NIH/NICHD) has redefined the criteria using ultrasound, clinical as well as biochemical means. According to the new criteria, the prevalence of PCOS was found to be 4% in a population of 369 unselected women of reproductive age.

Definition

The classic symptoms of amenorrhea, obesity, infertility and hirsutism do not all need to be present to diagnose PCOS. Most clinicians nowadays use a working definition from a 1990 US NIH/NICHD consensus conference. To fit this definition, a patient must have ovulatory dysfunction and evidence of hyperandrogenism either clinically or by laboratory means, in the absence of other causes of hyperandrogenism (Table 24.1).

Mechanism

The mechanisms of PCOS are not completely understood but certainly multifactorial. Recently, it has become apparent that insulin resistance and compensatory hyperinsulinemia are present in a majority of women with PCOS. Growing evidence indicates that high insulin mediates the development of hyperandrogenemia with resulting anovulation and infertility (Fig. 24.1). Insulin resistance is also central to the development of hypertension, low high-density-lipoprotein-cholesterol, and obesity. Indeed, women with PCOS appear to be at increased risk for cardiovascular disease.

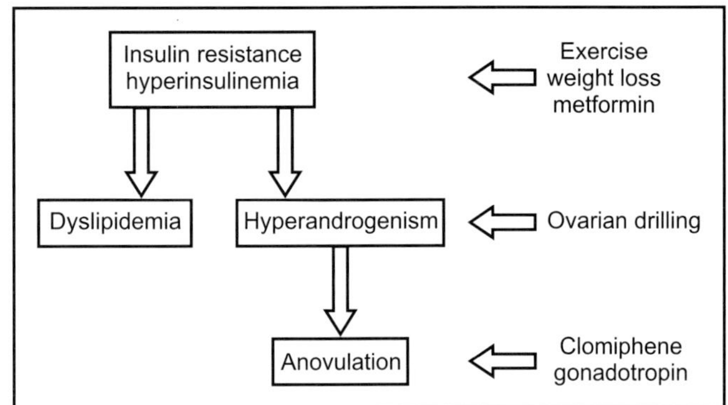

Figure 24.1: A putative paradigm of the pathophysiology of polycystic ovary syndrome

While this paradigm is not universally accepted and cannot explain each individual case of polycystic ovary syndrome, it is useful as a summary of our current understanding of the syndrome and it provides a framework for presenting currently available therapeutic options. The column on the right hand side represents various treatment available for PCOS.

Clinical Signs and Symptoms

- *Menstrual irregularity and infertility*
  66% of patients with PCOS will present with menstrual irregularity, in the form of oligomenorrhea

Table 24.1: The spectrum of clinical manifestation of polycystic ovarian syndrome[10]

Symptoms	% patients affected	Endocrine manifestation	Possible late sequelae
Obesity	38	↑ androgen (testosterone and androstenedione)	Diabetes mellitus (11%)
Menstrual disturbance	66	↑ LH	Cardiovascular disease
Hyperandrogenism	48	↑ LH: FSH ratio	Hyperinsulinemia
Infertility	73	↑ serum estrogen	Endometrial cancer
Asymptomatic	20	↑ fasting insulin	Hypertension
		↓ Sex Hormone Binding Globulin (SHBG)	

or amenorrhea. The irregular menses reflects anovulation, which in turn leads to infertility. Menstrual disturbance may occur shortly after menarche, or later on in life with increasing obesity. In women with anovulatory cycles the action of estradiol on the endometrium is unopposed because of the lack of cyclical progesterone secretion. In long term, it may result in the development of endometrial hyperplasia or malignancy.

- *Obesity*
  Obesity defined as a body mass index (BMI) greater than 25 kg/m^2 is found in 35 to 50% of women with PCOS.[6] Obesity is associated with the following alterations that interfere normal ovulation:
  a. Increase peripheral aromatization of androgens to estrogen
  b. Decreased levels of sex hormone binding globulin (SHBG) leading to a rise in free estradiol and testosterone levels
  c. Deleterious effect on glucose tolerance and increased insulin levels that can further stimulate ovarian stroma tissue production of androgens

- *Hyperandrogenism*
  One of the earliest signs of excess androgen levels is acne. Later, hirsutism develops and may lead to an increase in male hair patterns, such as alopecia. In extreme cases of androgen excess, as seen with testosterone producing tumor, virilism may occur. Virilisation may be accompanied by clitoromegaly, breast atrophy and increased muscular mass.

Investigations

- *Ultrasonography*
  The ultrasonographic description of polycystic ovaries are as follows: the presence of 10 or more cysts, 2-8 mm in diameter arranged either peripherally around a dense core of stroma (necklace sign) or scattered throughout a hyperplastic stroma, together with a increase in ovarian volume. It is important to bear in mind that *polycystic ovary is a sign, not a disease.*

- *Laboratory findings*
  Typically, serum luteinizing hormone (LH) is elevated relative to follicle stimulating hormone (FSH), often

at a ratio of 2:1. Elevated serum LH (>10 iu/l) and serum testosterone levels are commonly seen. Adrenal androgen, such as dehydroepiandrosterone sulfate (DHEA-s) may also be mildly elevated (Table 24.1).

Free testosterone accounts for 1% of total testosterone in normal women but rises to 2% of total testosterone in PCOS women. SHBG is the transport protein produced by the liver that binds testosterone and estradiol. Estrogen increases the amount of SHBG while androgen decreases SHBG levels. The increase in testosterone concentrations may reduce SHBG binding sites for the androgens, further resulting in the increased levels of free testosterone, which further decrease SHBG levels.

In addition, women with PCOS may develop insulin resistance, with elevated serum insulin. Lipid profiles are adversely affected, with increased triglycerides and LDL cholesterol and decrease in HDL cholesterol.

Management

Menstrual irregularity: The simplest way to control the menstrual cycles is to prescribe low dose combined oral contraceptive pills. This will result in an artificial cycle with regular shedding of the endometrium, hence reducing the long-term risk of endometrial cancer. An alternative is progestogens (such as medroxyprogesterone acetate or dydrogesterone) for 5 days every 1-3 months to induce a withdrawal bleed.

Obesity: Weight loss in obese patients with PCOS results in a striking improvement in ovulatory function and hyperandrogenism, largely related to amelioration of obesity-related hyperinsulinemia. Even a relatively minor loss of 5% of body weight often leads to the restoration of normal cycles. Weight loss also results in improved pregnancy rates. Exercise is independently effective in improving insulin sensitivity.

Insulin resistance: There is increasing evidence that PCOS and insulin resistance are intimately related. Metformin inhibits the production of hepatic glucose and thereby decreases insulin secretion. It would appear that Metformin does ameliorate hyperandrogenism and abnormalities of gonadotropins secretion in women with

PCOS and, thus, helps restore menstrual cyclicity and fertility.

Infertility: Ovulation can be induced with the use of anti-estrogens, such as clomiphene citrate or tamoxifen. The primary site of action is the hypothalamus where it binds to estrogen receptors, blocks the negative feedback effect of circulating estrogen and leads to an increase in gonadotropin-releasing hormone secretion.

Clomiphene citrate treatment is started on days three to five of a cycle following either spontaneous or induced bleeding with an initial daily dose of 50 mg for 5 days (Fig. 24.2). If ovulation is not achieved in the first cycle of treatment, dosage is increased to 100 mg. Thereafter, dosage is increased by increments of 50 mg up to a maximum daily dose in the range of 250 mg until ovulation is achieved. Once ovulation is achieved, conception is attempted for four to six cycles without further increasing the dose. If ovulation does not occur in three to four cycles using high doses of clomiphene citrate, the patient is considered Clomiphene resistant and should undergo gonadotrophins treatment or laparoscopic ovarian drilling.

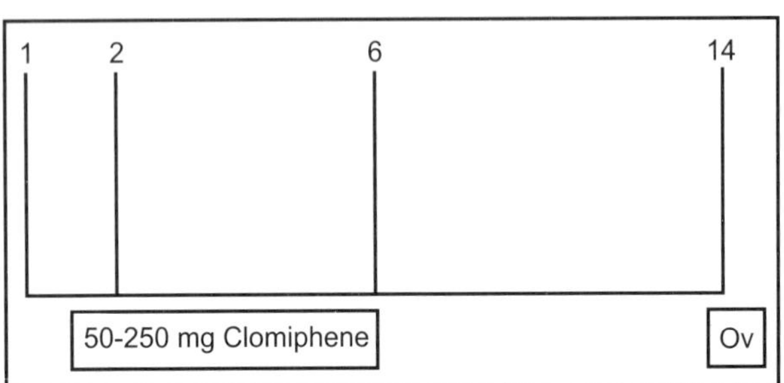

Figure 24.2: Clomiphene citrate treatment is started on days three to five of a cycle following either spontaneous or induced bleeding with an initial daily dose of 50 mg for 5 days. Ovulation (Ov) may be documented by basal body temperature charts, mid-luteal progesterone levels, or ovulation detection kits. Follicle growth may also be monitored by using ultrasound

Urinary human menopausal gonadotropin (hMG), which contains both FSH and luteinizing hormone (ratio of 1:1), is the oldest type of gonadotrophin available. In view of the batch to batch variability commonly seen in urinary preparation, the possible risk of cross infection by the use of human product and the high LH contamination, new technology have been developed to produce FSH that is produced in-vitro, under fully controlled conditions, by genetically engineered Chinese Hamster ovary cell, now called recombinant FSH (r-FSH).

Gonadotropins, while effective, are associated with a significant incidence of multiple pregnancy and ovarian hyperstimulation syndrome (OHSS). It is, therefore, extremely important to start with very low doses of gonadotropins and follicular development must be carefully monitored by ultrasound scans in order to reduce the incidence of these risks.

Laparoscopic ovarian drilling

In the initial report from Stein and Leventhal, seven women with polycystic ovaries, amenorrhea, hirsutism, and infertility were treated by bilateral ovarian wedge resection, removing one half to three quarters of each ovary. All seven women resumed menstrual cycles following surgery and three pregnancies occurred in two of these previously infertile women. However, bilateral ovarian wedge resection carried a highly significant postoperative morbidity. Many physicians had abandoned the procedure in view of the ovarian adhesion formation.

The development of operative laparoscopy has resulted in the introduction of new minimally invasive techniques designed to replace bilateral ovarian wedge resection and to reduce the incidence of post-operative morbidity. Laparoscopic ovarian drilling is introduced in an effort to decrease ovarian mass by approximately 0.5-1.0 cm^3 of tissue.[7] Electro-cautery is the modality used at laparoscopy to create thermal damage and necrosis of ovarian stroma. This technique consists of stabilizing the ovary by grasping the utero-ovarian ligament and applying unipolar needle coagulating current until the capsule has been penetrated for a total of 4-10 times in each ovary. Alternatively, laparoscopic laser delivery systems were also used successfully for the treatment of PCOS.

According to a comprehensive review,[7] the calculated ovulation rate of 84.2% and a pregnancy rate of 55.7% were obtained after laparoscopic ovarian drilling in patients with PCOS.

Primary Failures

Premature Ovarian Failure

In this condition, the ovarian follicles are depleted from the ovary before the normal age of menopause. This condition affects 1% of women under the age of 40. In majority of cases, the etiology is often unknown. Among the identifiable causes, genetic disorders (Turner's syndrome XO) predominate in those cases which present early and autoimmune disorders are more common in later onset presentation. The other causes include chemotherapy or pelvic radiotherapy.

The clinical history is usually of progressive oligomenorrhea proceeding to amenorrhea. The presence of hot flushes and night sweats may provide the only clue to the true diagnosis. The diagnosis may be confirmed by the persistent elevation of FSH and LH (>15 iu/l) and low levels of estradiol. One must bear in mind that elevated FSH and LH levels occur physiologically during the mid-cycle. Hence, at least 2 samples should be taken at 6 weeks intervals in order to make the diagnosis.

Women with premature ovarian failure are at increased risk of cardiovascular disease, cerebral vascular disease, and osteoporosis. Because of their young age, they are more likely to suffer the consequences of lack of estrogen as they will spend more years in the post-menopausal state. It is important that these patients are offered hormone replacement therapy. They should be informed that they are likely to be infertile; pregnancy, however, can be achieved by IVF using donated ovum.

Resistance Ovarian Failure

In resistance ovarian failure, the clinical presentation is very similar to those seen in premature menopause. Despite persistently raised gonadotropins, open biopsy of ovarian tissue will reveal a large number of primordial follicles, this feature distinguishes it from premature ovarian failure. In clinical practice, ovarian biopsy is not helpful; because the management and treatment is as for premature ovarian failure.

Gonadal Agenesis

Patients with this problem have chromosomal abnormalities, such as Turner's syndrome (XO) or Turner's mosaics. Women with gonadal dysgenesis have abnormal ovarian development leading to absent or streak ovaries. The number of germ cells that migrate to the ovaries during intrauterine life is reduced. These patients present with primary or secondary amenorrhea, and have persistently elevated gonadotropins.

Disorder of Anterior Pituitary

Disorder of pituitary must first focus on the problem of pituitary tumor. Pituitary tumors are usually benign. These tumors may arise from the hypothalamic area (gliomas, meningiomas, craniopharyngioma) or from the pituitary gland (pituitary adenoma) which grow in a confined space, hence, causing symptoms by compressing on the surrounding tissue and structures. Functional pituitary tumors may exert effects because of the hormones they release. The commonest of these are prolactin secreting pituitary tumors, accounting for 50% of all pituitary adenomas. The control of prolactin secretion is summarized in Figure 24.3.

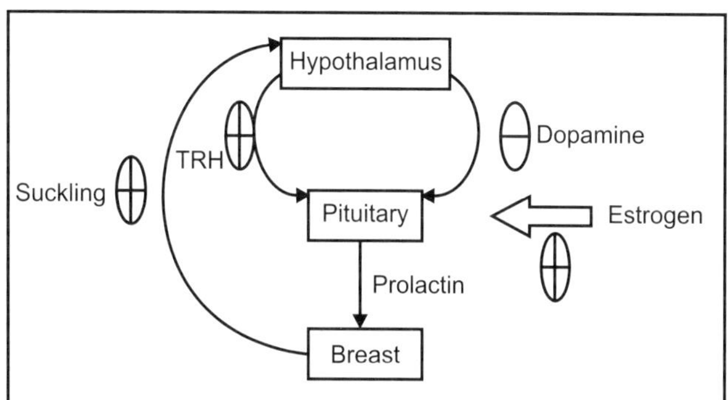

Figure 24.3: Control of prolactin release
Prolactin is controlled by the inhibition from the hypothalamus (by dopamine). Stimulatory factor of prolactin secretion includes thyroid-releasing hormone (TRH), peripheral estrogen (especially in pregnancy) and nipple reflex in response to suckling.

Hyperprolactinemia

Prolactin is secreted from the anterior pituitary gland. The pathological causes of hyperprolactinemia are summarized in Table 24.2.

Table 24.2: Pathological causes of hyperprolactinemia

1. Prolactin secreting adenoma		
2. Primary hypothyroidism	Thyroid releasing hormone (TRH) is increased in primary hypothyroidism. TRH stimulates the release of pituitary prolactin, (hyperprolactinemia).	
3. Drugs	Phenothiazines eg:	Chlorpromazine (Largectil) Prochlorperazine (Stemetil)
	Butyrephenones:	Haloperidol
	Benzamides:	Metoclopramide Cimetidine Methydopa
4. Tumor compressing the pituitary stalk or hypothalamus		

Hyperprolactinemia accounts for about 20% of patients with amenorrhea and 2% with oligomenorrhea. In amenorrheaic women, there appears to be a relationship between the degree of hyperprolactinemia and that of secondary ovarian dysfunction. High prolactin levels interfere with ovarian function by indirectly suppressing gonadotrophin secretion, hence leading to anovulation (Fig. 24.4). Galactorrhea, a typical symptom of hyperprolactinaemia, is not a reliable index. It occurs in half the patients with hyperprolactinaemic amenorrhea.

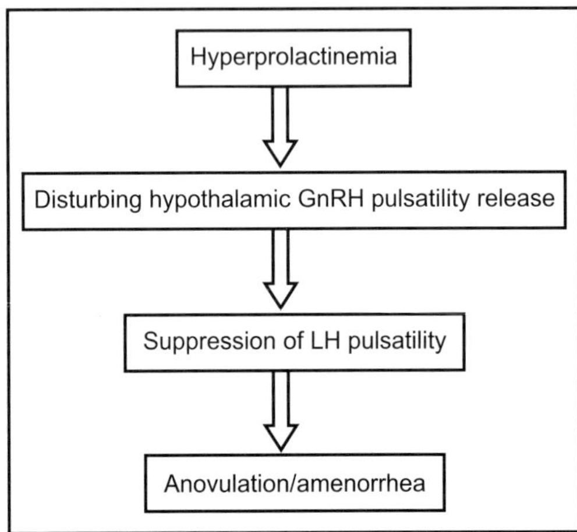

Figure 24.4: Mechanism of anovulation and amenorrhea in hyperprolactinemia

Plasma prolactin measurement is critical in assessing all women with amenorrhea. In the presence of oligomenorrhea/amenorrhea, a plasma prolactin of 800 iu/l or greater is considered to be of pathological significance. In the absence of other alternative causes, radiological examination such as computerized tomography (CT) scanning or magnetic resonance imaging (MRI) should be performed to exclude a pituitary tumor.

The treatment of choice is a dopamine agonist like bromocriptine. It is an ergot alkaloid that works in the same manner as dopamine (which is believed to be a prolactin-releasing inhibitory factor) in opposing prolactin secretion. Bromocriptine is effective in regulating menses, restoring ovulation, suppressing galactorrhea and achieving pregnancy.

The aim of treatment is to suppress prolactin to 200-300iu/l. The starting dose is 2.5 mg from once daily to three times a day. Side effects include nausea and giddiness. Side effects may be minimized by commencing medication before bedtime with small dose of drug (1.25 mg daily).

There are a few other alternative dopamine receptor agonists that can be used in cases of idiosyncratic intolerance to bromocriptine. They are Lysuride, Carbergoline and Quinagolide.

Transnasal-transphenoidal microsurgery may be used to resect micro- and macroadenoma. However, excision is often incomplete, and therefore, fails to cure the condition although prolactin levels are lower than before. Symptoms of hypopituitarism, especially diabetic insipidus, is a long-term consequence of surgery. Surgery and radiotherapy are therefore, reserved for very large tumors with suprasellar and frontal extension.

Disorder of Hypothalamus

Hypogonadotrophic Hypogonadism

Patient with hypothalamic disorder (hypogonadotrophic hypogonadism) have a deficiency in GnRH pulsatile secretion, a functional suppression of secretion, often a reflection of psychological response to stressful life events. Hypothalamic disorder is frequently seen in athletes and women with eating disorder (such as anorexia nervosa or bulimia). Women with a body mass index of less than 19 are likely to be anovulatory.

The degree of GnRH suppression determines how these patients present clinically. Mild suppression can be associated with a marginal effect on reproduction, especially inadequate luteal phase. Moderate suppression can lead to anovulation and menstrual irregularity, and profound suppression results in amenorrhea.

This hypothalamic disorder is often diagnosed by excluding pituitary and ovarian lesions. It is often characterized by low or normal gonadotrophins, normal prolactin levels, and a negative progesterone challenge test.

Patient with weight loss-related amenorrhea and anovulation should be encouraged to restore to normal reproductive function by dietary measures to increase their weight rather than resort to pharmacological stimulation of ovulation. The patients should also be counselled regarding the importance of weight by appreciating the serious endocrinological and other physical consequence of being underweight. Ovulation induction agents may only be used when the weight is increased to an optimal range.

Obesity

Body mass index of greater than 30, without any relevant pathological causes, can cause menstrual disturbance and anovulation in about 30% of over-weight women. Body fat can increase the peripheral aromatisation of androgen into estrogen, as well as decrease the levels of SHBG, resulting in the increase in free estrogen and testosterone. All these changes lead to a suppression of gonadotropins and anovulation.

There is evidence to show that weight reduction leads to improvement in menstrual function and ovulation.[8] Moreover, weight loss in obese infertile women results in better reproductive outcomes of all forms of fertility treatment.[9] Hence, weight loss should be seriously encouraged before resorting to the use of pharmacological agents to induce ovulation.

Hormonal Test

The most common method of detecting ovulation is to measure single midluteal plasma progesterone. Progesterone is secreted by corpus luteum and elevated levels are only seen in the luteal phase. Normally, progesterone levels peak at the mid luteal phase (1 week prior to the expected period). The minimal level of plasma progesterone taken to indicate ovulation within 95% confidence interval is usually accepted as

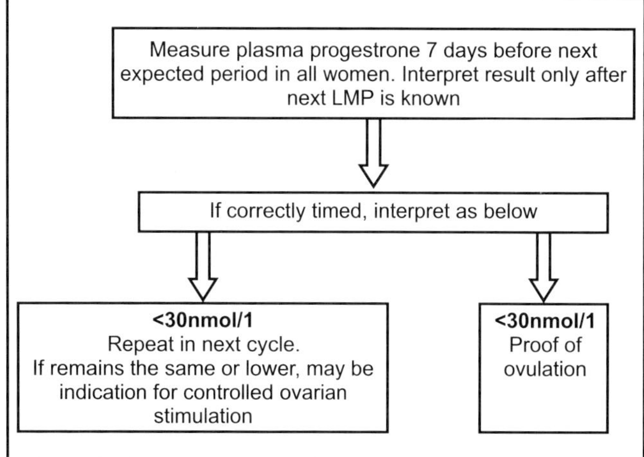

Figure 24.5: Plasma progesterone interpretation

30nmol/l. The interpretation of plasma progesterone is summarized in Figure 24.5.

REFERENCES

1. Stein IF, Leventhal ML. Amenorrhea associated with bilateral polycystic ovaries. Am J Obstet Gynecol 1935; 29:181-191.
2. Swanson M, Sauerbrei EE, Cooperberg PL. Medical implications of ultrasonically detected polycystic ovaries. J Clin Ultrasound 1981; 9:219-222.
3. Jacobs HS. Polycystic varies and polycystic ovarian syndrome. Gynecol. Endocrinol (1987); 35-44.
4. Clayton RN, Ogden V, Hodgkinson J, et al. How common are polycystic ovaries in normal women and what is their significance for the fertility of the population. Clin Endocrinol 1992; 37:127-134.
5. Adams J, Polson DW, Franks S. Prevalence of polycystic ovaries in women with anovulation and idiopathic hirsutism. Br Med J Clin Res 1986; 293:355-59.
6. Dunaif A, Segal KR, Futterweit W, et al. Profound peripheral insulin resistance, independent of obesity, in polycystic ovary syndrome. Diabetes 1989; 38: 1165-74.
7. Donesky BW, Adashi EY. Surgically induced ovulation in the polycystic ovary syndrome: wedge resection revisited in the age of laparoscopy. Fertil Steril 1995; 63:439-63.
8. Kopelman PG, White, N, Pilkington TRE, Jeffcoate, SL (1981) The effect of weight loss on sex steroid secretion and binding in massively obese women. Clinical Endocrinology 15: 113-16.
9. Clark AM, Thornley B, Tomlinson L, et al. Weight loss in obese infertile women results in improvement in repro-ductive outcome for all forms of fertility treatment. Hum Reprod 1998; 13:1502-05.
10. Balen AH, Conway GS, Kaltsas G, et al. Polycystic ovarian syndrome: the spectrum of the disorder in 1741 patients. Hum Reprod 1995; 8:2107-11.

25.
Polycystic Ovarian Disease

Pratap Kumar

INTRODUCTION

Polycystic ovarian syndrome (PCOS) is the most common endocrine disorder in women of reproductive age group, affecting 5 to 10% of women exhibiting, the full blown syndrome of hyperandrogenism, chronic anovulation and polycystic ovaries.[1] We now know that approximately 75% of anovulatory women of any cause have polycystic ovaries and 20 to 25% of women with normal ovulation demonstrate ultrasound findings typical of polycystic ovaries.[2] Chronic anovulation accompanied by hyperandrogenism and clinical manifestations including, hirsutism, acne, elevated testosterone and androstenedione, and frequently but not always obesity is seen in PCOS.[3]

PATHOPHYSIOLOGY

When compared with levels found in normal women, patients with persistent anovulation have higher mean concentration of LH, but low or low normal levels of FSH. The elevated LH levels are partly due to increased sensitivity of the pituitary to gonadotropic releasing hormone stimulation. Because the FSH levels are not totally depressed, new follicular growth is continuously stimulated, but not to the point of full maturation and ovulation, and they are in the form of multiple follicular cysts 2 to 10 mm in diameter. These follicles are surrounded by hyperplastic theca cells, often luteinized in response to high LH levels. As various follicles undergo atresia, they are immediately replaced by new follicles of similar limited growth potential.

PUBERTY AND PCOS

PCOS originates in puberty. Clinical observation teaches that PCOS often develops during adolescence. Excessive hair growth usually originates from before the onset of menstrual cycles. Menarche tends to be delayed. Irregular cycles, although considered a normal phenomenon during the first gynecological years, frequently continues into adulthood.

Mechanism of Onset of PCOS during Puberty (Fig. 25.1)

Taking into account the above remarks, the following hypothesis is postulated.[5]

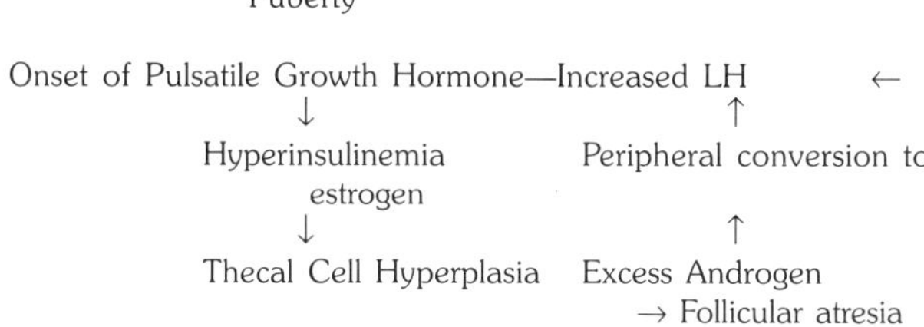

Figure 25.1: Mechanism of onset of PCOS

The onset of pulsatile growth hormone (GH) secretion during early puberty induces the release of IGF-1 (Insulin like growth factor-1) by the liver and most other tissues. GH also provokes insulin resistance, which selectively affects peripheral glucose. The resulting hyperinsulinemia acting on IGF-1 causes ovarian hyperstimulation inducing thecal cell hyperplasia and excessive androgen production. The increased androgens cause follicular atresia and increased circulating estrone levels because of peripheral conversion in adipose tissues.[5] The altered endocrine milieu provokes increased pituitary LH secretion, which aggravates the theca cell stimulation.

After puberty the insulin and IGF-1 levels progressively decline in most patients, resulting in normalization of clinical and morphological picture. Only in a few cases PCOS persists.

Insulin and the Mechanism of Anovulation in Polycystic Ovarian Syndrome

There is growing evidence that hyperinsulinemia may stimulate P 450c 17 enzyme resulting in hyperandrogenism. P 450c 17 is the key enzyme that regulates androgen synthesis.

The characteristic feature of anovulation in PCOS is the arrest of growth of antral follicles after reaching a diameter between 5 and 8 mm. This may be caused by premature activation of LH. It is well known that the syndrome is clustered in families. The sister of a woman with PCOS in such a family has a 50% risk of PCOS compared with a population prevalence of only 5 to 10%. There is evidence from family studies to support a genetic predisposition to develop PCOS[6] and insulin resistance that seem to co-exist in this syndrome.

Role of Hyperinsulinemia in the Pathogenesis of PCOS (Fig. 25.2)

Obesity, genetic predisposition and insulin receptor disorders lead to insulin resistance. Insulin resistance leads to abnormal glucose tolerance raising the blood sugar, and hyperinsulinemia. This hyperinsulinemia acts on the liver and reduces SHBG (Sex hormone binding globulin) and also increases IGF-1 (Insulin like growth factor-1). Reduction of SHBG increases the testosterone, whereas the increased IGF-1 will cause increased androgen production from ovaries. Hyperinsulinemia itself causes the theca cell hyperplasia and increased androgens.

Considering these clinical observations and invivo/ in vitro studies, it was proposed that hyperinsulinemia and hyperandrogenism, regardless of which is the primary event, is connected to PCOS.

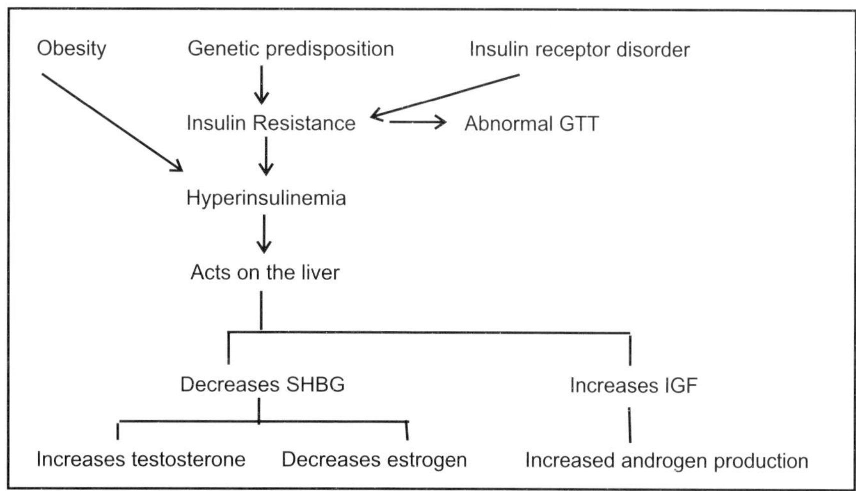

Figure 25.2: Role of hyperinsulinemia in the pathogenesis of PCOS

DIAGNOSIS

The diagnosis of PCOS is usually made on the basis of a combination of clinical, ultrasonographic and biochemical criteria. A woman presenting with oligomenorrhea is likely to have the problem of PCOS if she has one or more of these three features: polycystic ovaries on utrasound, hirsutism and hyperandrogenemia. Many women have high LH, although normal LH do not rule out the diagnosis.

In its fully developed form, PCOS is characterized by menstrual abnormalities, hirsutism, obesity, hyperandrogenemia, elevated plasma luteinizing hormone (LH) and ultrasonographic evidence of polycystic ovaries. However, thin women can also have the problem. Ultrasonographically, there should be more than 10 cysts 2 to 8 mm in diameter, scattered either around or through an echodense, thickened central stroma.[6] Indeed many women with polycystic ovaries detected by sonography do not have symptoms of the PCOS. Ovarian morphology appears to be the most sensitive marker for the PCOS compared with the classic endocrine features of a raised serum LH and /or testosterone concentration. Currently, if two of the three features of polycystic ovaries, biochemical endocrine aspects described with PCO or clinical features (of hyperandrogenesis) that are described are present, then the diagnosis of PCOS is made.

Important Clinical Features

- Hirsutism
- Oligomenorrhea
- Obesity
- USG showing
  - Subcapsular cysts

APPROACH TO INFERTILITY IN A PATIENT WITH PCOS

Women with PCOS often present to gynecologists and reproductive endocrinologists for treatment of infertility caused by anovulation. The approach to the patient with PCOS should involve the use of progressively more aggressive treatment strategies until ovulation is established and pregnancy can be achieved. Barbieri et al[8] suggested a step by step approach to ovulation induction in women with PCOS (Table 25.1).

Table 25.1: Stepwise approach to ovulation induction in PCOS

Step	Approach
1	If BMI is elevated loss of at least 5% of current body weight.
2	Ovulation induction with clomiphene citrate
3	Insulin sensitiser as a single agent (Metformin)
4	Insulin sensitiser in combination with clomiphene citrate
5	Gonadotrophin therapy
6	Insulin sensitiser in combination with gonadotrophin therapy
7	Ovarian Surgery- Laparoscopic ovarian puncture
8.	In vitro Fertilization

Weight Loss

Although obesity is not a prerequisite for the diagnosis of PCOS, it is a common feature. Almost 50% of women with PCOS have an android type of phenotype characterized by waist: hip ratio greater than 0.85(9). Obesity may induce hyperandrogenism by increasing the production of androgens, reducing sex hormone binding globulin levels (SHBG), thereby increasing free testosterone levels[10] causing hyperestrogenemia. This causes pulsatile LH secretion and/or insulin resistance and therefore, insulin secretion which could amplify the LH dependent regulatory mechanisms that regulate ovarian androgen secretion.

Increase of LH can cause a vicious cycle of hyperandrogenemia and follicular atresia. Even moderate obesity (BMI>27 kg/m^2) is associated with a reduced chance of ovulation. Obese women with PCOS (BMI>30 kg/m^2) should therefore be encouraged to lose weight. Weight loss improves the endocrine profile and a likelihood of ovulation and healthy pregnancy. Achieving weight reduction, however, is extremely difficult.

Insulin Sensitizing Agents

Improving the action of insulin is a relatively new concept in therapy. It is demonstrated that reduction of hyperandrogenism in women with PCOS may be achieved by interventions which improve insulin sensitivity and reduce circulating insulin.[11] Such measures might include, but are not limited to weight loss, dietary modifications and insulin sensitizing agents like Metformin.

Metformin[12]

Metformin (dimethyl biguanide) is an orally administered drug used to lower blood glucose concentrations in patients with NIDDM (Non insulin dependent Diabetes Mellitus) and is now also being used for infertile patients with PCOS.

Mechanism of Action of Metformin

Metformin therapy improves insulin sensitivity shown by a reduction in fasting plasma glucose and insulin concentrations. It is not effective in the absence of insulin. It decreases basal hepatic glucose output in patients

Ovulation Induction Methods

Clomiphene Citrate[13]

It acts by binding with the estrogen receptor, thus modifying the hypothalamic pituitary activity by an antiestrogen effect. This in turn diminishes the negative feedback of estrogen, activates GnRH secretion and raises the amplitude of gonadotrophin pulses.

The first line drug for the treatment of PCOS induced anovulation is clomiphene citrate. After spontaneous or progesterone induced withdrawal bleeding, the starting dose of 50 mg is given for 5 days starting on day 2, 3, 4, or 5. The patient's ovulation is usually monitored by transvaginal ultrasound from day 11, but may also be documented by basal body temperature charts, midluteal progesterone levels or ovulation detection kits. If there is a mature follicle (> 18 mm) as seen by Ultrasound, the patient can either ovulate spontaneously or it can be triggered by 5000/10,000 I.U. of hCG. The maximum dose of Clomiphene citrate should not exceed 150- mg/day. If the dose required is more than this, it is generally considered as a clomiphene non responder.

Human Menopausal Gonadotrophin[14]

This is the second line of treatment. Purified FSH has a theoretical advantage of avoiding additional LH in PCOS, which often have elevated LH levels. The complications of ovarian hyperstimulation syndrome has to be borne in mind when gonadotrophins are used which could lead to enlargement of ovaries with ascitis, vomiting and electrolyte imbalance and may progress to severe problems. The dose of 75 IU per day is used for about a week, which also requires monitoring, by Ultrasound for the response.

GnRH Therapy

Women with elevated baseline or mid follicular LH levels have higher rates of anovulation, ovulation without conception, and early pregnancy loss than normal controls.[15] It has been hypothesized that by suppressing the pituitary with a GnRH analogue before ovulation induction it will reduce the LH. But both LH and FSH will get reduced. Hence more of gonadotrophins have to be given for ovulation induction later.

Surgical Induction of Ovulation

In 1939 after removing wedges of ovarian tissue for pathologic analysis, Stein and Cohen observed that ovulatory function and regular menses were restored. For years, ovarian, wedge resection via laparotomy was standard therapy for infertile women with PCOS until it was observed that, although ovulation was restored, postoperative adhesions were high and this caused mechanical infertility. Medical treatments replaced surgery for PCOS induced infertility. With the development of laparoscopic and microsurgical techniques, the possibility of a single minimally invasive operation as a potential treatment for PCOS restored interest in surgical operations. Techniques such as multiple biopsies and ovarian "drilling" by laparoscopic cautery or laser vaporization on one or both ovaries have been used to restore ovulation and a more normal hormonal environment. Other potential benefits of surgical treatment are lower cost, avoidance of risk of ovarian hyperstimulation and lower rates of pregnancy loss (~15%) and multiple gestation (~2% twin pregnancies) in comparison with pharmacologic treatment.[16] The rates of ovulation and pregnancy with surgical treatment are at least comparable with the rates achieved medically (approximately 80% and 50% respectively). Surgical treatment is probably most effective in the first year after operation when conception rates are highest.

SUMMARY

Polycystic Ovarian Syndrome is a disorder of unknown cause characterized by anovulation, hyperandrogenism, hyperinsulinemia and/or obesity. There is a great individual variation. Restoring fertility can be challenging since not all patients with this problem respond satisfactorily to ovulation induction. Weight loss and the use of insulin sensitizers may benefit the individuals.

REFERENCES

1. Dunaif A. Hyperandrogenic anovulation (PCOS): A unique disorder of insulin action associated with an increased risk of non-insulin-dependent diabetes mellitus. Am J Med 1995; 98(IA): 33S-39S.
2. Polson DW, Adams J, Wadsworth J, Franks S. Polycystic ovaries—a common finding in normal women. Lancet 1988; 16:1(8590): 870-72.
3. Franks S: Polycystic ovary syndrome N Engl J Med 1995; 333: 853-61
4. Frank Nobels, MD, Didier Dewailly, MD. Puberty and polycystic ovarian syndrome: the insulin/insulin-like growth factor I hypothesis. Fertil Steril 1992; 58: 655-66.
5. Joseph T McKenna. Current concepts: Pathogenesis and treatment of Polycystic Ovary Syndrome. N Eng J Med 1988; 318(9):558-62.
6. Anna Krook, Sudhesh Kumar, Ian Laing, Andrew Jm, M Boulton, John AH. Wass and Stephen O'Rahilly. Molecular scanning of the insulin receptor gene in syndromes of insulin resistance. Diabetes 1994;43:357-68
7. Adams J, Franks S, Polson DW et al. Multifollicular ovaries: clinical and endocrine features and response to pulsatile gonadotrophin-releasing hormone. Lancet 1985;ii:375-84
8. Lena H Kim, Ann E Taylor, Robert L Barbieri. Insulin sensitizers and polycystic ovary syndrome: Can a diabetes medication treat infertility? Fertil and Steril 2000; 73(6): 1097-98.
9. Lefebvre P, J Bringer, E Renard, F Boulet, S Clouet, C Jaffiol. Influences of weight, body fat patterning and nutrition on the management of PCOS. Hum Reprod 1997; 12 Suppl 1: 73-81.
10. Stephen R Plymate, Bruce L Fariss, Martin L Bassett, Louis Matej. Obesity and its role in polycystic ovary syndrome. J Clin Endocrinol Metab 1981; 52: 1246.
11. John E Nestler. Insulin regulation of human ovarian androgens. Hum Reprod 1997; 12 Suppl 1: 53-61.
12. Clifford J Bailey, Robert C Turner. Metformin. N Eng J Med 1996; 334(9): 574-578.
13. John D Isaacs, Jr, Stephen R Lincoln, Bryan D Cowan. Extended clomphene citrate (CC) and prednisone for the treatment of chronic anovulation resistant to CC alone. Fertil Steril 1997; 67: 641-43.
14. Loughlin T, S Cunningham, A Moore, M Culliton, PPA Smyth, TJ. Mckenna. Adrenal abnormalities in polycystic ovary syndrome. J Clin Endocrinol Metab 1996; 62: 142-47.
15. Stefano Venturoli, Roberto Paradisi, Raffaella Fabbri, Otello Magrini, Eleonora Porcu, Carlo Flamigni. Comparison Between Human Urinary Follicle-Stimulating Hormone and Human Menopausal Gonadotropin Treatment in Polycystic Ovary. Obstet Gynecol 1984; 63: 6.
16. Damario MA, Barmat L, HC Liu, Davis OK, Rosenwaks Z. Dual suppression with oral contraceptives and gonadotrophin releasing-hormone agonists improves in-vitro fertilization outcome in high responder patients. Hum Reprod 1997; 12 (11): 2359-65.

26. *Hirsutism*

Muralidhar V Pai

DEFINITION

Hirsutism is defined as conversion of villus hair to terminal hair in a masculine pattern on the upper lip, chin, chest, back and/or thighs of female. Androgens promotes the conversion of villus hair, which is fine and lightly pigmented, to terminal hair, which is coarse and darkly pigmented. Non-sexual terminal hair occurs in both men and women in the scalp, eyebrows and eyelashes. During puberty, villus hair is converted to terminal hair in the axilla, legs, forearms and lower pubic triangle (ambo-sexual hair) in both sexes. In adult men, androgens cause terminal hair growth in other areas such as the upper lip, chin and inter-gluteal region.

HYPERTRICHOSIS

Hypertrichosis is the term reserved to describe androgen-independent growth of hair, which is villus, prominent in areas, such as the forehead, forearms or legs, and does not grow in a male pattern of distribution. It is most commonly congenital or caused by metabolic disorders (e.g. hypothyroidism, anorexia nervosa, porphyria cutanea tarda), or medications (e.g. phenytoin, minoxidil, cyclosporine, diazoxide, excess of glucocorticoids) or by starvation.

Excess hair in a non-androgen dependent distribution may have an ethnic or racial basis for which medical treatment is inappropriate.

PATHOPHYSIOLOGY

The pathophysiology of hirsutism is best understood in the context of the physiology of normal hair growth. The number of hair follicles is fixed before birth. They cover the entire body except for the palms, lips, and the soles.

Normal women rarely have terminal hair on the upper back or upper abdomen. Thus, the type and distribution of the excess hair is important in the diagnosis of hirsutism. The amount of terminal hair increases with age. Women gradually develop more facial and body hair with age.

Hirsutism in itself is not a disease but rather a cutaneous manifestation of hyperandrogenism. It may rarely be a manifestation of a serious underlying disorder, most often resulting from a combination of increased androgen production (compared to non-hirsute women) and increased sensitivity to androgens. Hirsutism is usually associated with other hyperandrogenic conditions like alopecia, seborrhea and acne. Obesity is a common but not universal finding in women with hirsutism caused by the polycystic ovary syndrome. It may be associated with *acanthosis nigricans*, a consequence of marked insulin resistance. In this condition, the skin is thickened and hyperpigmented, characteristically in the neck and axilla and also in flexures, over the knees, elbows and vulva. Hyperandrogenism (HA), insulin resistance (IR), and acanthosis nigricans (AN) is together termed as *HAIR-AN syndrome.*

The major androgens of biological importance are Testosterone (T) and its metabolite dihydrotestosterone (DHT); this metabolite is more potent and is produced in the skin by conversion of T by the enzyme 5-α reductase. Dihydrotestosterone is more potent than T primarily because of its higher affinity for and slower dissociation from the androgen receptor.

Most hirsute patients have elevated androgen levels upon thorough evaluation. If only urinary 17-ketosteroids are measured; only 15% of hirsute women will have elevated values. If total plasma testosterone is measured, about 40% of hirsute patients are found to have an elevated level. If total plasma levels of several androgenic hormones and prehormones-testosterone, DHT, DHEAS, androstenedione, and 17-hydroxyprogesterone are measured, approximately 90% of hirsute women will have elevated values of one or more hormones. Free testosterone is elevated in about 50% of cases.

Hirsute women with polycystic ovary syndrome have higher insulin levels than those with polycystic ovary syndrome alone, and there is a significant correlation between plasma insulin concentration and plasma testosterone or androstenedione levels.[1]

Prolactin may increase adrenal androgen secretion. Hirsutism and acne have been reported in about 20% of women with prolactin-secreting microadenomas. Hyperprolactinemia also affects androgen metabolism.[2]

Hirsutism and virilisation occurring during menopause or pregnancy involve a somewhat different differential diagnosis. Androgen levels generally fall during the menopause, so estrogen deficiency may play a role in these cases. Postmenopausal virilisation may be due to hyperthecosis or hilar cell hyperplasia. Virilisation during pregnancy is usually due to various manifestations of ovarian over-stimulation by HCG[3]

ETIOLOGY

Hyperandrogenism may result from multiple causes. They may be divided into endocrine and non-endocrine causes as follows.

Endocrine Causes

	FUNCTIONAL	NEOPLASTIC
OVARIAN	Polycystic ovary syndrome (PCOS)	Sex cord stromal tumor Arrhenoblastoma Lipoid cell tumor Luteoma
ADRENAL	Congenital adrenal hyperplasia Idiopathic adrenal hyperandrogenism	Adrenal adenoma Adrenal carcinoma
PITUITARY	Cushing's disease Acromegaly Hyperprolactinemia	

Non-endocrine Causes:

1. Racial
2. Familial
3. Idiopathic
4. Iatrogenic (drugs):

Functional hirsutism

Phenytoin
Diazoxide cause **hypertrichosis**
Minoxidil
Cyclosporin
Androgenic progestins e.g.: norethisterone, levonorgestrel
Danazol
Corticosteroids

The most common cause of hirsutism is idiopathic or polycystic ovary syndrome (PCOS). Androgen-producing ovarian tumors are an uncommon cause of hirsutism and virilization. The underlying defect leading to hyperandrogenism in idiopathic hirsutism remains to be identified.

DIAGNOSIS

The medical evaluation should be directed at ruling out serious underlying disorder. This can often be

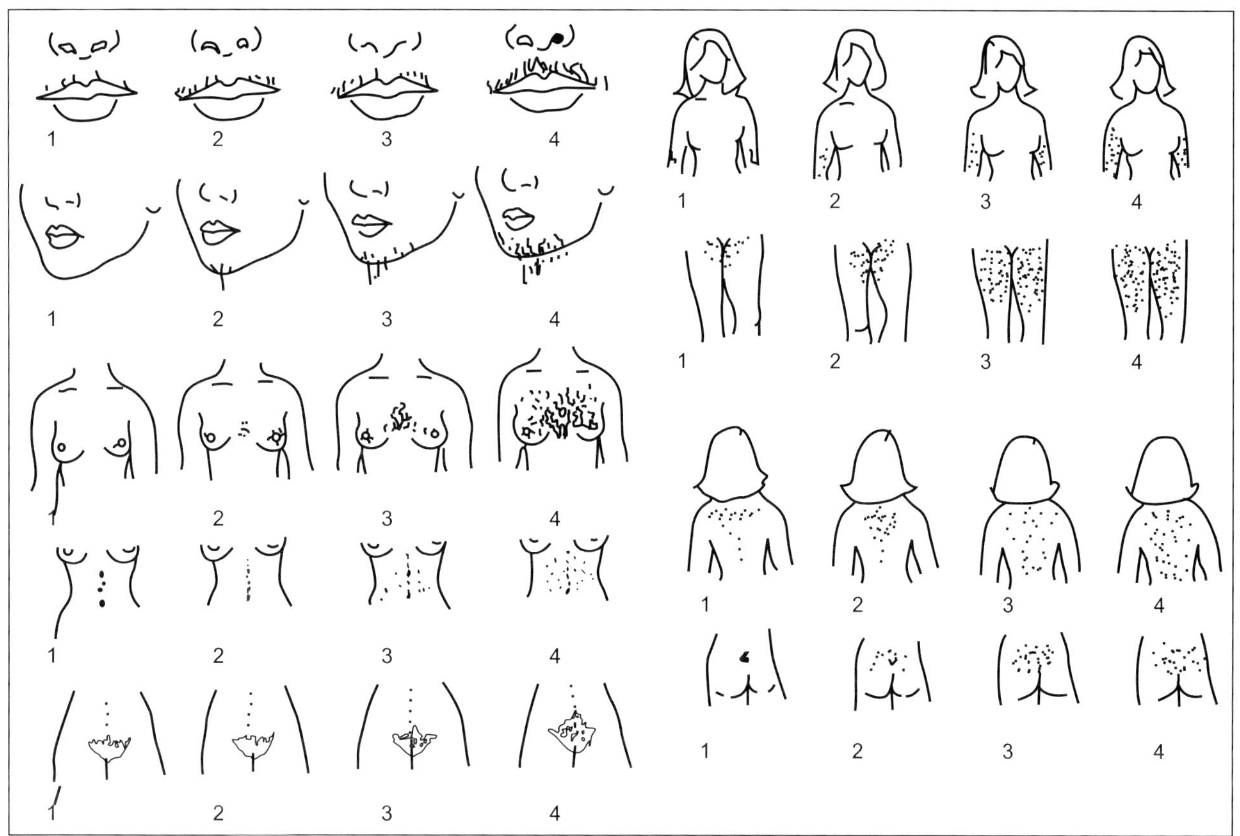

Figure 26.1: Ferriman and Gallwey scoring system

accomplished by evaluating patient's history, clinical examination and few basic hormonal investigations.

History of familial hirsutism, oligomenorrhea, amenorrhea, galactorrhea, symptoms of thyroid dysfunction, intake of drugs such as androgens, anabolic agents, Danazol or 19-nortestosterone derivatives should be noted.

The *severity of hirsutism* is determined according to modified Ferriman and Gallwey scoring system[4] (Fig. 26.1). With this system 9 body areas that contain hormone-sensitive hair were graded from 0 (no terminal hair) to 4 (frank virilisation). The grade for each area is added (maximum possible score = 36). A score of 8 or more was established as the threshold for hirsutism. A total score of 8 or more is seen in only 5% of premenopausal women.

Other signs of hyperandrogenism like acne, alopecia, seborrhea or acanthosis nigricans should be looked for.

The *presence of virilisation*, which may include clitoromegaly, temporal baldness, breast involution, hoarseness of voice and male-pattern muscular development, alerts the clinician to the possibility of a neoplastic etiology. In general, neoplasm can be excluded when masculinization is absent.

Hyperprolactinemia may be suspected by demonstrating galactorrhea.

Drug-induced hirsutism (other than that caused by androgens) consists of an increase in lanugo-like hair that is not restricted to androgen-dependent areas of the body.

Other signs on physical examination may indicate a specific endocrine disorder such as *Cushing's syndrome*.

An abdominopelvic examination should be done to look for any palpable ovarian or adrenal tumor. Although adrenal adenomas can be quite small, most adrenal carcinomas are large by the time they cause symptoms; half are palpable abdominally. About half of ovarian tumors are palpable on pelvic examination. *Functioning ovarian tumors* are almost always palpable.[5]

Abdominopelvic ultrasound is the key investigation when PCOS is suspected. Routine MRI, selective venous catheterization, or extensive hormonal analysis is not required. More extensive investigation is required only if an androgen secreting tumor is suspected by history or basic investigations.

Estimation of FSH, LH, PRL, Testosterone (T) and TSH are advocated routinely in all cases of hirsutism. Measurement of serum DHEAS is not required, because its concentration does not change the therapeutic approach as long as T levels are within 2 ng/ml.[6] Urinary 17-ketosteroids (KS) are of little or no use in the evaluation. Although DHEAS is its major contributor, nonandrogen steroids and nonsteroid chromogens also contribute significantly to urinary 17-KS production. Only gross elevations of 17-KS (>30 ng/24 hr) reliably reflect pathology.

Urinary free cortisol level is measured only if Cushing's disease is suspected. If elevated, an overnight dexamethasone suppression test is indicated. Basal insulin level and the insulin response to a glucose load should be measured if insulin resistance is suspected.

TREATMENT

Patients' distress is the prime indication for therapy. Apart from the rare circumstance when a tumor is present, surgery does not play a role in the management of hirsutism. Most women respond to medical therapy. It is easier to prevent hair growth than to treat established hirsutism. Adolescent girls who are beginning to develop hirsutism and who have a family history of excessive hair growth are excellent candidates for medical therapy.

Non-surgical treatment can be classified as:
1. Cosmetic
2. Weight control
3. Pharmacological treatment
4. Psychological management

Cosmetic measures like bleaching, depilation, epilation (plucking, shaving) and electrolysis are of great value. It is possible, but unsubstantiated, that such treatments are more beneficial overall than endocrine manipulation. Medical method does not remove hair already present, nor does medical therapy completely prevent hair growth.

Weight control is essential for the control of hirsutism. Weight loss has been shown experimentally to lower insulin resistance and consequently to reduce serum insulin concentrations.[7]

Pharmacological intervention slows the growth of new hair but does not lead to loss of established hair. It is a preventative measure and is thus, most effective when initiated in the younger patient and combined with cosmetic measurers.

The selection of a pharmacological agent depends on the severity of the hirsutism, patient preference and the need to treat associated conditions such as hypertension or oligomenorrhea. The latter will require correction either because of the development of endometrial hyperplasia or because induction of ovulation is needed to treat infertility. The dosage of drugs used to treat hirsutism should be the lowest, which is effective, although high doses of medication may be required initially to induce remission of hair growth. Most drugs, nevertheless, have a shallow dose-response relationship, and maximal doses are often only slightly more effective than midrange doses.

Women must have a clear understanding that medication does not offer a permanent cure and benefit may be lost when treatment is stopped. Women should also be aware that antiandrogen medication couldn't be used while fertility is being pursued.

Typically, long standing facial hirsutism responds slowly to medical treatment even if androgens are suppressed to undetectable levels. When starting a medication, it may take as long as 6 months for a woman to note an improvement, especially if she is not mechanically removing hair at the same time. If after 6 months of medical therapy no improvement is seen or unacceptable hirsutism remains, either a higher dose or a second medication should be used.

Most pharmacological therapies fall into two major categories:
1. Suppression of androgen secretion.
   Ovarian
      Combined oral contraceptive pill
      GnRH analogues
      Ketaconazole

Adrenal
> Glucocorticoids

2. Antiandrogens
> Androgen receptor antagonists
>> Cyproterone acetate
>> Spironlactone
>> Flutamide
> 5α-reductase inhibitors
>> Finasteride

Suppression of androgen excess alone does not cure hirsutism, but must be coupled with an anti-androgen.[8]

Treatment with OCP is unsatisfactory in several hirsute women, including PCOS patients, because it only partially inhibits gonadotropin secretion.[9] The GnRH-a is too cumbersome and expensive to find a role as first line therapy in the treatment of hirsutism. Moreover, use of GnRH-a can be complicated by side effects such as headache, depression, breast tenderness and fatigue. Glucocorticoid therapy (dexamethasone, prednisolone or betamethasone) decreases serum androgen concentrations by suppressing ACTH-mediated adrenal secretion. But the clinical efficacy of glucocorticoids in hirsute women has been a subject of much debate.

The imidazole derivative, ketoconazole, in addition to its antifungal properties, was found to inhibit several enzymes involved in adrenal and gonadal steroid synthesis. This causes a fall in gonadal androgen synthesis without an associated fall in adrenal cortisol. There is also serum testosterone fall along with SHBG rise. On this basis, ketoconazole would seem a rational choice of drug to use for the treatment of hirsutism. Doses of ketoconazole ranging from 400-1200 mg/day were used. Although antiandrogen effects are dose dependent, starting with a low dose is recommended because of side effects.[10]

Spironolactone is a steroid and its use is widespread in North America. The clinical efficacy of spironolactone is dose dependent.[12] It is generally used in doses of between 25 and 200 mg daily with treatment being commenced at 25-50 mg. Most patients require at least 100 mg to achieve a satisfactory response. Spirono-lactone works best in ovulatory women with normal testosterone levels. In women with PCOS, the addition of an oral contraceptive improves response rates. Side effects are also dose-related.

Cyproterone acetate is one of the most commonly used antiandrogen in European countries. Cyproterone acetate is a potent progestogen that is derived from 17α-hydroxyprogesterone and has moderately potent antiandrogenic peripheral activity and is a weak glucocorticoid.[12] It is generally well tolerated, but can be associated with gastrointestinal upset and breast engorgement.

Flutamide (4'-nitro-3'-trifluoromethylisobutyranilide) is a potent, nonsteroidal antiandrogen devoid of hormone agonist activity,[13] which compete with the binding of testosterone and dihydrotestosterone to the target tissues. Because of its antiandrogen activity, Flutamide recently has been proposed for women as a therapeutic approach to hirsutism.

Motta et al[14] were among the first one to suggest that **250 mg of Flutamide once a day** for 6 months could be effective for most patients with hirsutism. They found a reduction of up to 50% in hair growth. No side effects were noted, and there were no abnormalities in hepatic, renal, or hematological function.

Finasteride inhibits 5α -reductase activities, blocking dihydrotestosterone production, thus peripherally decreasing the amount of hormone available for interaction with androgen receptors without altering ovarian and adrenal testosterone secretion. The drug has a good safety profile. Doses of up to 400 mg daily have been given to men without serious adverse effects, but also with no greater reduction in serum dihydrotestosterone levels.

The educational and psychotherapeutic aspects of treating hirsutism should not be under valued. The presence of unwanted hair in a masculine distribution may conflict with a woman's concept of her femininity and so distort her self-image. Fears regarding gender identity may need to be addressed and dispelled.

The patient's perception of the severity of her hirsutism should be assessed. Even mild degree of hirsutism can undermine confidence and lead to disproportionate self-consciousness. This may lead to social withdrawal and interfere with interpersonal relationships to such an extent that psychotherapeutic intervention may be warranted. It has been documented that anxiety and depression are common in the polycystic ovary syndrome. Associated fears regarding potential fertility may remain unexpressed and it is important to address this issue if appropriate to the clinical context.

REFERENCES

1. Barbieri RL, Makris A, Randall RW, Daniels G, Kistner RW, Ryan KJ. Insulin stimulates androgen accumulation in incubations of ovarian stroma obtained from women with hyperandrogenism. J Clin Endocrinol Metab 1985; 62:904.
2. Barnes RB. Adrenal dysfunction and hirsutism. Clin Obstet Gynecol 1991; 4: 827.
3. Braithwaite SS, Erkman-Balis B, Avila TD. Postmenopausal virilization due to ovarian stromal hyperthecosis. J Clin Endocrinol Metab 1978; 46: 295.
4. Ferriman D, Gallwey JD. Clinical assessment of hair growth in women. J Clin Endocrinol Metab 1961; 21: 1440.
5. Speroff L, Glass RH, Kase NG. Hirsutism. In Charles Mitchell (Eds): Clinical Gynecologic Endocrinology and Infertility, 5th edn. Williams and Wilkins, 1994; 501.
6. Rittmaster RS. Medical Treatment of Androgen-Dependent Hirsutism. J Clin Endocrinol Metab. 1995; 80: 2559.
7. Franks S. Polycystic ovary syndrome: A changing perspective. Clin Endocrinol. 1989; 31: 87.
8. Eden JA. Hirsutism. In: John Studd (Ed): Progress in obstetrics and gynecology. Churchill Livingstone 1991; 9: 319.
9. Hancock KW, Levell MJ. Use of estrogen/progestogen preparation in the treatment of hirsutism in female. J Obstet Gynecol Br Commonwealth 1974; 81: 804.
10. Schriock EA, Schriock ED. Treatment if Hirsutism. Clin Obstet Gynecol 1991; 4: 852.
11. Lobo RA, Shoupe D, Seafini P, Brinton D, Horton R. The effects of two doses of spironolactone on serum androgens and anagen hair in hirsute women. Fertil Stril 1985; 43: 200.
12. Belisle S, Love EJ. Clinical efficacy and safety of cyproterone acetate in severe hirsutism: results of a multicentric Canadian study. Fertil Steril 1986; 46: 1015.
13. Sogani PC, Vagaiwala MR, Withmore WF. Experience with Flutamide in patients with advanced prostatic cancer without prior endocrine therapy. Cancer 1984; 54: 744.
14. Motta T, Maggi G, Perra M, Azzolari E, Casazza S, D'Alberton A. Flutamide in the treatment of hirsutism. Int J Gynecol Obstet 1991; 36: 155.

27.

Muralidhar V Pai

Intersex

INTRODUCTION

One of the responsibilities of the obstetrician is the assignment of sex to the newborn. Sexual differentiation and subsequent normal development are fundamental to the continuation of the human species. If the external genitalia of the newborn are ambiguous (with respect to complete male or female development), a profound dilemma is faced. An incorrect assignment of sex threatens grave psychological and social problems for the baby and family. So every obstetrician must be well versed with the problem and be able to establish the diagnosis.

SEXUAL DIFFERENTIATION OF THE FETUS

Genetic sex is determined by the presence or absence of the Y chromosome. The Y chromosome determines the development of testes and maleness (Fig. 27.1). The Y chromosome contains a *sex-determining region* (the SRY gene), which encodes the *testis-determining factor* (TDF). The genetic sex is independent of the ovum. If the ovum is fertilized by an X spermatozoa (22 + X-chromosomes) the offspring is XX, a female and if it is fertilized by a Y spermatozoa (22 + Y-chromosomes) the offspring is XY, a male.

Phenotypic sex is genital sex whether apparent female or apparent male.

Gonadal sex is determined by the presence of normal *ovaries* or *testes*. It is clear that male phenotype sexual differentiation is directed by the function of the fetal testis. In the absence of the testis, female differentiation ensues irrespective of the genetic sex.

Sex differentiation in the embryo usually hormonises with the *sex genotype*, but hormonal disturbances can lead to abnormalities. Proliferation of non-germinal and germinal cells in the *genital ridge* creates the gonadal *primordia*, which develops into a cortex surrounding the medulla. Until the 7th week of gestation, each sex has a bipotential system (the sexual indifferent stage) with both Wolffian and müllerian ducts. The *urogenital sinus* develops into the external genitals in both females and males.

Around the 7th week, the medulla of the primitive gonad begins to differentiate into a *testis,* if a *Y chromosome* is present. As the testes grow and their Leydig cells start to produce testosterone, the *Wolffian ducts* develop into the male reproductive tract (epididymis, vas deferens, seminal vesicles and the ejaculatory ducts), whereas the *müllerian ducts* regress. Testosterone stimulates the growth and differentiation of the Wolffian ducts in the male. The regression of the müllerian ducts is caused by the *antimüllerian hormone* from the Sertoli cells.

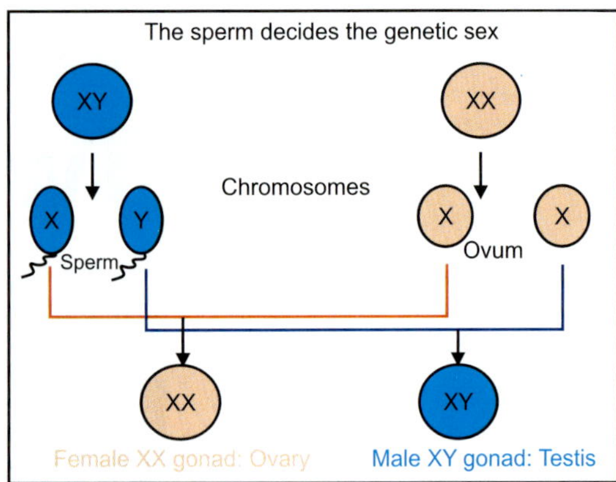

Figure 27.1: The sperm decides the genetic sex

Conversely, in the female, the cortex of the indifferent gonads differentiate into *ovaries*, if only two X chromosomes are present and no Y. In the female fetus, where there is a developing ovary and no antimüllerian hormone, the müllerian ducts develop into the female reproductive tract (the uterine tubes, uterus and the upper vagina), and the Wolffian ducts degenerate because the ovary does not secrete testosterone. When a normal female fetus is exposed to androgens during the period of differentiation of the external genitalia, an *apparent male* can result.

Visible differentiation of the gross anatomy does not appear until late in the second month of embryonic life. Testosterone causes the *differentiation* of the fetus to a male. The fetal genital tract will always develop into female genitals, if unexposed to embryonic testicular secretion. The *genital sex* is a phenotypic female. If testosterone is present, male external sex organs develop and the *genital tubercle* elongates to form the male phallus. If testosterone is absent, female organs develop instead. It is the action of *testosterone* and 5-α-dihydrotestosterone on the urogenital sinus that is behind the normal development of the male external genitalia. In the last months of gestation the growth of the external genitalia depends upon fetal pituitary luteinizing hormone (LH).

DEFINITION OF INTERSEX

Intersexuality may be defined as the presence of both male and female external and or internal genital organs in the same individual causing confusion in the diagnosis of true sex. The incidence is about 2 per 1000.

Intersex problems may be grouped under following subdivisions.

Genetic Sex Disturbances

Turner's Syndrome

In 1938, Turner described a syndrome in small persons, retarded in growth and in sexual development. They are apparent females with small or no ovaries and a *XO chromosomal karyotype*. Since they have only one sex chromosome (X), their total chromosome number is 45. The *Turner patient* lacks the inputs from two active X chromosomes and from a Y chromosome. The lack of anti-müllerian hormone and testosterone leads to müllerian duct development and female genitals, but the ovary is just a fibrous streak devoid of germ cells. The Turner patients have no sex chromatin and no drumstick (Fig. 27.2).

The syndrome is characterized by short stature (mean adult height 141 + 0.6 cm) and poor development of secondary sex characters. They are mentally retarded. Other physical findings associated with classical forms of gonadal dysgenesis include: epicanthal folds, high arched palate, low nuchal hairline, webbed neck, shield chest, coarctation of the aorta, ventricular septal defect, renal anomalies, pigmented nevi, nail hypoplasia, cubitus valgus, and short fourth metacarpal. These patients usually will have primary amenorrhea. Hypertension is relatively common in adults with the disorder. They also frequently have autoimmune thyroid disorders (Hashimotos thyroiditis).

The disorder is a result of accelerated oocyte atresia in which these women undergo menopause before they enter puberty. Both X chromosomes are required for female germ cell survival. Because of oocyte atresia ovarian development is altered and sex steroid secretion is deficient resulting in elevated FSH levels consistent with menopause. Additionally, the deficiency of the X chromosome results in abnormalities of skeletal structures; epiphyses, teeth, and skull. These patients also have an unusual cognitive defect, which renders them unable to appreciate the shapes and relationships of objects to each other (space-form blindness). While Turner's syndrome (45, X) is the sine quo non of

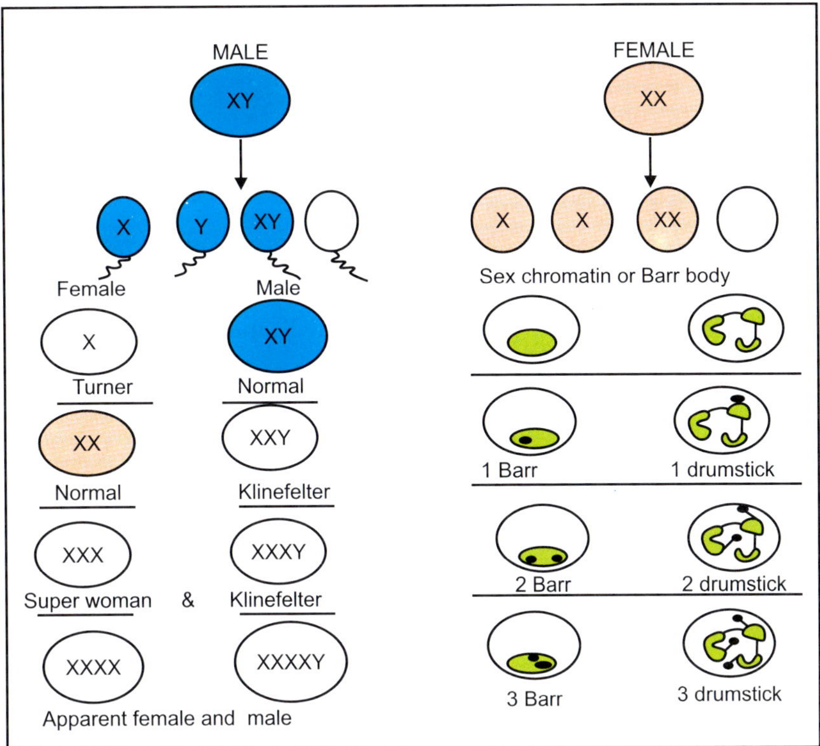

Figure 27.2: Intersex syndromes

gonadal dysgenesis and is the chromosomal-complement found by pediatricians in 80% of young women manifesting these signs and symptoms, only 40% of women presenting with primary amenorrhea have the 45, X complement. The remainders are divided between 46, XX or 46, XY (40%) or X-chromosome structural abnormalities or mosaicism (20%). Approximately 20-30% of patients with 46, XY gonadal dysgenesis develop a dysgerminoma or gonadoblastoma; therefore gonads should be removed from individuals with 46, XY gonadal dysgenesis.

Klinefelter Syndrome

In 1942, Klinefelter described a syndrome in persons appearing as men. These males are tall, have long extremities, and an eunuchoidal appearance with gynecomastia, have small dysgenetic testes, and they are sterile. Their cells contain XXY chromosomes (47 instead of the normal 46). Thus, Klinefelter patients must have one sex chromatin and one drumstick just like normal females (Fig. 27.2). These *phenotypic XXY-males* have significantly higher LH and FSH, and lower blood (testosterone) than matched XY controls. The

seminiferous tubule development and spermatogenesis are deficient in Klinefelter males. The XXY-males did not show more feminine behavior than matched controls. A similar group of tall males with *XYY chromosomes* were not extraordinarily masculine. Some XYY-males have significantly higher (testosterone) in their blood than matched XY controls.

Hermaphrodites

A very small number of individuals end up being of *indeterminate gonadal sex* (i.e. has both ovarian and testicular tissues present). Some persons have an ovary on one side and a testis on the other—a *true hermaphrodite*. In the Greek mythology *Hermaphrodites* was the child of Hermes and the beautiful Aphrodite. *Pseudo-hermaphrodites* have external genitals from both sexes, but only one gonadal sex. Males have normal XY chromosomes, but small testes with poor sperms (poor spermatogenesis). An enzyme defect that blocks the conversion of testosterone to *5-a-dihydrotestosterone* disturbs the development of the external genitals. Female hermaphrodites have ovaries, female ducts, XX chromosomes, and varying degrees of masculine differentiation of the external genitals. Any XY individual with a genetic defect in testosterone synthesis develops testes due to the presence of the Y chromosome, and müllerian duct regression due to the presence of antimullerian hormone. The Wolffian duct does not develop normally, because of the testosterone deficiency.

True hermaphroditism is a rare condition and makes up less than 10% of all intersex cases. More than 400 cases have been reported worldwide.

True hermaphrodites have ambiguous genitalia at birth. The majority of affected individuals have been reared as males. However, because of functioning, normal ovarian tissue, most true hermaphrodites experience breast development at puberty, and 40% with a 46, XX peripheral karyotype menstruate. Some of these genetic (XY) boys are born as apparent girls, but they may change from female to male at puberty if the penis grows.

Aside from the physical and emotional consequences associated with genital ambiguity, patients with true hermaphroditism usually do not possess other developmental malformations. These individuals usually possess average intelligence and in general have a normal life expectancy.

Gonadal tumors with malignant potential occur in 2.6% of all true hermaphrodites. Dysgerminomas, seminomas, gonadoblastomas, and yolk sac carcinomas have been reported. Benign tumors including mucinous cystadenomas, benign teratomas, and Brenner tumors have also been reported.

Cryptomenorrhea, hematometra, and lower abdominal pain associated with endometriosis may occur in those individuals with cervical atresia or other forms of müllerian duct anomalies.

Because of malposition of the gonads, gonadal torsion may occur. A variety of organs have been encountered within the inguinal canal, and inguinal hernias. Complications associated with undescended or partial testicular descent may also be encountered.

Testicular Feminization Syndrome

Other XY individuals lack the androgen receptor. They develop testes (Y chromosome presence) and the so-called *X-linked testicular feminization syndrome*. These XY persons show müllerian duct regression because of the presence of antimüllerian hormone. The lack of androgen receptors and the effects of androgens on the Wolffian ducts prevent masculinization. The external genitals are feminine.

Other Intersex Syndromes

Some small *super women* have an extra X chromosome: XXX, making a total of 47 chromosomes. They have two sex chromatin and two drumsticks. The XXX females have deficient germ cell development and often a short reproductive life.

Apparent men with XXXY (48) chromosomes have Klinefelter *characteristics* with testes, and also two sex chromatin and two drumsticks (Fig. 27.2).

Individuals with *four* X-chromosomes are extremely rare. They are *apparent females* with XXXX (48), and *apparent males* with XXXXY (49). Cells with 4 X-chromosomes contain a maximum of 3 sex chromatin (Barr bodies) and 3 drumsticks, regardless of whether the cells come from apparent females or males (Fig. 27.2).

Hormonal Differentiation Disturbances

The virilising effect of testosterone on the *urogenital sinus* in early life causes the *adrenogenital syndrome* in XX individuals. They have ovaries (XX chromosome presence) and the müllerian duct develops normally, because of the absence of antimüllerian hormone. The androgen hyper secretion results in variable development of male external genitalia. The *adrenal hyperplasia* is caused by enzyme defects.

In XY individuals with testes, but deficient testosterone synthesis ability to convert testosterone to dihydrotestosterone develop, the Wolffian duct structure are underdeveloped to a varying degree ranging from a partial to a complete female pattern.

XY individuals who lack estrogen receptors or have a mutant gene for aromatase, lack estrogen effects. The functional lack of estrogen results in unfused epiphyseal zones, so these males are tall, and they have high plasma concentrations of LH although testosterone is normal.

Androgen Insensitivity

Patients have an XY chromosomal complement, lack of müllerian structures and a blind vaginal pouch and absence of sexual hair. The syndrome is a result of an inability to respond to testosterone through a target organ androgen receptor defect (60-70%) or a post-receptor signaling defect (30-40%).

Müllerian structures are absent because the gonads secrete müllerian inhibiting substance.

The gonads may be located in the abdomen, inguinal canal, or labia. The development of gonadal neoplasia is thought to be increased to approximately 5%, however, the incidence is very low before the age of 30. Routinely, orchiectomy is performed after puberty, to allow full pubertal development. Some of these patients show clitoral enlargement and labioscrotal fusion. Their condition is referred to as incomplete (partial) androgen insensitivity. These entities (complete and incomplete androgen insensitivity) are a result of mutations of genes located on the long arm of the X chromosome.

Kallman's Syndrome

Hypogonadotropin eunuchoidism or Kallman's syndrome is the most common form of isolated gonadotropin deficiency. Recent studies demonstrate that GnRH neurons originate in olfactory tissues and migrate to the hypothalamus. Thus, hypogonadism and anosmia are classic presentations for this disorder.

This disorder of sexual differentiation results in delayed puberty and primary amenorrhea. Deletions of the Kallman's gene (KALIG-1) on the short arm of X have been identified with subjects demonstrating an X-linked form of Kallman's syndrome. This gene encodes a cell adhesion protein, which participates in the migration of the GnRH neurons from the medial olfactory placode to the hypothalamus.

Congenital Adrenal Hyperplasia

Congenital adrenal hyperplasia (CAH) is due to a group of enzyme defects, which are inherited in an autosomal recessive fashion. The 21-hydroxylase deficiency is the most common (95%). Because patients with this disorder cannot form cortisol in normal amounts, there is a compensatory increase in ACTH, leading to hyperplasia of the adrenal gland. The excess ACTH drives steroid production to the point of the enzymatic block, with a resultant increase in 17-hydroxyprogesterone production and testosterone. This results in virilization of female neonates and/or salt-wasting, secondary to a lack of aldosterone production (salt wasting CAH).

Affected girls are born with some degree of virilization of their external genitalia, while the internal genital structures derived from the müllerian ducts (fallopian tubes, uterus and cervix) are unaffected. Postnatally, both sexes may experience rapid somatic growth, accelerated skeletal maturation and premature development of sexual and body hair. Affected boys present with premature sexual maturation.

A third form of the 21 hydroxylase deficiency is referred to as "nonclassic" or "late onset" and results in virilization in childhood or adolescence and in females subsequent hirsutism, acne and infertility. Most of the patients with the nonclassic form do not demonstrate over activation of the hypothalamic pituitary axis, as do the other forms. Glucocorticoid therapy suppresses the over activity of the HPO axis in the severe forms and mineralocorticoid replacement is necessary in the salt wasting form.

About two-thirds of patients with the severe classic variant of 11-beta-hydroxylase deficiencies have early-onset hypertension. This hypertension generally is mild to moderate but, in as many as one-third of cases, is associated ultimately with left ventricular hypertrophy, retinopathy, and macrovascular events. The exact cause of the hypertension is unclear and is presumed to be due to excessive secretion of DOC, a mineralo-corticoid.

Rarely, patients with 11-beta-hydroxylase deficiencies may have salt wasting, especially during infancy. The exact pathophysiology of this is unclear. In some cases, excess glucocorticoid administration appears to play a role through suppression of deoxycorticosterone (DOC) secretion.

CAH is estimated to occur in 1/14,000 births, and is much higher in the Ashknazic Jewish and Eskimo population. The enzyme defects, which can result in virilization of the female in utero, are 11-beta hydroxylase deficiency, and 3-beta hydroxysteroid dehydrogenase deficiency.

PCOS is one of the most important differential diagnoses of late-onset or nonclassic variants of virilizing CAH. CAH is far less common than PCOS.

Variant of CAH

The rare variant of congenital adrenal hyperplasia (CAH) known as 17-hydroxylase deficiency was first described in the 1960s in patients with sexual infantilism and hypertension. The disorder reportedly is very rare. It comprises less than 1% of all patients with CAH.

Patients with 17-hydroxylase deficiencies have reduced secretion of cortisol, androgen, and estrogen, with both adrenal and gonadal steroidogenesis impairment. Although patients with 17-hydroxylase deficiencies have decreased cortisol production, they do not have signs or symptoms of adrenal insufficiency due to elevations of corticosterone and glucocorticoids.

CAH due to 17-hydroxylase deficiencies is associated with hypertension and an excess of deoxycorticosterone (DOC), which is the second most common naturally occurring mineralocorticoid after aldosterone.

The major morbidities and mortality associated with the condition mainly stem from delayed or nonrecognition of hypertension. The long-term sequelae of myocardial infarction, cerebrovascular accident, renal failure, heart failure, and peripheral vascular disease may occur if blood pressure is not well controlled.

Psychosocial Sex-deviations

Sex identity is the individual *perception* of herself or himself as a female or a male. Sex identity is established early, and is not lost by castration. Both psychological and social factors can interfere with normal sexual development on the psychological plane. An imminent urge to change sex (operative sex shifts) characterises *trans-sexual persons*.

The *sex role* is the social behavior or cultural role played by or forced upon each individual. Some male homosexuals wish to *express their femininity* while other males clearly signal that they are men. *Transvestites* love to dress like the opposite sex. Transvestites are heterosexual, homosexual or asexual just as others.

Cryptorchidism

Cryptorchidism is the most common genital problem encountered in pediatrics. Cryptorchidism literally means hidden or obscure testis and generally refers to an undescended or maldescended testis. Despite over 100 years of research, many aspects of cryptorchidism are not well defined and remain controversial. If the testes do not descend from the abdominal cavity to the scrotum, heat destroys the sperm-producing seminiferous tubule cells. Heat does not harm the Leydig (testosterone-producing) interstitial cells. Untreated cryptorchidism clearly has deleterious effects on the testis over time.

Understanding the abnormalities of morphogenesis and the molecular and hormonal milieu associated with cryptorchidism is critical to contemporary diagnosis and treatment of this extremely common entity.

Overall, cryptorchidism is seen in 3% of full term, newborn boys, decreasing to 1% at 1 year of age. Prevalence is 30% in premature boys. Predisposing factors include prematurity, low birth weight, small size for gestational age, twinning, and maternal exposure to estrogen during first trimester. A 7% incidence is seen in siblings of boys with undescended testes. Spontaneous descent after the first year of life is uncommon.

Clinically the most useful classification is whether testes are palpable upon physical examination. Accordingly there may be;

Non-palpable testes	*Palpable testes*
Intra-abdominal	Undescended
Absent	Ectopic and retractile

Non-palpable testes occur in about 20-30% of the cryptorchid population. The absent testis is thought to occur from an intrauterine or perinatal vascular event. It is likely a late gestational event since most of these testicular nubbins are found below the internal inguinal ring. Only 20-40% of non-palpable testes will be absent at surgical exploration.

Ectopic testes exit the external inguinal ring and then are misdirected. Retractile testes may be palpated anywhere along the natural course of the testis, although most are inguinal. Though not truly undescended, these testes may be suprascrotal due to an active cremasteric reflex. This reflex is usually weak during infancy and most active at five years. These testes can be manipulated into the scrotum where they will remain without tension.

V. Castration

Certain cultures castrate boys to preserve their tenor voices. Puberty and natural sex development does not take place. Adult males retain their *secondary* sex characteristics and *erection* but they often lose libido. The effects of castration of adult females are surprisingly trivial, as long as the pituitary is working well. Castration, of course, stops their menstrual periodicity (*artificial menopause*), and they are *sterile*.

DIAGNOSIS OF INTERSEX

Most cases of ambiguity of sex detected at birth are due to either congenital adrenal hyperplasia or to androgenic drugs administered to the mother in early pregnancy. Cases presented at puberty are late manifestations of congenital adrenal hyperplasia, those of gonadal dysgenesis and rarely male Intersex (testicular feminization syndrome). In these conditions, the child is reared up as girl and she is brought either for poor development of secondary sex characters or for primary amenorrhea with or without hirsutism.

The diagnosis is made on careful general physical and abdominopelvic examination of clinical presentations. Chromosomal studies to find out genetic and chromosomal defects are essential to confirm genetic disorders. Hormonal evaluation is essential in diagnosing conditions caused by hormonal disturbances. Pelvic/abdominal ultrasound may aid in the identification of gonads and duct structures. A scrotal ultrasound may pick up occult gonads. A genitogram is used to evaluate the structure of the urethra and to confirm the presence of a vagina. An intravenous pyelogram is important to rule out any associated urinary tract anomalies. Cystoscopy may be used to determine the position of entry of the urethra into the vagina or urogenital sinus. Laparoscopy and gonadal biopsy may be necessary to confirm true hermaphroditism.

MANAGEMENT OF INTERSEX

It is always better to diagnose the correct nature of intersex at birth or as early as possible not only to correct the underlying disorders promptly but to avoid the adverse psychological effect on the child and the family. If the diagnosis remains uncertain or the corrective surgery is deferred for the future, the baby is to be reared as female.

Gonadal Dysgenesis

If karyotyping shows presence of Y chromosome removal of gonads is necessary as there is chance of dysgerminomas or gonadoblastoma in such ovaries. Substitution therapy with estrogen and progesterone will help develop secondary sex characters.

Testicular Feminization

The individual should be reared up as girl. The Ectopic gonads are to be removed, for fear of malignancy, along with vaginoplasty after the growth is completed with development of secondary sexual characters. After gonadectomy long-term estrogen replacement therapy should be considered.

Hermaphrodite

With the exception of 46, XX individuals with congenital adrenal hyperplasia or documented maternal androgen excess, most patients with genital ambiguity will require surgical exploration for diagnostic confirmation and removal of contradictory gonadal tissue. This should be done to allow for maximal gender specific development and to increase fertility potential. True hermaphroditism can only be confirmed with gonadal biopsy. Clitoral recession, vaginoplasty, and labioscrotal reduction will be necessary for true hermaphrodites given a female sex assignment. Ideally this should occur at 3-6 months of age.

Congenital Adrenal Hyperplasia

This can be life-threatening in the neonatal period secondary to sodium depletion, hyperkalemia, and dehydration. Newborn female babies with ambiguous genitalia and males with dehydration must be evaluated for CAH immediately and treated with corticosteroids, mineralocorticoids, and sodium chloride if the salt wasting form is diagnosed. Treatment of the 17-hydroxylase deficiencies is also on similar lines.

Glucocorticoid replacement is vital because it reduces ACTH secretion and thus, reduces the production of ACTH-dependent androgens and mineralocorticoids. Oral hydrocortisone is the ideal glucocorticoid for replacement therapy in children. A typical dose is 12-25 mg/m^2/d in 2-3 divided doses. If the response to hydrocortisone is poor, dexamethasone may be used in adults.

Antihypertensive therapy is often needed. Potassium-sparing diuretics, such as spironolactone or amiloride, with or without a calcium channel blocker, such as nifedipine, are used.

Prenatal treatment is an option for fetuses known to be at risk for classic 11-beta-hydroxylase deficiency. The only setting in which this therapy should be considered is if both parents are known carriers of virilising CAH. Dexamethasone may be used in mothers during pregnancy at a dose of 20 mcg/kg initiated as soon as the pregnancy is confirmed, starting at 4-5 weeks' gestation. However, the long-term effects on the child are unknown. Genetic testing is performed on the fetus, typically via chorionic villus sampling. Dexamethasone is discontinued if the fetus is XY or unaffected XX.

Surgical care generally is limited to reconstruction of ambiguous genitalia in female patients and this is the subject of continuing debate. The surgical procedure usually involves both clitoroplasty and vaginoplasty in infancy or clitoroplasty in infancy with vaginoplasty in late adolescence. Use of vaginal dilators sometimes is necessary to prevent restenosis and hence the preference to do it when the girl is going to be sexually active.

Cryptorchidism

Indications for hormonal or surgical correction of cryptorchidism include improved fertility, early detection of testis mass (cancer), correction of associated hernia, prevention of testicular torsion and psychological effects of empty scrotum.

The appropriate time for treatment is approximately 1 year of age. This age has decreased over the recent decades and is based on (1) the rarity of spontaneous descent after 1 year of age and (2) the possible salvage of improved fertility by earlier intervention. The choice of initial treatment is a reflection of both physician and patient (parents) preference.

Primary hormonal therapy with hCG or gonadotropin-releasing hormone has been used for many years, especially in Europe. The action of hCG is virtually identical to that of pituitary LH although hCG appears to have a small degree of FSH activity as well. It stimulates production of gonadal steroid hormones by stimulating the Leydig cells to produce androgens. The exact mechanism of action of the increased androgens in testicular descent is not known but may involve effects on the testicular cord or cremaster muscle. This medication is administered by intra-muscular injection.

Successful placement of the testis in the scrotum by surgery is based on the principles originally described by Bevan in 1899. These include adequate mobilization of the testis and spermatic vessels, ligation of the associated hernia sac, and adequate fixation of the testis in a dependent portion of the scrotum. Many different techniques have been described and can be read from surgical textbooks.

REFERENCES

1. Textbook in Medical Physiology And Pathophysiology Essentials and clinical problems. Copenhagen Medical Publishers 1999—2000. http://www.mfi.ku.dk
2. Human reproduction, clinical, Pathologic and Pharmacological correlations,1997, http://utah.edu
3. Medicine World Medical Library, 2001, http://www.emedicine.com,.
4. Dc Dutta Text Book of Gynecology, 2nd edn, New Central Book Agency (P) Ltd, 1994.

28.

Prashant Nadkarni

Infertility

INTRODUCTION

Infertility is a worldwide phenomenon and is prevalent in every community. The psychological trauma of prolonged infertility on the couple is enormous. This chapter will explain some of the mechanisms involved in establishment of a pregnancy, and the investigation of the infertile couple. Common treatment modalities are discussed.

Infertility is defined as the inability to conceive a pregnancy after two years of unprotected intercourse (i.e. without contraceptive precautions). It can either be primary, where no previous pregnancy has occurred, or secondary where there has been a previous documented pregnancy. The previous pregnancy may be a live birth, or even a failed pregnancy, e.g. miscarriage or ectopic pregnancy.

Infertility is a common condition, occurring in approximately 10 to 15% of couples worldwide. The prevalence is similar across racial and ethnic groups and, apart from certain parts of sub-Saharan Africa, is the same worldwide.

CAUSES OF INFERTILITY

The main causes of infertility can be subdivided as shown in the pie chart (Fig. 28.1):

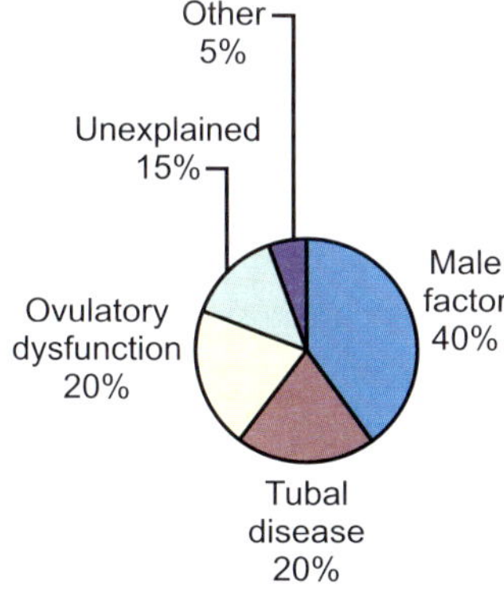

Figure 28.1: Causes of infertility

Male Factor Infertility

This is an often underestimated cause of infertility. Current statistics show that abnormalities of seminal parameters represent the single most important cause of infertility, accounting for approximately 40% of infertility in couples. There has recently been controversy regarding whether sperm parameters (especially sperm counts) have been deteriorating in recent years due to environmental pollutants commonly referred to as endocrine disrupters (ED).[1] If this is proven, the contribution of the male factor to infertility may be even greater in years to come.

Spermatozoa are produced in the testicles under the influence of the anterior pituitary hormones, luteinizing hormone (LH) and follicle stimulating hormone (FSH). The former acts on Leydig cells in the testicle to stimulate production of Testosterone, which in conjunction with FSH, stimulates spermatogenesis in the seminiferous tubules. It takes an average of 74 days for the functionally competent spermatozoa to develop and when mature, they are stored in the epididymis prior to ejaculation. Any insult to the developing spermatozoa during this relatively long development time can potentially damage the spermatozoa. Damage from excessive cigarette smoking, alcohol intake or high local temperature is thought to work in this way.[2]

While up to 70% of men with subnormal semen may have no demonstrable cause, a detailed history, physical and genital examination of the male partner is mandatory as clues to the diagnosis may be evident.

In congenital absence of the vas deferens (CAVD) linked to cystic fibrosis, or occlusion due to previous infection and scarring by gonorrhea, spermatogenesis is present but the obstruction of vasa deferens prevents sperm from being released in the ejaculate. These men have normal sized testes but the vasa may be absent (CAVD). Conversely, in testicular failure, where there is complete absence of spermatogenesis, examination shows small soft testicles due to lack of spermatogenic tissue. If doubt exists, assessment of serum follicle stimulating hormone (FSH) is helpful. Where spermatogenesis is present, the levels are in the normal range, whereas elevated levels characterize absent spermatogenesis. Testicular biopsy and histological examination of the tissue give a definitive diagnosis. Impaired spermatogenesis due to hypogonadotrophic hypogonadism is characterized by very low or even undetectable serum FSH and LH levels, and treatment with exogenous hormones is beneficial in restoring sperm production.

While the role of a varicocoele in the pathogenesis of the subnormal semen assessment is controversial it should be looked out for, and if detected, referral to the urologist sought to discuss the potential benefits of correction of the anomaly.

Tubal Factor

The fallopian tube retrieves the oocyte either from the ovulatory follicle or from the peritoneal fluid post-ovulation. It then nourishes the oocyte and spermatozoa, facilitates fertilization and subsequently transports the embryo into the uterus, where it reaches approximately 96 to 120 hours post ovulation (4 to 5 days). It is thus easy to imagine that any disease process, which interferes with the structure or function of this vital organ, would seriously compromise fertility.

Ascending infection from the cervix, commonly chlamydial or gonococcal, results in pelvic inflammatory disease, which damages the delicate ciliated columnar epithelial cells of the fallopian tube as well as resulting in the formation of peri-tubal adhesions. These sequelae prevent both the retrieval and transport of the oocyte.

Other causes of adhesions include peritonitis (e.g. after a ruptured appendix), endometriosis and post-pelvic surgery (e.g. for an ovarian cyst or uterine myoma).

Ovulatory Dysfunction

The normal menstrual cycle results in the ovulation of usually a single mature oocyte approximately once a month. On average, therefore, a woman releases only twelve oocytes a year.

Any dysfunction of this regular ovulatory mechanism compromises fertility potential and this occurs in approximately 20% of couples. These disorders are among the easiest to diagnose and have the best prognosis for fertility, as they are often the easiest to treat.

The disorders of ovulation are discussed in another chapter.

Unexplained Infertility

Sometimes called idiopathic infertility, this is a diagnosis of exclusion after full assessment of the infertile couple.

Despite the lack of a definite diagnosis of cause, they often have a good prognosis with treatment.

Other Causes

This heterogenous group of causes includes sexual dysfunction, immunological or anatomical disorders, chronic illness, etc. A good history from the couple will often reveal the root cause.

ASSESSMENT OF THE INFERTILE COUPLE

It is often the case that only the female partner attends a consultation, but as the problem of infertility involves the couple, the presence of both the partners is essential. Not only is the male partner a significant cause of infertility, he is also involved in the treatment. The psychological impact of infertility and its treatment on the couple may also be readily assessed if the couple are together. A joint consultation with both partners also allows discussion of diagnosis, further evaluation necessary and the planned treatment so that any questions from the husband can be addressed. Treatment of infertility can sometimes be a long process and getting the male partner's cooperation and trust at the outset is of great benefit.

A full history from both partners is imperative. Each partner's age, general health, duration of the union (including previous unions) and previous pregnancy is elucidated. Frequency of coitus and any difficulty thereof may also be gently questioned.

Important information from the woman includes a detailed menstrual history encompassing premenstrual and menstrual symptoms, previous pelvic infections, usage of an intrauterine contraceptive device and previous pelvic surgery. A full general and pelvic examination, including a cervical smear is undertaken. Ultrasonography of the pelvic organs may also be helpful.

Similarly, a detailed history and examination of the male partner is obtained, including any previous history of genital injury or sexually transmitted disease. Genital examination includes the assessment of testicular size, the presence of vasa deferens and the absence of a palpable varicocoele or hernia.

INVESTIGATION OF THE INFERTILE COUPLE

This should include assessment of :
- The sperm
- The oocyte
- The fallopian tubes and uterus

Investigation of the Sperm Factor

The basic laboratory assessment of the male factor is the semen analysis. As it is easily obtained and assessed, this should be done early in the investigative process. The man should be asked to abstain from ejaculation for two to three days prior to the test, as recent ejaculation gives falsely low sperm counts. Additionally, he should be advised to collect the semen by masturbation and into a clean, sterile container. The specimen should be taken to the laboratory within an hour of collection.

The WHO criteria for assessment are most commonly used in assessing normality.[3] Normal parameters are as follows:

Volume	2-6 mls
Viscosity	liquefaction within 1 hour
pH	7-8
Count	20 million/ml or more
Motility	50% or more
Morphology	30% normal forms or greater

Investigation of the Egg Factor (ovulation)

A good history will invariably identify the woman with ovulatory dysfunction. Ovulation is characterized by regular cycles and premenstrual symptoms such as breast tenderness and low abdominal bloating as well as primary dysmenorrhea. Nevertheless, as ovulation is essential to conception, it is important to confirm its occurrence objectively. Many means are available to do so, and are described below:
- *Basal body temperature*

  This is an easy and inexpensive method, which the patient performs at home. On waking, a specially graduated thermometer is used to determine her body temperature and the reading recorded on a graph. This is done daily over the whole menstrual cycle. As progesterone is a thermogenic hormone, the post-ovulatory half of the cycle (luteal phase) is characterized by an elevated basal temperature of about 0.2 to 0.4 °C in the last twelve to fourteen days of the cycle. A biphasic graph with a lower temperature in the first half and an elevated temperature in the second half of the cycle indicates ovulation. The patient is also asked to mark coital encounters and this also serves to objectively assess coital frequency.

- *Luteinizing hormone monitoring*
  Commercially available home testing kits now make it easy to determine the presence of the LH surge, which triggers ovulation. The early morning urine is tested in the days leading to ovulation and a positive test is an indicator of impending ovulation.
- *Midluteal serum progesterone*
- After ovulation, a corpus luteum is formed from the ovulatory follicle and this secretes progesterone. The level peaks between seven and nine days after ovulation and the finding of an elevated serum level at this time confirms ovulation. However, the timing of the test can be difficult given that menstrual cycle length can vary month to month, and a negative test may be a signal that the test was mistimed.
- *Ultrasound monitoring*
  The developing ovarian follicle can be monitored over a period of days until evidence of ovulation is seen. However, one drawback is that the patient needs to attend the doctor's surgery repeatedly as the developing follicle is ultrasonically tracked over the days leading to ovulation.
- *Endometrial biopsy*
  Progesterone causes the development of a secretory endometrium and accurate histological confirmation is possible with an endometrial biopsy. However as this is an invasive test and may also disrupt an early implanted pregnancy. It is seldom used.

Investigation of the Uterus and Fallopian Tubes

As discussed previously, tubal damage results in mechanical disruption of the process of fertilization and embryo transport. Similarly, a space occupying lesion in the uterus (e.g. fibroid or endometrial polyp) disrupts the process of implantation of the embryo. There are currently two commonly performed investigations to assess normality:

- *Hysterosalpingography(HSG)*
  This is a radiological procedure, which involves the injection of a radiopaque dye through the cervix. The dye courses through the uterus and tubes and into the peritoneal cavity. Blocked tubes are characterized by obstruction to this flow into the peritoneum. Additionally, filling defects in the uterus may delineate intrauterine lesions discussed above. To reduce X-ray exposure to the ovaries, the procedure is performed under continuous fluoroscopy and two or three X-rays are taken as a permanent record of the outcome. It is performed prior to ovulation to prevent accidental irradiation of an embryo.
- *Laparoscopy*
  This is the gold standard in tubal and peritoneal assessment. A telescope is inserted into the peritoneal cavity to allow direct visualization of the pelvic organs. Any abnormality, including endometriosis and pelvic adhesions which would not be visualized by ultrasonography or hysterosalpingography, would be readily diagnosed. An inert colored dye such as methylene blue is injected into the cervix and its passage freely through the fimbrial ends of the fallopian tubes confirms patency.

  Occasionally, a *hysteroscopy* may also be performed at the same time. In this procedure, a telescope is inserted intracervically into the uterus to assess the uterine cavity.

  Disadvantage of this method of assessment are the need for a surgical incision to insert the laparoscope, as well as the need for general anesthesia.

TREATMENT OPTIONS

Once the tests are completed, the physician is in a better position to make a diagnosis and plan treatment. Even in unexplained infertility, good pregnancy rates can be achieved with available treatment. It is important to remember that apart from total bilateral tubal obstruction or azoospermia, pregnancies occur in the infertile even without treatment, although with a lowered frequency. While treatment increases the chance of pregnancy in any one cycle, it does not guarantee success.

Induction of Ovulation

This is beneficial in ovulatory dysfunction and unexplained infertility with high odds ratios for pregnancy.[3,4]

The commonest agent used is Clomiphene citrate, an anti-estrogen agent which acts as a competitive inhibitor at the hypothalamic level. In anovulatory women, ovulation rates of up to 80% have been reported with its usage. It is taken usually from days 2 to 6 of the menstrual cycle and results in an increased secretion of pituitary FSH resulting in ovulation. Occasionally, multiple ovulation may occur, resulting in multiple pregnancy, generally twins (5-8% of conceptions).

Where Clomiphene citrate has failed, in hypogonadotrophic hypogonadism and in assisted reproductive technology (e.g. in vitro fertilization), more potent agents are required. Gonadotropins are the agent of choice. They may either be derived from the urine of postmenopausal women or more recently, synthetically derived from recombinant technology. They are administered parenterally and as they contain FSH, act directly on the ovary to recruit multiple ovarian follicles for ovulation. They are potent stimulators of folliculogenesis, and their use must be combined with strict patient monitoring if complications are to be avoided. The two most common adverse effects are multiple gestation and the ovarian hyperstimulation syndrome.

The reported incidence of multiple gestation can be up to 30%, and while most of these are twins, higher order gestations such as triplets and quadruplets (quintuplets, sextuplets) are reported.

The ovarian hyperstimulation syndrome is a consequence of ovulation following gonadotropin usage, especially if pregnancy occurs. It is directly related to the number of follicles stimulated; the greater the number of follicles, the higher the risk. It is characterized by ovarian enlargement, ascitis, hemoconcentration, hypercoagulability, and in severe cases, even pleural and pericardial effusion. Death can occur in the severe case.

Intrauterine Insemination

This involves the injection of a small volume of concentrated spermatozoa into the uterine cavity at the time of ovulation, thus optimizing the process of natural fertilization. Ovulation is usually stimulated with Clomiphene citrate, gonadotropin therapy or a combination of the two, and the semen has been previously prepared in the laboratory to yield highly active spermatozoa and to remove dead cells, debris and prostinoid substances found in the raw semen. This method is widely practiced and has good results in unexplained infertility, ovulatory dysfunction and mild male factor infertility. Pregnancy rates are approximately 15% per cycle.[5]

In Vitro Fertilization (IVF, "test tube treatment")

Fertilization takes place outside the human body, in the laboratory environment. This process allows the fallopian tubes to be bypassed and is especially useful in tubal infertility although it is increasingly being used for all forms of infertility. Once again, multiple oocytes development is induced, but just prior to ovulation, the ovarian follicles are punctured and the oocytes retrieved. These are then inseminated with the spermatozoa in the laboratory, where the embryos are nurtured before transfer into the uterus at 48-72 hours usually. At this time, the embryo is at the 4 to 8 cell stage of division. More recently, embryos are being transferred at day 5 or 6 (blastocyst stage) but no advantage in pregnancy rates has been demonstrated.[6] The delivery rate per treatment cycle (i.e. the chance of having a live delivery after each completed treatment cycle) is almost 30%.[7]

Intracytoplasmic Sperm Injection (ICSI)

Until very recently, the majority of men with severe male factor infertility were virtually untreatable and even with in vitro fertilization, embryos could not be generated because of the inability of the spermatozoa to penetrate the oocytes. With the advent of ICSI, single spermatozoa can now be introduced directly into the oocytes resulting in fertilization in the majority of patients. This has opened a whole new avenue of treatment for couples previously considered untreatable except by donor sperm insemination of the female partner. ICSI is an offshoot of in vitro fertilization, and the procedure is very similar to IVF, except for the laboratory aspects. Pregnancy rates and delivery rates are similar to IVF.

CONCLUSION

As the fields of medicine and embryology develop, newer and more sophisticated treatment modalities become available to the infertile couple. However, the principles of management remain the same as in any other field of medicine: a good history and physical examination from both partners, relevant investigations and proper diagnosis are essential for treatment and counseling. Infertility is a complex problem and despite advances in treatment, not all couples will achieve their desired family size. In managing these couples, the clinician needs to bear in mind the emotional pressures that they face and try to minimize further stresses. A sympathetic and caring attitude helps to ease the pressures of treatment, given that even with the most advanced treatment modalities, there is a high failure rate.

REFERENCES

1. Skakkebaek NE, Rajpert-De Meyts E, Main KM. Testicular dysgenesis syndrome: an increasingly common developmental disorder with environmental aspects. Human Reproduction 2001; 16(5): 972-8.
2. Hruska KS, Furth PA, Seifer DB, Sharara FI, Flaws JA. Environmental factors in infertility. Clinical Obstetrics and Gynecology 2000; 43(4): 821-9.
3. World Health Organisation. Laboratory Manual for the examination of human semen and sperm cervical interaction. Cambridge University Press, 1992
4. Hughes, E. Collins, J. Vandekerckhove, P. Clomiphene citrate for ovulation induction in women with oligo-amenorrhea Cochrane Database of Systematic Reviews. Issue 3, 2002.
5. Hughes, E. Collins, J. Vandekerckhove, P. Clomiphene citrate for unexplained subfertility in women. Cochrane Database of Systematic Reviews. Issue 3, 2002.
6. Hughes EG. The effectiveness of ovulation induction and intrauterine insemination in the treatment of persistent infertility: a meta-analysis. Human Reproduction 1997; 12: 1865-72
7. Blake D Proctor, M Johnson, N Olive D. Cleavage stage versus blastocyst stage embryo transfer in assisted conception. Cochrane Database of Systematic Reviews. Issue 3, 2002
8. Society for Assisted Reproductive Technology /American Society for Reproductive Medicine. Assisted reproductive technology in the United States: 1998 results. Fertility and Sterility 2002; 74(1): 18-31

29.
Premitha Damodaran

Menopause and Hormone Replacement Therapy

INTRODUCTION

Menopause is the last menstrual period and marks the end of the reproductive phase of a woman. She may experience symptoms such as bleeding irregularities, hot flushes, tiredness, aches and pains, mood swings, urinary incontinence and vaginal dryness. The long-term effects of menopause are mainly cardiovascular disease and osteoporosis.

Every woman should be aware of the changes that can occur with menopause and be informed about the benefits of HRT. Presently HRT is widely advocated for a woman who is experiencing perimenopausal symptoms such as vasomotor symptoms and urogenital atrophy. It is not indicated for prevention and treatment of primary and secondary cardiovascular disease. HRT has been shown to be beneficial in decreasing the risk of an osteoporotic fracture. An individual risk profile is essential for every woman contemplating any regimen of HRT. A woman is endowed at birth with a finite number of oocytes which are steadily lost at differing rates from her ovaries, at different times in her life. When these oocytes fall below a certain threshold level, she reaches menopause. Thus, menopause denotes the end of reproductive aging in a woman. However, a woman is said to have only attained menopause when she has not had her menstrual periods for twelve months, making it a retrospective diagnosis.[1]

DEFINITIONS

Menopause is not an abrupt event for most women and the gradual process to reach menopause can last many years. Various nomenclature have been used to define the various stages of menopause. The STRAW classification has recommended the following:[1]

Menopausal transition: The period of time which begins with a variation in the menstrual cycle length, in a woman with a raised Follicular Stimulating Hormone (FSH) and ends with her final menstrual period.

Perimenopause or climacteric: Literally means "around or about the menopause". It begins with the menopausal transition and ends one year after the last menstrual period.

Early postmenopause: The first five years since the last menstrual period.

Late post menopause: More than five years since the last menstrual period.

Life expectancy has increased worldwide over the past century. Men and women are living beyond the age of 80 years in most parts of the world. However, the average age of menopause remains around 50 years. This would mean that the average woman would spend one-third of her life in the menopause. In Malaysia, two separate studies have confirmed the average age of menopause to be 50.7[2] and 49.6 years.[3] There appears to be no difference in the age of menopause amongst the various ethnic groups.

Among factors that can effect the age of menopause are

- current and prior cigarette smoking
- family history of early menopause
- low body weight
- living in high altitudes
- vegetarianism
- malnourishment in women[4]

Premature menopause occurs when there is cessation of periods before the age of 40 years. This occurs in about 1% of women and could be caused by genetic factors, autoimmune processes or medical interventions such as chemotherapy or radiotherapy. The effects of premature menopause is usually severe with a higher incidence of long-term problems such as osteoporosis and heart disease.

If both the ovaries are removed before the age of menopause, the woman is then surgically menopaused. She usually experiences acute vasomotor and physiological symptoms at this time.

ENDOCRINOLOGY OF MENOPAUSE

The basis of reproductive aging in a woman is the loss of oocytes from her ovary. At birth, a female child is born with 1-2 million follicles. This depletes to around 500,000 follicles at menarche. At every menstrual cycle thereafter, a certain number of follicles are recruited by the ovary. One follicle is selected for ovulation, the others undergo atresia and are lost. The rate of uptake and loss of follicles vary with time and in different women. In addition to providing the egg, these follicles secrete the sex hormones. At menopause, the number of ovarian follicles fall below a certain threshold. The ovaries then are unable to produce estrogen, progesterone, and to a lesser extent testosterone.[5]

The climacteric is the phase from the decline of the reproductive capacity. This is signified by a decrease in the number of ovarian follicles around 37.5 years of age, about 10 years before menopause.[5]

Serum inhibin is a marker of the ovarian follicular activity. Inhibin levels drop in the perimenopause causing a corresponding increase in the levels of serum follicular stimulating hormone(FSH). FSH levels, thus may increase despite a normal estrogen level. This increase in FSH levels is the cause of irregular cycles in the perimenopause. Estrogen levels which are higher than normal can be seen during the perimenopause, however, these are transient and due to episodic burst of ovarian activity. The increase in serum luteinizing hormone (LH) only occurs when both the estrogen and progesterone levels drop due to the disruption of the LH feedback mechanism.

The levels of testosterone also start declining, however not at the same rate as estrogen and progesterone. This leads to an imbalance in the ratio of estrogen to testosterone which is responsible for problems such as hirsutism (over the face and chin) and loss of scalp hair in the postmenopausal woman.

SIGNS AND SYMPTOMS OF MENOPAUSE

The falling levels of estrogen bring about certain changes to the menopausal woman. These changes could be classified into short term, medium term or long term changes (Table 29.1).

Table 29.1: Signs and symptoms of menopause

Short term	Medium term	Long term
Irregular menses	Urogenital changes	Heart
Vasomotor symptoms	Skin changes	Bone
Psychological symptoms		Brain

Short-term Problems

The menstrual periods become irregular. This is due to the rise in the FSH levels. The periods may be longer, shorter, heavier or lighter before ceasing altogether.

Vasomotor symptoms such as hot flushes, night sweats and palpitations are features of declining estrogen levels. Hot flushes are feelings of heat a woman experiences when there is a sudden gush of blood to the upper chest wall and face. Hot flushes are usually felt in the perimenopause and early postmenopausal period though in rare instances may extend for a longer period of time. Surgically menopaused women have severe and more long lasting hot flushes than women who undergo natural menopause. The community based Swan study in the US showed a lesser incidence of hot flushes in Asian women.[6] However in the local Malaysian setting, 2 studies have shown the incidence of hot flushes to be about 57%.[2,7]

The psychological symptoms associated with menopause are insomnia, memory loss, mood swings, anxiety, loss of libido, difficulty in concentration and irritability. Serotonin has a positive effect on the mood and is dependant on estrogen levels. Declining estrogen levels cause a decrease in the serotonin levels leading to the emotional disturbances seen at the menopause.

Medium-term Problems

The medium-term problems are to the genitourinary tract and the skin. There is atrophy to the vagina and lower urinary tract. The vaginal epithelium begins to loose its glycogen content resulting in a change in the vaginal ecosystem. The vagina loses its tone and contractility becoming short and narrow with a surface which is vulnerable to infection and ulceration. Common vaginal complaints are dryness, irritation, discharge and post coital bleeding.

The urethra and bladder trigone undergo similarly atrophy. As the vagina shrinks, the urethral meatus becomes anatomically closer to the vagina. Infections in the vagina can lead to urinary tract infections and vice versa. Estrogen deprivation also leads to weakening of the connective tissue and muscles supporting the uterus, bladder and rectum which can result in uterine prolapse, cystocoele, rectocoele and enterocoele. All this contributes to incontinence and pelvic pressure.[8]

Menopause affects a woman's sexuality. The shortening and loss of elasticity of the vagina, along with vaginal dryness can cause dyspareunia. There is also decreased blood flow to the vulva and other reproductive organs such as the breast and skin resulting in reduced sexual arousal. A fall in the androgen levels results in a loss of libido, as testosterone is important for desire, motivation and fantasies in both men and women.

Type 1 collagen which is predominant in both the skin and bone decrease with menopause. About 30% of collagen is lost in the first five years of menopause after which there is a 2% decrease yearly. As skin collagen correlates strongly with skin dermal thickness, the skin becomes thin with menopause. External factors such as sun and toxins causes further damage to the skin.[9]

Long-term Problems

Though recent literature has changed the standard view on cardiovascular disease (CVD) and estrogen, cardiovascular disease still remains the leading cause of death in a postmenopausal woman. The frequency of myocardial infarction begins to rise in the perimenopausal period and is approximately similar to the man by 70 years. However, women have different initial symptoms, are not as aggressively treated and have a higher mortality and morbidity than men. Other risk factors towards CVD should also be considered in the management of the postmenopausal woman (Table 29.2).

Table 29.2: Risk factors for coronary heart disease[10]

Unmodifiable risks	Modifiable risks
Family history of MI or sudden death in male relative before the age of 55 years or female relative before the age of 65 years.	Elevated serum cholesterol levels (>6.2 mmol/l)
Male > 45 years	Low plasma HDL—C levels (<0.9mmol/l)
Female > 55 years or premature menopause	Obesity Hypertension Smoking Excessive alcohol intake Sedentary lifestyle

The lipid profile is adversely altered with menopause. Total cholesterol levels increase; high density lipoproteins (HDL), a good predictor for coronary heart disease risk in women decreases, while the level of low density lipoproteins (LDL) increase. Even a 1% increase in total cholesterol levels have been shown to increase the risk of CVD significantly.[11] The main culprit seems to be the formation of the atheromatous plaque which is caused by the reversal of the HDL/LDL ratio. These plaques also lead to thrombus formation and complications such as strokes.

Osteoporosis or the "brittle bone disease" is a serious, long term complication of menopause. It is characterized by low bone mass and structural deterioration of bone tissue leading to fragile bones and an increased susceptibility to fractures of the spine, wrist and hip. It has been established that the peak bone mass in men and women is achieved in the thirties after which there is slow bone loss. This bone loss is exaggerated with menopause and estrogen deprivation. In the first 5 to 7 years after menopause, a woman might lose about 20% of her bone, while an average woman loses half her bone by the age of 70 years.[12]

Osteoporosis is twice more common in women than men. The factors that determine peak bone mass are genetic heritage, physical activity and diet. Bone loss is highest in a small built, fair skinned woman (Table 29.3). In 1997 alone the women from the Chinese ethnic group in Malaysia accounted for 44.8% of hip fractures in Malaysia.[13]

Table 29.3: Risk factors for osteoporosis[14]

Non-modifiable	Modifiable
Advancing age	Low calcium intake
Ethnic group (Oriental and Caucasian)	Cigarette smoking
Female gender	Sedentary lifestyle
Premature or early menopause	Excessive alcohol intake
(<45 years) or surgical menopause	
Slender build	Excessive caffeine intake
Fair skinned	
Family history of osteoporosis in a first degree relative	

Other Effects of Estrogen Deprivation

Alzheimer's disease, a neurodegenerative disease of the brain is more common in the woman than man and has been said to be associated with estrogen loss.[15]

Macular degeneration, a leading cause of blindness has been shown to be more common in those with early menopause as opposed to women with late menopause.[16]

In line with osteoporosis, alveolar bone also undergoes resorption leading to loose teeth. Bone mineral density in post menopausal women is directly correlated with the number of teeth.[17]

MANAGEMENT OF A POSTMENOPAUSAL WOMAN

A woman approaching menopause should be aware of the changes that are to take place in her body. Primary prevention is very important in this age group and simple lifestyle measures should be emphasized.

Key lifestyle changes for a menopausal woman are:
- to normalise weight
- to initiate dietary interventions
- to carry out regular exercise
- to stop smoking
- to control hypertension/diabetes
- to control excessive alcohol intake
- to control lipid levels

The menopause serves a focal point for a woman to review her health for the postmenopausal years. Risk factor scoring for gynecological and non gynecological cancers should be carried out along with assessment towards risk for cardiovascular disease and osteoporosis. Every woman should be counseled regarding HRT treatment.

Hormone Replacement Therapy

Hormone replacement therapy (HRT) consists of replacing lost or diminished hormones in the body. Though applicable for any form of hormones produced by the body, it remains synonymous for postmenopausal hormone replacement.

HRT was first introduced in the 1950s. At that time the postmenopausal woman, despite the presence of a uterus was only given estrogen. When the lack of opposing progestogen was shown to increase the risk of endometrial hyperplasia, both estrogen and progestogen was then introduced. Women without a uterus require only estrogen.

Types of estrogen available:

- *Estradiol valerate*, a synthetic natural estrogen given at a dose of 2 mg/day
- *Estradiol,* a micronised version of natural estrogen given at a dose of 2 mg/day
- *Conjugated equine estrogens*, estrogens distilled from the urine of pregnant mares given at the dose of 0.625ug/day.[18]

Progestogens (progestins) refer to all steroids used as a substitute for endogenous progesterone. Natural progesterones can be either micronised or in the form of dydrogesterone. Unfortunately, natural progesterones have low bioavailabilty and increasing its dose may lead to unpleasant side effects. The progestogens available are either derivatives of the 17 α-hydroxyprogesterone or the 19-nortestosterone.[19]

Treatment Modalities

Postmenopausal women without a uterus only require estrogen replacement therapy (ERT). If the ovaries have been left behind at surgery, a woman does not require ERT until she reaches menopause. She could await the normal transitional symptoms or carry out a blood test to determine the levels of FSH and LH at this stage.

Women with a uterus require both estrogen and progestogen. Progestogens are added to reduce the risk of endometrial hyperplasia and endometrial carcinoma. Progestogens given for ten days or more offers an endometrial protective effect with an odds ratio of less than 1.0.[20]

Sequential HRT: Progestogens are added for at least 10 to 14 days of every cycle. This causes a withdrawal bleed every month. Sequential HRT is recommended for women who are in the perimenopausal phase when bleeding irregularities are common.

Continuous combined HRT: Progestogens and estrogen are given daily. This causes suppression of the endometrial lining of the uterus. This regime is recommended for women in the post menopause phase. Though irregular bleeding may be common in the first six months of use, thereafter this treatment regime does not cause any withdrawal bleeding if correctly taken.

For long-term use, the continuous combined HRT regime is preferred to the sequential regime, as a higher rate of endometrial carcinoma was found in the latter when taken for more than 5 years.[21]

Delivery Systems

HRT may be delivered in various ways.

- Oral tablets are available in both estrogen (E) and estrogen and progestogen (E/P) combinations. Though widely accepted, they have a first pass effect through the liver which may contribute to certain side effects such as pigmentation and thrombosis. However, oral tablets remain the most popular although different regimes, dosages and combinations are available.
- Transcutaneous patches are available both in E and E/P preparations. It produces similar effects as the oral form though metabolic changes related to it's effect on the heart are said to be less. A significant side effect is the irritation around the edge of the patch and premature detachment which is more common in the tropical climate. Transcutaneous estrogen gel is also available.
- Subdermal implants (estrogen only) are available in various sizes containing 20, 50, 100 mg of estradiol so as to provide different durations of action. Taccyphylaxis is the biggest disadvantage. Testosterone implants given in conjunction with estradiol implants help with lowered libido levels in postmenopausal women.
- Transvaginal estrogen cream has very minimal systemic absorption and is recommended in women with vaginal dryness.[22]

Action of Estrogen

The action of estrogen is mediated through receptors. The two distinct types of receptors, ERα and ERβ are similar but functionally different as they are expressed differently in the various parts of the body. ERα is predominant in the breast, uterus and vagina and is mainly involved in reproductive events. ERβ is more general and is found in the ovary, brain, cardiovascular system and skin. When estrogen or any other compound bind with these receptors, it causes a conformational change that then predicts the response in the various end organs. Depending on the predominant receptor found in the end organ, differing responses may then be obtained.[23]

The principal aim of HRT is to restore healthy levels of estrogen so as to reduce the effects of estrogen deprivation. HRT can be started at the perimenopausal or post menopausal phase. Prior to starting HRT, a full examination which includes a detailed history, general examination, blood pressure reading, breast examination, Pap smear and a gynecological examination is important. Screening mammograms should be encouraged in women over the age of fifty. Bone mineral density testing should be carried out in women with a high risk of osteoporosis. Every woman should be counseled in detail regarding HRT. Her individual benefits and risks towards HRT should be evaluated.

Benefits of HRT

Conventional benefits of HRT include:
- Relief of vasomotor symptoms
- Relief of urogenital arophy
- Relief of skin atrophy
- Prevention and treatment of osteoporosis[24]
- Improvement in mood and cognition.[25,26]

Newer Benefits of HRT

- Decreased risk of colorectal cancer by 37%[24]
- Decreased age-related tooth loss[17]
- Decreased age-related macular degeneration[16]
- Delay of onset and progression of Alzheimer's disease when started early postmenopausal.[15, 26]

Side Effects of HRT

Breast tenderness and bloating are common when HRT is initiated. These initial side effects can be minimized by altering the dose and type of estrogen and progestogen. Allergic reactions are usually rare. An increase in pigmentation may occur.

Weight gain is always assumed to be due to HRT use. However, no evidence exists that either ERT or HRT contributes towards body weight. The increase in weight is usually due to a decreased metabolic rate which occurs at perimenopause and menopause.

HRT and Bleeding

Unscheduled vaginal bleeding is worrying and should be investigated. The commonest reason for unscheduled vaginal bleeding is the missed HRT pill or irregular HRT intake. Irregular bleeding is also common in the first 4-6 months of continuous combined HRT use. If this persists, a detailed investigation in the form of pelvic ultrasound with endometrial thickness measurement and possibly an outpatient endometrial sampling should be carried out. The latter may be difficult with a post menopausal stenosed cervix. Alternatively diagnostic hysteroscopy and curettage, the gold standard in investigation for post menopausal bleeding can be done.

HRT and the Vascular System

The cardiovascular benefits of HRT were initially believed to be through the following factors:
- Favourable actions on the lipid profile i.e. decrease in total cholesterol levels and reversal of HDL: LDL ratio
- Vascular effects leading to vasodilatory effects,
- Decrease in fibrinogen, plasminogen activator inhibitors and homocysteine levels,
- Antioxidant and anti inflammatory properties.

However, since the HERS (Heart and Estrogen Replacement Study)[28,29] and WHI (Women's Health Initiative)[24,30] study results, HRT has not been shown to be favorable in the prevention of primary or secondary cardiovascular disease.

The HERS study was a randomized, blinded placebo controlled trial of continuous combined estrogen—progestin use in postmenopausal women with documented coronary heart disease (CHD). HERS I[28] ended at 4.1 years when it was shown that during the study period, there was no significant decrease in CHD events (non fatal myocardial infarction plus CHD related death) or in any secondary cardiovascular outcomes when compared to the placebo group. The first year of HERS 1 actually showed an increase in coronary events. However, post-hoc analyses suggested a significant time trend decrease in CHD and thus 93% of the initial HERS participants continued treatment for an additional 2.7 years (HERS II).

However, despite a longer time frame, the risk of cardiovascular events in a post menopausal women with established heart disease was still found to be not significantly decreased with HRT use when compared to placebo (RR0.9, CI 0.84—1.17).[29]

The WHI study was on the use of HRT in over 27000 apparently healthy postmenopausal women aged 50 to 79 years. These women were divided based on their HRT or ERT usage. The continuous combined progestin therapy arm (CCEPT) which studied the effects of conjugated equine estrogen (CEE) and medroxyprogesterone acetate (MPA) in women with a uterus was terminated at 5.2 years,[24] whilst the estrogen only arm which studied the effect of CEE in hysterectomised women was stopped at 6.8 years.[30]

The CCEPT arm of the WHI showed an increased risk of coronary heart disease (CHD) by 29% (RR 1.29 CI 1.02-1.63) and stroke by 41% (RR 1.41 CI 1.07-1.85). These results were despite significantly improved lipid profiles. The estrogen only arm on the other hand, showed a decrease in CHD events, however, this did not reach clinical significance (RR 0.91 CI 0.75-1.12). The increase in stroke was similar (RR 1.39 CI 1.10-1.77).

This increased risk in CHD events are now thought to be due to the prothrombotic, proinflammatory and proarrhythmic effects of hormones, possibly progestins rather than estrogen. This is still being investigated. In view of these figures, estrogen or estrogen/progestin combinations are presently not recommended for prevention of primary and secondary coronary heart disease

Venous thromboembolism (VTE) is a known complication of HRT. There is a 2 to 3 fold increase in VTE events with HRT use.[31] This has been corroborated by the HERS and WHI studies.[29,24]

HRT and the Breast

Though cardiovascular disease is the leading cause of death in women, breast cancer appears to be more the primary health concern. Multiple studies and meta analyses have previously alternated between showing either a significantly increased or decreased risk of breast cancer in HRT users when compared to placebo.

Risk factors for breast cancer should also be considered in evaluating one's risk in developing breast cancer. The non-modifiable factors are early age of menarche, late menopause, first child birth after the age of 30 years and breast cancer in a first degree relative before the age of 50 years. Modifiable factors are a body mass index (BMI) >25 kg/m^2 or consuming more than 10 alcoholic drinks a week.

In 1997, the Collaborative Group on Hormonal Factors in Breast Cancer study[32] showed a small but significantly increased risk in breast cancer risk in current users when compared to never users (RR1.14, CI 1.08-1.2). This relative risk increased by a factor of 1.02 with each year of use. However, there was no significant increase in risk in the first five years of use and after 5 years of cessation of therapy. The stage and tissue type of the cancer also appeared to be more favorable in the current users. HRT use has also not shown to increase breast cancer risk in women with prior breast disease[33] and in women with family history of breast cancer.[34]

Mammographic density is known to decrease with age when the ratio of fatty tissue to glandular and fibrous tissue increase. Estrogen has been shown to increase breast density and this has translated into fears that increased density may miss an underlying breast cancer.

The CCEPT arm of the WHI study was halted prematurely after 5.2 years of use as the incidence of invasive breast cancer was found to exceed the boundaries set at the beginning of the study.[24] This increased risk was not significant (RR 1.26 CI 1.00-1.59) and was comparable to the non-significant increase in HRT users of the HERS study. This increased risk was noted after 4 years of use and is higher in women who had been on HRT previously and leaner in body mass (BMI <25 kg/m^2). Fortunately, women who were on HRT for premature menopause did not show an increased risk towards breast cancer.

Soon to follow were the results of the Million Women Study (MWS), a large observational study of one million women between the ages of 50 and 64 and followed up for 5 years in the UK.[35] The MWS showed that current use of either estrogen alone or estrogen/progestin combination increased the risk of breast cancer, with the risk being higher in the latter. Varied delivery methods i.e. transdermal, oral and estrogen implants as well as the use of tibolone showed a similar increased risk of breast cancer.

The estrogen only arm of the WHI was halted in 2004 after 6.8 years, due to an increase in stroke events. This arm, however, showed a decreased risk towards breast cancer by 33% which just missed clinical significance (RR0.77 CI 0.59-1.01). This decrease in risk was apparent from the beginning of the second year.

Estrogen has always been thought to be a procarcinogenic which has till recently explained the slight increased risk of breast and endometrial cancer. However with the WHI data and extrapolating form the MWS, more thought is now on progestins being the main culprit. The secretory phase of the menstrual cycle is under progestogenic influence and has been shown to be high in mitotic activity. Though this could explain the increase in breast cancers in those on a combined estrogen and progestin therapy, more research is still needed in this area.

Estrogen and Bone

Estrogen is an anti-resorptive agent and helps prevent postmenopausal osteoporosis. Though earlier evidence promoted ERT/ HRT at any stage of postmenopausal life with respect to osteoporosis prevention and treatment, present data support the use of estrogens at the onset of menopause; i.e. when bone loss is supposedly maximum.

Both arms of the WHI data support the use of HRT in the prevention of fractures. The CCEPT arm showed a 34% reduction in hip fractures (RR 0.39, CI 0.45-0.98) whilst the estrogen arm showed a 39% decrease (RR 0.69 CI 0.41-0.91).There was also a reduction in total fractures in both arms of the study.[24,30]

Estrogen and Brain

The association of dementia and Alzheimer's disease with estrogen deprivation has been inconsistent. Post menopausal women have·a greater risk than men of developing Alzheimer's disease. A subset of the WHI, i.e. the women's health initiative memory study showed that in women above the age of 65 years, either ERT

or HRT was not beneficial. However, it did prevent mild cognitive impairment in this group.[26]

Contraindications to HRT Use

Contraindications to HRT use are:
- Known or suspected pregnancy or breast cancer
- Presence of estrogen dependant neoplasia
- Undiagnosed abnormal genital bleeding
- Active thromboembolic disorders.[27]

Tibolone

Tibolone is a synthetic steroid with weak estrogenic, progestogenic and androgenic effects. It is advocated for use in a post menopausal woman who has not had her period for one year. Due to its tissue specific action, tibolone can be used for relief of vasomotor symptoms, vaginal dryness and prevention of osteoporosis. Its effect on the heart is mediated via a reduction in apolipoprotein A. Tibolone has an androgenic effect and may be used to improve libido in post menopausal women.

In contrast to estrogens, tibolone does not stimulate the breast and does not cause an increase in breast density. Endometrial stimulation is also absent and the incidence of genital bleeding is very low. However, the incidence of VTE is similar to that of estrogen.[36]

Role of Calcium

Adequate calcium intake has been shown to prevent bone loss and reduce fracture risk in peri and post menopausal women. Though not as effective as other antiresorptive agents, doses between 1000 and 1500 mgs of calcium per day have been shown to be effective. Vitamin D (400-600 IU/day) to aid calcium absorption, is supplemented in women who are unable to get enough sunlight or those who are institutionalized.[37]

Non-HRT Treatment for Menopausal Symptoms

The use of HRT relieves menopause related symptoms. However for women who are unable or refuse to take HRT, other modalities are required. Hot flushes may be treated with central acting anti hypertensives or clonidine. The use of lubricants is popular for vaginal dryness. Abundant herbal remedies are available for vasomotor symptoms.

Women with risk for cardiovascular disease are advised to start lipid lowering agents under the advice of their physician. This should be carried out in combination with healthy lifestyle measures. Various antiresorptive drugs are available for the treatment of osteoporosis. Bisphosphanates significantly increases bone mineral density and reduces the incidence of hip and non-hip fractures. The major side effect is an increase in gastro-esophageal reflux.[38] Raloxifene, a selective estrogen receptor modulator has shown to have a sustained effect on the bone with a decrease in the incidence of vertebral fractures. It also has a positive effect on lipids and has been shown to decrease the risk of developing breast cancer.[39]

Present Recommendations for HRT

The era of promoting ERT or HRT use in every woman is over. In light of the recent data, i.e. mainly the women's health initiative, recommendations towards the use of estrogen and estrogen/progestin combination in the postmenopausal woman is made with careful consideration of each individuals benefit and risk ratio.

Though not directly comparable, the two arms of the WHI have shown interesting results.

Table 29.4: The women's health initiative (WHI)[24,30]

	CEE* + MPA** (CCEPT)	CEE (Estrogen only)
Number of years	5.2	6.8
Coronary Heart Disease	+ 29% (1.02-1.63)	-9% (0.75-1.12)
Stroke	+ 41% (1.07-1.85)	+39% (1.10-1.77)
Breast cancer	+ 26% (1.00-1.59)	-33% (0.59-1.01)
Hip fractures	- 34% (0.45-0.98)	-39% (0.41-0.91)

* conjugated equine estrogen
** medoxyprogesterone acetate

The risk of stroke is clearly increased in ERT and HRT users while hip fracture reduction is seen in both arms. Opposing results are seen in CHD events and breast cancer. The risk of coronary heart disease appears to be increased in the CCEPT arm while showing a reduction which does not reach clinical significance in the estrogen only arm. The risk of breast cancer is higher with the E/P users and lower in the estrogen only users, however, both arms did not reach clinical significance. Progestins seem likely to cause this increased risk.

The present recommendations towards HRT use are:[40-42]

- An individual risk profile is essential for every woman contemplating any regimen of HRT. Women should be informed of the risks.
- The primary indication of HRT is the treatment of menopausal symptoms (vasomotor and urogenital).
- Women with an intact uterus should be given progestin for more than 10 days while women without a uterus should only have estrogen
- Either estrogen or combined estrogen—progestin therapy should NOT be used for primary or secondary prevention of CHD. Dietary and lifestyle changes and lipid lowering agents should be considered.
- These recommendations may not be applied to women with premature or early menopause
- The use of estrogen or combined estrogen—progestin therapy should be limited to the shortest duration consistent with treatment goals, benefits and risks.
- Low dose preparations should be considered and have been shown to have symptomatic relief and preservation of bone density without an increase in endometrial hyperplasia.
- Other estrogen—progestin combinations and a transdermal therapy should be considered.[37-39]

In practice, HRT is the drug of choice for women with vasomotor symptoms and is advised to be given "short term". "Short term" was previously considered at 5 years, however with the increased risk of breast cancer after 4 years in the WHI study, "short term" seems now more in the region of 3 to 4 years.

Women already on HRT for long term should evaluate their individual risks and benefits and consider alternative therapy. For women planning to discontinue HRT, there is no definitive guide to this process. Some patients might develop vasomotor symptoms and bleeding problems if HRT is stopped abruptly. Alternative therapy in the form of herbal medication may help the vasomotor symptoms at this stage.

REFERENCES

1. Executive Summary: Stages of Reproductive Aging Workshop (STRAW). Medscape Ob/Gyn and Women's Health 2002;7(1);1-6.
2. NN Ismael. A study of menopause in Malaysia. Maturitas 1994;19:205-09.
3. Premitha D, P Nadkarni, ST Nathan, S Raman, SZ Omar, RK Nadason. Malaysian women with regards to menopause and hormone replacement therapy. Abstract. 9th Malaysian Congress of Obstetrics and Gynecology. 1999: 29.
4. Torgerson DJ, Avenell A, Russell IT, Reid DM. Factors associated with onset of menopause in women aged 45-49. Maturitas 1994;19:83-92.
5. Faddy MJ, Gosden RG, Gougeon A. Accelerated disappearance of ovarian follicles in mid life: implications for forecasting menopause. Human Reproduction. 1992;7:1342-46.
6. Grisso JA, Freeman EW, Maurin E, Garcia-Espana B, Berlin JA. Racial differences in menopause information and the experience of hot flashes. Journal of General Internal Medicine 1999;14(2):98-103.
7. P Damodaran, R Subramaniam, SZ Omar, P Nadkarni, M Paramsothy. Profile of a Menopause Clinic in an urban population in Malaysia. Singapore Medical Journal, 2000;41(9):431-35.
8. Hajji SN. Pelvic relaxation and procidentia. In: Hajji SN, Evkans WJ (Eds) Clinical Reproductive Gynecology. Norwalk, Conn: Appleton and Lange,1993 pp 112-117.
9. Brincat MP, Galea R. Collagen: The significance in skin, bone and carotid arteries. In: Lobo RA (Ed). Treatment of the Postmenopausal Woman: Basic and Clinical Aspects, 2nd edn. Philadelphia, Pa; Lippincott Williams & Wilkins 1999; 203-12.
10. 2nd Consensus Statement on Management of Hyperlipidemia. Ministry of Heath, Malaysia. Academy of Medicine of Malaysia. 1998.
11. Gorodeski GI, Utian WH. Epidemiology and risk factors of cardiovascular disease in post menopausal women. In: Lobo RA (Ed). Treatment of the Postmenopausal Woman: Basic and Clinical Aspects, 2nd edn. Philadelphia, Pa;Lippincott Williams & Wilkins 1999; 315-26.
12. Hologic Inc. Normative data base. Waltham, Mass. 1995.
13. Lee JK, Khir ASM. Incidence if hip fracture in Malaysia above 50 years of age - variation in different age groups. Osteoporosis International. In press.
14. Clinical Practice Guidelines on Management of Osteoporosis. Ministry of Health, Malaysia. Malaysian Osteoporosis Society. Academy of Medicine 2001.
15. Jorm AF, Korten AE, Henderson AS. The prevalence of dementia: a quantitative integration of the literature. Acta Psychiatry Scandinavia 1987;76:465-79.
16. Vingerling JR, Dielemans I, Witterman CM. Macular degeneration and early menopause: a case control study. British Medical Journal 1995;310:1570-71.
17. Jeffcoat MK, Chesnut CH. Systemic osteoporosis and oral bone loss. Journal of American Dental Association 193;124:49-56.
18. Hollihn Uwe-K. Hormone Replacement Therapy. In: Hormone Replacement Therapy and the Menopause. Schering AG, 1997;84-116.
19. Lobo RA. The role of progestins in hormone replacement therapy. American Journal of Obstetrics and Gynecology 1992;166:1997-2004-2008.
20. The wrting group for the PEPI trial. Effects of hormone replacement therapy on endometrial histology in post menopausal women. Journal of the American Medical Association 1996;275:370-75.
21. Beresford S, Weiss NS, Voight L, McKnight B. Risk of endometrial cancer in relation to use of oestrogen combined with cylic progestogen therapy in post menopausal women. Lancet 1997;349:458-61.
22. Fraser IS, Wang Y. New delivery systems for hormone replacement therapy. In: Progress in the Management of Menopause. The Proceedings of the 8th International Congress on the Menopause. Wren BG (Ed). Parthenon Publishing Group. 1986;58-67.
23. Scughrus PJ, Lane MV, Scrimo PJ. Comparative distribution of estrogen receptor α(ERα) and β (ERβ) mRNA in rat pituitary, gonad and reproductive tracts. Steroids 1998;63:498-504.
24. Writing Group for the Women's Health Initiative Investigators. Risks and benefits of estrogen plus progestin in healthy post menopausal women: principal results from the Women's Health Initiative randomized controlled trial. Journal of the American Medical Association 2002; 288:321-33.
25. Kaunitz AM, Shulman LP. The hormone continuum. A disease preventive strategy during the 5th and 6th decades. Medscape Dec 2000.
26. Shumaker SA, Legault C, Rapp SR. Estrogen plus progestin and the incidence of dementia and mild cognitive impairment in postmenopausal women; the Women's Health Initiative Memory Study: a randomized controlled trial. Journal of the American Medical Association 2003; 289:2651-62.
27. Hammond CB. Confronting Aging and Disease: The role of HRT. Medscape, July 1999.
28. Hulley S, Grady D, Bush T for the Heart and Estrogen/ Progestin Replacement Study (HERS) Research Group. Randomised trial of estrogen plus progestin for secondary prevention of coronary heart disease in post menopausal women. Journal of the American Medical Association 1998; 280:605-13.
29. Grady D, Herrington D, Bittner V for the HERS Research Group. Cardiovascular disease outcomes during the 6.8 years of hormone therapy: Heart and Estrogen/Progestin Replacement Study follow up (HERS II) Journal of the American Medical Association 2002;288:49-57.

30. The Women's Health Initiative Steering Committee. Effects of Conjugated Equine Estrogen in Post Menopausal Women with Hysterectomy. The Women's Health Initiative Randomised Controlled Trial. Journal of the American Medical Association 2004: 291:1701-12.

31. Daly E, Vessey MP, Hawkins MM. Risk of venous thromboembolism in users of hormone replacement therapy. Lancet 1996;348:977-80.

32. Collaborative Group on Hormonal Factors in Breast Cancer. Breast Cancer and HRT: collaborative reanalyses of data from 51 epidemiological studies of 52, 705 women with breast cancer and 108,411 women without breast cancer. Lancet. 1997;350:1047-1059.

33. Dupont WD, Page DI, Parl FF. Estrogen replacement therapy in women with a history of proliferative breast disease. Cancer 1999;85(6):1277-83.

34. Sellers TA, Mink PJ, Cerhan JR. Role of HRT in the risk for breast cancer and total mortality in women with a family history of breast cancer. Annals of Internal Medicine 1997;127(11):973-80.

35. Garton M. Breast Cancer and Hormone Replacement Therapy: The Million Women Study. Lancet 2003; 362:1328-31.

36. Ginsburg J, Prelevic GM. The place of tibolone in menopausal therapy. In: The Management of the Menopause: The Millenium Review. John Studd (Ed).The Parthenon Publishing Group. 2000: 59-68.

37. Consensus Opinion. Role of calcium in peri and post menopausal women: consensus opinion of the North American Menopause Society. Menopause 2002;8(3): 84-95.

38. Black DM, Thompson DE, Bauer DC, Ensrud K for the Fracture Intervention Trial. Fracture risk reduction with alendronate in women with osteoporosis: the Fracture Intervention Trial. Journal of Clinical Endocrinology and Metabolism 2002;85:4118-24.

39. Barrett-Connor E, Grady E, Sashegyi A for the MORE investigators (Multiple Outcomes of Raloxifene Evaluation). Raloxifene and cardiovascular events in the osteoporotic post menopausal women: four year results from the MORE randomized trial. Journal of the American Medical Association 2002;287:847-57.

40. Response to the Women's Health Initiative Study Results by the American College of Obstetrician and Gynecologists. Statement from the American College of Obstetricians and Gynecologists, August 2002.

41. Report for the NAMS Advisory Panel on Post menopausal Hormone Therapy. Statement from the North American Menopause Society, October 2002.

42. Hormone Replacement Therapy (HRT) and Women's Health Initiative (WHI) Report: The Position of the Ministry of Health Malaysia. October 2002.

30.

V Sivanesaratnam

Gynecological Cancer Screening

INTRODUCTION

The genital tract is one of the commonest situations of primary malignant disease in women. Such malignancies continue to be a major cause of mortality amongst women worldwide. The aim of screening is to detect the disease before symptoms occur, i.e. at the pre-invasive or more curable stage, when timely treatment can avert disability and mortality. The screening test is not intended to be diagnostic, but rather to differentiate the population likely or not likely to have the disease; the former will subsequently require further tests to confirm the diagnosis. A suitable screening test should have high specificity, sensitivity and positive predictive value and should not be costly.

The three most prevalent gynecological cancers in the Asia-Oceania region are cervical, ovarian and endometrial cancers. Methods of screening these cancers will now be discussed.

CERVICAL CANCER

The uterine cervix is the most frequent site in the genital tract affected by cancer. It is important to note that all pre-invasive and very early invasive lesions of the cervix are completely asymptomatic. Cervical cancer is easily detected in the pre-invasive or cervical intra-epithelial neoplasia (CIN) phase by cervical cytology; *cervical cancer is, thus, perhaps the only cancer that is preventable.* Yet in many parts of the developing and underdeveloped world cervical cancer is diagnosed in a late stage and as a consequence results in a high mortality. About 50% of all women in the industrialized countries would have had at least one Pap smear test during a 5-year period, compared to only 5% in developing countries.[1] Thus, in the industrialized world cervical cancer is uncommon, ranking 10th after more common cancers, such as breast, lungs, colon, etc.[1] Data from several Scandinavian studies showed that organised screening programs resulted in sharp reductions in incidence and mortality from cervical cancer; an 80% reduction in mortality was observed in Iceland, whilst a reduction in mortality of 50 and 34% occurred in Finland and Sweden. Similar reductions have been observed in the US and Canada.[2]

In contrast cervical cancer continues to be a leading cause of mortality and morbidity in developing countries. In Malaysia it is the second most common cancer in females (after breast cancer). The peak incidence is 60 to 69 years; the disease is more common

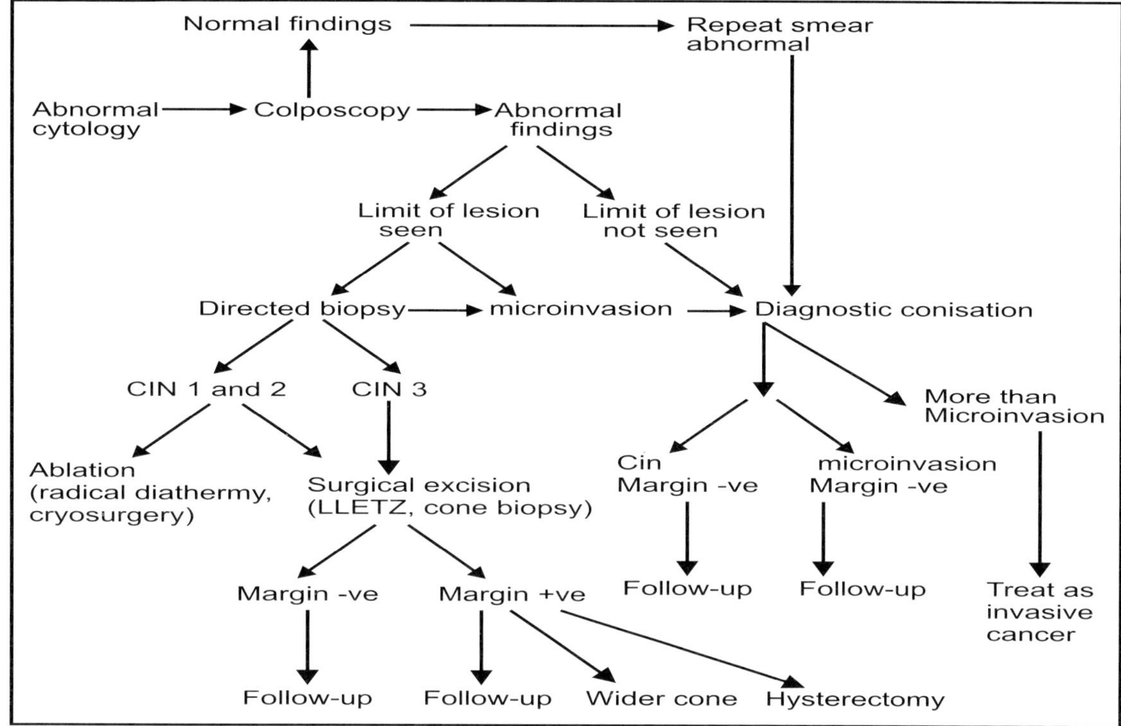

Figure 30.1: Cervical cancer age—standardized incidence per 100,000 population (*Source* - First Report of the National Cancer Registry—Malaysia 2002)

amongst Chinese compared to Malays and Indians[3] (Fig. 30.1).

Papanicolao Smear

The Papanicolao (Pap) smear fulfills the most important criteria of a useful screening test: good sensitivity and specificity, low cost, and little risk or discomfort to the patient. Furthermore, effective modes of therapy are available when abnormal cells are detected.

Taking a Cervical Smear

Invasive cervical cancer begins in the transformation zone, the area at or just outside the squamo-columnar junction, which was originally lined by columnar epithelium, and which by the process of metalplasia becomes covered by squamous epithelium. It is this area that is at risk of carcinogenic attack and which may show abnormal changes. As these changes may occur in just small foci of the transformation zone, sweeping the sampling device a full 360° to cover the whole transformation zone is essential for proper sampling. It is obvious that the cervix must be well visualized first,

as occasionally obvious carcinoma may give "negative" smears because blood, necrotic material and leucocytes may obscure the often poorly preserved malignant cells.

The use of traditional lubricants to aid speculum examination is best avoided as these may induce artifact and interfere with the interpretation of the smear. If necessary water can be used as a lubricant.

Whilst various techniques have been used for obtaining a cervical smear, we have found the use of a wooden spatula to scrape the ectocervix and moist cotton tip application to obtain an endocervical sample, will adequately sample the whole transformation zone. Such combined endocervical and ectocervical samples halves the false negative rate. Slides should be immediately fixed to avoid drying artifact resulting in loss of staining specificity and morphological detail.

Significance of Endocervical Cells in Smear

The importance of the presence of endocervical cells in cervical smears has been stressed; the use of the cytobrush does significantly increase the yield of endocervical cells. It is often said that the presence of endocervical cells in a cervical smear implies that the squamo-columnar junction has been adequately sampled. It appears that the pursuit of endocervical cells as an indication of an adequate smear has been over emphasized. In 10% of pre-menopausal and 50% of postmenopausal women, endocervical cells may not be obtained even on repeat smears. There is no doubt that complete sampling of the transformation zone where CIN begins is essential to reduce the number of false negative smears; thus, the importance of visualization of the cervix and taking an adequate ectocervical smear should not be overlooked. In postmenopausal women an additional smear with a cytobrush will be of help as the transformation zone usually recedes into the cervical canal.

False Negative Smears

This may arise from:
- A sampling error by the clinician
- A screening error by the cytotechnician who has failed to recognize the abnormal cells
- An error in interpretation

Clinician sampling errors accounts for two-thirds of false negative smears, primarily due to failure to obtain an adequate smear from the transformation zone. Screening errors of 17 to 58.5% have been reported.

Liquid-based Cytology

This test (Thinprep) aims to reduce the incidence of false negative results by optimising the cell collection and preparation by removing mucus, protein and red blood cells from the preparation; this allows for cells to be uniformly distributed, improves fixation and preserves cellular architecture. This is new technology requiring technicians and cytopathologists to be retrained. Other disadvantages include difficulty in assessing glandular abnormalities.

Automated Cytological Screening

As most Pap smears do not contain atypical cells, a semi-automated system such as PAPNET might help minimise the tedious aspects of the cytotechnician's tasks. The use of PAPNET may facilitate identification of high grade squamous intraepithelial lesions missed during standard cytological screening. Whilst this method of screening is more accurate than the Pap smear, this is very expensive and may not be cost-effective in developing countries.

The Bethesda System (TBS)

Recently, the terms low- and high-grade squamous intraepithelial lesion (SIL) have emerged from the TBS system of reporting cervical/vaginal smears.[4] Under this system are defined:
- Atypical squamous cells of undertermined significance (ASCUS)
- Inclusion of changes associated with human papilloma virus (HPV) (i.e. koilocytosis) with CIN 1 as low-grade squamous intra-epithelial (LSIL) lesion
- Use of only two terms, LSIL and high-grade squamous intra-epithelial lesion (HSIL) to encompass the spectrum of squamous cell carcinoma precursors, in lieu of the degrees of dysplasia/CIS and the three grades of CIN

Low-grade precursor lesions usually regress, and in a compliant low-risk population, this can be managed by repeat cytology. However, whatever method of classification is used for reporting cervical smears, clinicians must take note that this does not confirm the diagnosis. Any form of atypia seen on the smear is significant and needs further evaluation.

ADENOCARCINOMA

Screening programs probably have little effect on detection of adenocarcinomas. At least 40% of adenocarcinoma or adeno-squamous carcinoma were not detected on cervical cytology in an Australian study.[6] In a case-control study in Japan,[7] the risk of adeno-carcinoma of the cervix was reduced by only 55% by cervical cytology compared to 86% reduction in the risk of squamous cell carcinoma.

Nevertheless, it is important to note that an increasing number of adenocarcinoma are now being seen, particularly in young women. An incidence of 26.9% of invasive adenocarcinoma has been reported by Sivanesaratnam et al.[8]

Who are the Women "at risk"?

There is no single ideal screening program at present. A balance of good medicine and practical/financial aspects needs to be considered. The population "at risk" needs to be screened. These include:

- Early age of coitus
- Experience with multiple sexual partners
- "High risk" males and their multiple exposures

The above factors would help promote the development and spread of sexually transmitted diseases. Epidemiological studies indicate that cervical cancer and its precursor are caused principally, if not exclusively, by HPV infection.[9] Of the more than 90 sub-types of HPV so far detected, about 20 infect the cervix. The "high risk" HPV types are 16, 18, 31, 33, 35, 39, 45, 51, 52, 56 and 58 and the "low risk" types are 6, 11, 42, 43 and 44. Reid *et al*[10] demonstrated that almost all patients who had HPV type 6 and 11 had CIN 1 or 2 lesions, whilst 90% of patients with CIN 3 and invasive lesions were infected with HPV 16, 18 or 31.

HPV infection is much more common in the younger than older patients. Recent evidence[9] suggests that in many women HPV infection is transient and is cleared within the first 12 to 24 months. Thus, whilst the presence of HPV infection in the young is an indication of sexual activity rather than a cervical cancer risk, in older women persistence of HPV is an indication of increased cervical cancer risk. A combination of *Pap smear* and *HPV DNA screening* can help detect 95% of patients with high grade lesions, 100% with invasive cancers and 70% with low grade lesions.[11] This method is being considered as a primary screening method in some countries.

Other "risk factors" include:

- Smoking—nicotine and cotinine were noted to be concentrated in the cervical mucus in patients with CIN 3; this may represent a mechanism for the association of cervical neoplasia and smoking.[12]
- Oral contraceptives—a firm statement on its role in cauzation of cervical cancer cannot yet be made.

Clearly, the multifactoral etiology of cervical carcinoma must be accommodated in screening programs.

What should the Pap Smear Screening Interval be?

As squamous cell carcinoma of the cervix is related to sexual activity, screening should commence at onset of sexual activity. There is no agreement as to how frequently it should be done. The Canadian Task force, noting that dysplasia may predate CIN 3 by a decade or so, suggested that in "low risk" women smears at 3-yearly interval may be adequate. The American Cancer Society and the American College of Obstetricians and Gynecologists similarly permit less frequent screening in a "low risk" woman after she has had 3 annual satisfactory cytological smears.

A large retrospective study on invasive cervical carcinoma by Morrell *et al*[13] found at least 2 negative smears in 20% of cases in the 3 years prior to diagnosis of cancer. Similarly, a Alaskan study[14] noted 52% of native women who developed invasive cervical cancer had a normal Pap smear 3 years prior to d ignosis. Although sampling error is a possibility, these developments suggest a rapidly developing carcinoma. This means that clinicians must deal with two groups of patients: one with rapidly growing CIN lesions and the other with slow growing ones. Annual screening would thus appear appropriate.

When should Screening Stop?

This is still under debate. For women who have had regular negative smears, 60 years has been suggested as a safe cut-off point. Ashley[14] pointed out the existence of two different forms of cervical cancer:

- Those with a recognisable pre-invasive stage occurring in young women
- A less common type occurring in older women which develops without a detectable pre-cancerous phase.

16.6% of women with early invasive carcinoma of the cervix undergoing radical hysterectomy were noted by us to be between 50 and 69 years.[8] Furthermore, the peak incidence of cervical carcinoma in Malaysia is between 60 and 69 years.[3] Age should, therefore, be no barrier for cervical screening, particularly when the woman has had no previous Pap smear.

The Abnormal Smear—What is the Next Step?

The cervical smear detects that an abnormal area exists and provides an estimate of its severity. Colposcopy would be the next step as it would help assess the site, extent and severity of the lesion, enabling "targeted" biopsies without resort to cone biopsy or more radical measures. Figure 30.2 outlines the plan of management.

When no lesion is visible and the whole transformation zone has been visualized, a false positive smear has to be considered. The time and expense involved in performing colposcopic evaluation makes colposcopy less effective than cytology for cervical cancer screening. It is, however, useful for following up women with an abnormal smear in pregnancy to help monitor the progression, if any, of the lesion; absence of appearance of invasion will allow a conservative approach leaving the definite treatment to be considered after delivery.

Other Methods of Screening for Cervical Cancer

- *Cervicography*

  This colpophotographic screening technique, which photographs the cervix after application of acetic acid, has a very high false positive rate and is costly compared with Pap smear; it is, thus, inappropriate as a primary screening tool.

- *'Down staging' for cancer of the cervix*

  Lack of laboratory facilities or resources for cytological screening is largely responsible for the late stage at diagnosis of cervical cancer in developing countries. An active attempt should be instituted to detect the cancer at an early stage when it is curable. This approach of "clinical down-staging" by visualization of the cervix with a speculum and recognising cervical abnormalities would require training of nurses and other pramedics. However, a recent evaluation found unaided visual inspection not very promising either as a preselection procedure

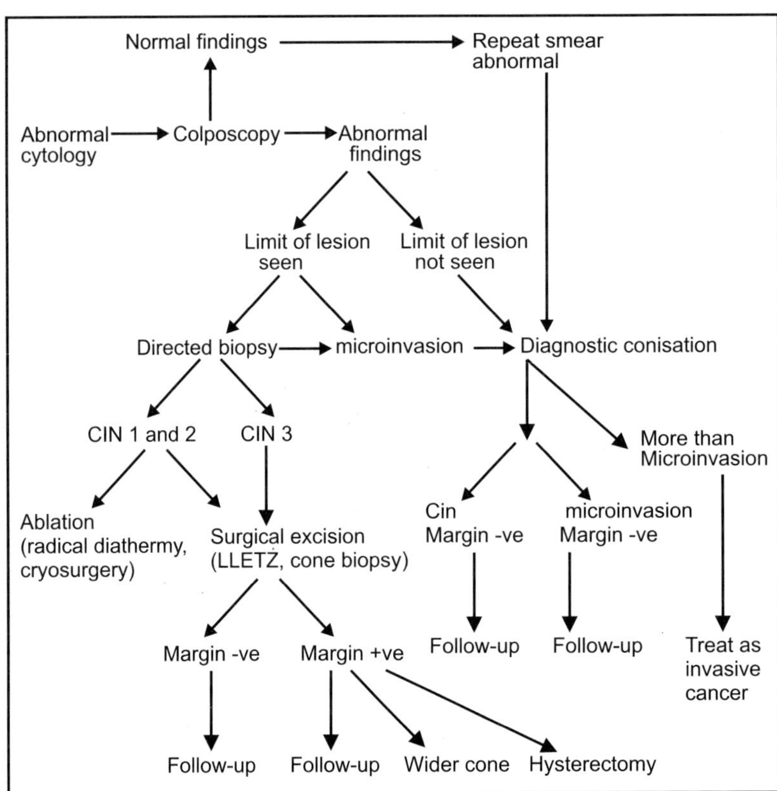

Figure 30.2: Outline of plan of management of patients with abnormal smear

for cytology or as a low-technology measure for cervical cancer screening.[15]

OVARIAN CANCER

Ovarian cancer is a leading cause of death amongst women both in the West and in the Asia-Oceania region, and other parts of the world. In spite of advances in surgical staging and debulking surgery and the use of modern chemotherapeutic regimes, the overall survival for ovarian cancer is only 41.6%.[16] The paucity of early symptoms and the intra-pelvic location of the ovaries which limits their accessibility to physical examination makes this an elusive disease. This results in the majority presenting in an advanced stage. A major reduction in mortality will not occur until patients can be identified with early stage disease; the 5-year survival in stage 1 disease is 80-90%.[16] A reliable screening test is, therefore, essential.

Attempts to screen the disease have often resulted in frustration; this is accounted for by several factors:

- The anatomic location of the ovaries is not amenable to any direct inspection
- Unlike cervical cancer, ovarian cancer lacks any defined precursor lesion
- Little is understood of the natural history, and time interval for progression from early to advanced disease is not known. Several reports in the literature of advanced ovarian cancer developing within months of a negative laparoscopy and peritoneal cytology, would suggest that ovarian cancer can develop quickly from normal-looking ovaries. Thus, the surveillance interval should not exceed 1 year in order to detect early stage of the disease.
- The incidence and prevalence of ovarian cancer are relatively low. The majority (90-95%) destined to develop ovarian cancer do not have a family history, and, thus, will not benefit from screening.

The screening techniques available include:
- Serum tumor markers
- Ultrasound
- Pelvic examination

Serum Tumor Markers

An ideal tumor marker for ovarian cancer does not exist. The marker most commonly studied is CA_{125}. This is an antigenic determinant on a glycoprotein shed into the blood stream by malignant cells derived from coelomic epithelium, i.e. müllarian ducts and cells lining the peritoneum, pleura and pericardium. The CA_{125} levels are increased in about 50% of patients with stage 1 and 90% of those with stage 2 epithelial ovarian cancers, more frequently the serous type. This marker is usually not elevated in mucinous, sex cord, germ cell and Brenner tumors. However, CA_{125} is not specific to ovarian cancer as it can be elevated in other malignancies and non-gynecological tumors as well as in benign disorders (Table 30.1)

Table 30.1: Conditions associated with elevated CA_{125} levels

Malignancies	Non-malignant conditions
Gynecological	*Gynecological*
• Epithelial ovarian carcinoma	• Uterine leiomyomata
• Endometrial carcinoma	• Pelvic inflammatory disease
	• Early pregnancy
Non-gynecological	• Benign ovarian cysts
• Carcinoma of pancreas	• Endometriosis
• Breast carcinoma	• Ovarian hyperstimulation
	Non-gynecological
	• Acute pancreatitis
	• Cirrhosis
	• Pericarditis
	• Colitis
	• Peritonitis
	• Abdominal tuberculosis

The serum CA_{125} levels may be influenced by various factors:
- It fluctuates during the menstrual cycle
- Menopausal status,
- Previous hysterectomy (in pre-menopausal women)
- Age (in postmenopausal women)

The reference limit of 35 U/ml needs to be adjusted for these conditions.[17] Most studies agree that CA_{125} levels is most helpful in the evaluation of post-menopausal women with pelvic masses. Vasilev *et al*[18] observed 80% of women > 50 years of age with pelvic masses and CA_{125} > 35 U/ml had malignancies compared to only 15% in those < 50 years of age. This is useful information in deciding on management by a gynecologic oncologist or general gynecologist.

Ultrasound

Transabdominal ultrasound has a poor specificity and sensitivity for detecting ovarian cancer. In one of the largest prospective studies on ovarian cancer screening of 5540 asymptomatic pre- and post-menopausal women, 65 laparotomies were performed for each case of ovarian cancer detected.[19]

Transabdominal ultrasound has now been largely replaced by transvaginal sonography (TVS) along with color Doppler techniques to improve specificity.

The advantages of TVS are:

- A full bladder which is both uncomfortable and time-consuming is not needed
- Obese patients can be easily scanned
- The transducer probe is close to pelvic organs resulting in better images

There can be difficulties associated with differentiating benign from malignant ovarian cysts on ultrasonography. De Priest *et al*[20] proposed a "morphology index"—based on tumor volume, cyst wall structure and structure of septa—that may increase the specificity of TVS as a screening tool. Van Nagell[21] recently reported on 57,214 patients who had annual TVS and 180 patients were subjected to surgical intervention. Of the 17 cases of ovarian cancer detected, 11 were in Stage 1, 3 in Stage 2, and 3 in Stage 3. In this study the use of TVS was associated with a sensitivity of 81%, specificity of 98.97%, positive predictive value of 9.4% and negative predictive value of 99.97%. Annual TVS screening appeared to achieve the primary objective of earlier detection of disease.

The risk of malignancy in a unilocular ovarian cyst <10 cm in diameter is essentially non-existent, whilst that in complex ovarian tumors is significant requiring their early removal.

The presence of neovascularization in malignant ovarian tumors has prompted the use of Doppler ultrasound as a screening tool. Malignant tumors on color Doppler have a low resistance index (RI) and low pulsatility index (PI) than benign tumors. However, low impedence flow are normal in the luteal phase and in

inflammatory process and some benign lesions and these should be kept in mind. Further, some carcinomas have high impedence flow. A recent European randomised study for ovarian cancer screening found that color Doppler did not reduce the false positive rate.

Whilst ultrasound has no hazards, the disadvantages to take note of are time, costly equipments and trained personnel needed to carry out the examination. The available data suggests that on its own ultrasonography does not exhibit adequate specificity for screening the general population.

Pelvic Examination

Routine pelvic examination for the early detection of ovarian cancer is disappointing and is of limited value in screening asymptomatic women. Despite the limitations, it is reasonable to examine the ovaries at any opportunity during cervical screening, antenatal booking, postnatal visits or family planning clinics. Physicians must have a high degree of suspicion especially on women with vague pelvic symptoms and perform a pelvic examination as part of routine gynecological examination. Ten percent of post-menopausal women with palpable ovaries have an ovarian neoplasm; palpable ovaries more than one year before menarche and in post-menopausal period are abnormal.

Multi-modal Strategy

A critical factor for ovarian cancer screening is achieving a predictive value that is sufficiently high because of the rarity of the disease and the need for invasive procedures to evaluate a positive test. A positive predictive value of less than 10% is unacceptable in clinical practice. The low predictive values obtained with either CA_{125} or ultrasound do not justify their individual use for population screening, particularly when data documenting a decrease in mortality because of screening is lacking.

Jacob *et al*[22] concluded after a large randomised trial that there was no significant difference in mortality rate between asymptomatic post-menopausal women subjected to annual CA_{125} followed by TVS (if CA_{125} was

> 30 U/ml for 3 years) and controls and stated there was no justification in this type of multimodal ovarian cancer screening of the general population.

What then is the Current Status of Ovarian Cancer Screening?

Screening techniques may be appropriate in patients with a documented significant family history of ovarian cancer; these, however, comprise < 1% of all ovarian cancers. The current screening modalities to identify highly curable early stage ovarian cancer in asymptomatic women have been rather disappointing. The high false positive tests can result in unnecessary investigations including surgical intervention in otherwise healthy women resulting in unnecessary morbidity and adverse psychological effects. No conclusion can be drawn as to the efficacy of any screening method at the moment; we have to await the results of several on-going large scale prospective randomised studies using multimodal strategy. At the current moment, in view of the low prevalence of the disease in the general population and the lack of scientific evidence that deaths from ovarian cancer are decreased by screening, routine screening for ovarian cancer cannot be recommended. It is, however, prudent to examine the adnexae when performing gynecological examination for other reasons; in fact, all women should have an annual recto-vaginal examination as part of medical care.

Attention should also be directed at prevention of ovarian cancer instead. All women should be encouraged to engage in risk reducing lifestyle: breast feeding, oral contraceptives and tubal ligation. Increased contraceptive usage in the UK had resulted in a parallel decrease in ovarian cancer incidence.[22]

ENDOMETRIAL CANCER

In Malaysia this constitutes 3.4% of all female cancers. Mortality from this disease is low largely because of the early development of symptoms; it primarily manifests as postmenopausal or abnormal uterine bleeding which triggers an evaluation with an endometrial sampling. Majority of cases are thus, diagnosed when the disease is confined to the uterus.

Risk factors associated with the development of endometrial carcinoma include:

- Obesity
- Use of estrogen after menopause
- History of anovulation and nulliparity
- Breast cancer and tamoxifen therapy
- Hereditary nonpolyposis colorectal cancer (Lynch type II syndrome)

Routine screening of women for endometrial cancer is not of any proven benefit. No screening test has been evaluated for its impact on endometrial cancer mortality, even amongst "high risk" women.

Cytology

The Pap smear test is too insensitive for detection of early endometrial cancer; occasionally this may pick up exfoliated endometrial cells. The presence of such cells in a Pap smear of a postmenopausal woman, not on exogenous hormones, is abnormal and requires further assessments. Endometrial cytology has not been evaluated in women who do not have symptoms of endometrial cancer.

Endometrial Biopsy

Pipelle endometrial sampling is a convenient office procedure; whilst the overall accuracy is high, the efficacy of the technique in asymptomatic women has not been evaluated.

Ultrasonography (TVS)

Whilst this has been used to evaluate women with abnormal vaginal bleeding, its efficacy in screening for endometrial cancer in asymptomatic women is unknown.

Thus, much remains to be done in developing a safe, sensitive and specific screening test for endometrial cancer.

CONCLUSION

The goal of screening programs is to make a diagnosis before invasive cancer develops. The only gynecological malignancy where cytological screening has proven its value is in cervical cancer, but as yet, there is no reliable, cost effective screening tests available for ovarian and endometrial cancers. An annual Pap smear test will not only allow for early detection of malignancies of the cervix, but will also give an opportunity to physicians to screen for breast lumps by palpation, for ovarian malignancies and pelvic abnormalities by bimanual and rectovaginal examinations, and for vulval neoplasm by careful inspection.

REFERENCES

1. Richart R. Screening—the next century. Cancer 1995; 76: 1919-27.
2. Benedet JL, Anderson MB and Matistic JP. A comprehensive program for cervical cancer detection and management. Am J. Obstet Gynecol 1992; 166: 1254-59.
3. Lim GCC, Yahaya H, Lim TO. The first report of the National Cancer Registry—Cancer incidence in Malaysia, 2002.
4. Kurman RJ, Soloman DJ. The Bethesda system for reporting cervical/vaginal cytological diagnosis. Definitions, criteria and explanatory notes terminology and specimen adequacy. New York: Springer Verlag, 1993.
5. Anderson GH, Boyes DA, Bendect JH, et al. Organization and results of cervical cytology screening program in British Columbia, 1955—85. MBJ 1988; 296: 975-78
6. Mitchell H, Medley G, Drake M. Quality control measures for cervical cytology laboratories. Acta Cytol 1988; 32: 288-92.
7. Makino H, Sato S, Yajima A, Fukao A. Case-control study of the effectiveness of mass screening in reducing invasive cervical cancer. Nippon Sanka Fujunka Gakkai Zasshi, 1991; 43: 1226-32.
8. Sivanesaratnam V, Sen DK, Jayalakshmi, Ong G. Radical hysterectomy and pelvic lymphadenectomy for early invasive cancer of the cervix—14 years experience. Int. J. Gynecologic Cancer 1993; 231-36.
9. Schiffman MH. Recent progress in defining the epidemiology of human papilloma virus infection and cervical neoplasia. J Nat Cancer Inst 1992; 84: 394-98.
10. Reid R, Greenberg M, Jenson et al. Sexually transmitted papillomaviral infection. 1. The anatomic distribution and pathological grade of neoplastic lesions associated with different viral types. Am J Obstet Gynecol 1987; 156: 212-222.
11. Meijer CJLM, Snijders PJF, Van der Brule AJC et al. Can cytologic screening be improved by HPV screening? In: J Monsenego and AB Miller (Eds). Papillomavirus in Human Pathology. Ares-Serono Symposia Publications, Paris, 493-498.
12. Hellberg D, Nilson S, Haley MJ, et al. Smoking and cervical intra-epthelial neoplasia: nicotine and cotinine in serum and mucus in smokers and non-smokers. Am J Obstet. Gynecol 1988; 158: 910.
13. Morell ND, Taylor JR, Synder RN, et al. False—negative cytology rates in patients in whom invasive cervical cancer subsequently developed. Obstet Gynecol 1982; 60: 41-44.
14. Davidson M, Schnitzer PG, Bulkow LR, et al. The prevalence of cervical infection with human papilloma-viruses and cervical dysplasia in Alaska native women. J. Infact Dis 1994; 169: 792-800.
15. Wesley R, Sankaranarayanan R, Mathew B, et al. Evaluation of visual inspection as a screening test for cervical cancer. Br J Cancer 1997; 75: 436-40.
16. Pecorelli S, Odicino F, Maisonneuve P. J Epidemiol Biostat 1998; 3:17.
17. Grover S, Guinn M, Weidman P, Koh H. Obstet Gyneco 1992; 79: 511.
18. Vasilev SA, Schlaerth J, Campeau J, Morrow CP. Obstet Gynecol 1998; 71: 751-56.
19. Campbell S, Bhan V, Royston P et al. Transabdominal ultrasound screening for early ovarian cancer. BMJ 1989; 299: 1363-67.
20. De Priest PD, Shenson D, Fried A et al. 24th Annual Meeting of the Society Gynecologic Oncologists. Abstract No 21. 1993.
21. Van Nagell JR, De Priest PD, Reedy MB, et al. The efficacy of transvaginal sonographic screening in asymptomatic women at risk for ovarian cancer. Gynecol Oncol 2000; 77: 350-56.
22. Dos Santos Silva I, Swerdlow AJ. Br. J. Cancer 1995; 75: 485.

31.

V Sivanesaratnam

Preinvasive and Invasive Cancer of the Cervix

INTRODUCTION

The female genital tract is one of the commonest sites for primary malignant disease and the cervix uteri is the most common site affected by cancer. As shown in Figure 31.1 more than 75% of invasive cancer of cervix occurs in developing countries.

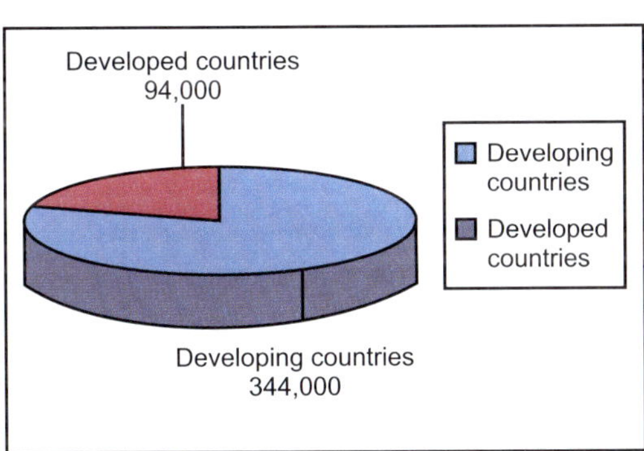

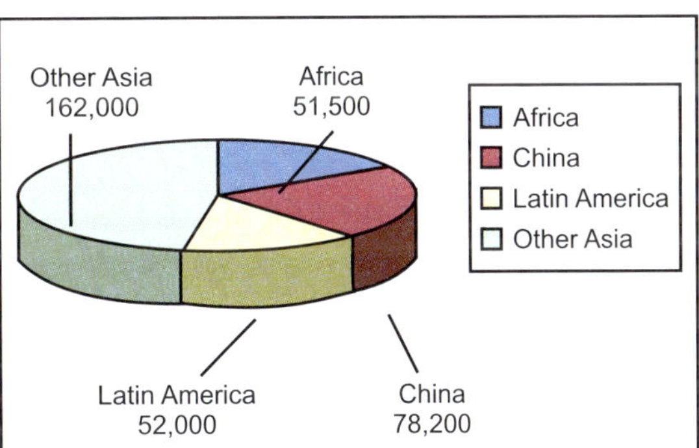

Figure 31.1: Estimated number of new cervical cancer cases per year, 1985 (Source-Parkin' et al, 1993)

In Malaysia it is the second most common cause of death from cancer amongst women after breast cancer (Fig. 31.2) and constitutes 12.0% of the total female cancers. In the West the incidence has decreased markedly as a result of effective screening programs; in many parts of Asia-Oceania, on the other hand, invasive cervical cancer is relatively high (Fig. 31.3) with most of the patients presenting in an advanced stage.

The reasons for the late presentation are:

- Fear of cancer
- Cultural taboos
- Ignorance
- Lack of appropriate facilities for early detection.

This is despite the fact that cervical cancer is the only preventable cancer. In Malaysia, the incidence of cervical cancer peaks at 60-69 years of age (Fig. 31.4). With changing trends,

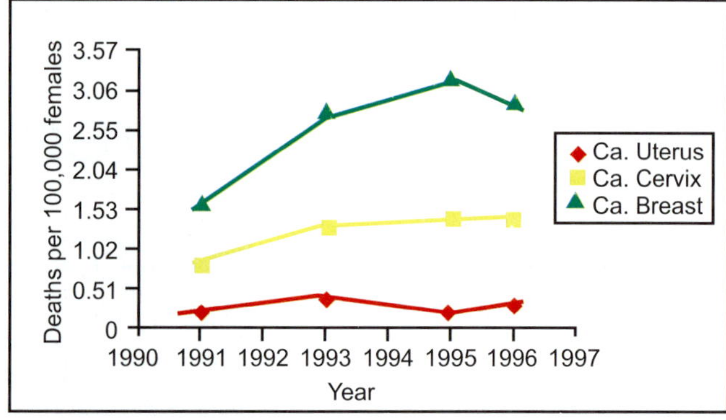

Figure 31.2: Death from gynecological cancer in Malaysia (per 100,000 females) (*Source:* SEAMIC Health Statistics 1991-1998)

this cancer is being seen in younger patients in many parts of the world, including the Asia-Oceania region.

Preinvasive Lesions of the Cervix

These by themselves are completely asymptomatic; only routine screening will help to detect these lesions (Details of screening for cervical cancer are discussed in the chapter on "Gynecologic Cancer Screening").

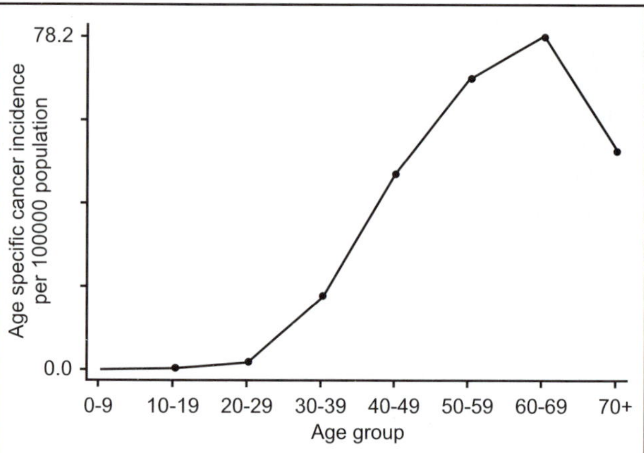

Figure 31.4: Carcinoma cervix: Age specific cancer incidence per 100,00 population, Peninsular Malaysia 2002. (*Source:* The first report of the National Cancer Registry. Cancer Incidence in Malaysia 2002)

The Concept of Cervical Intraepithelial Neoplasia

An active process of squamous metaplasia occurs within the transformation zone of the cervix in adolescence during periods of endocrine change; although this is a

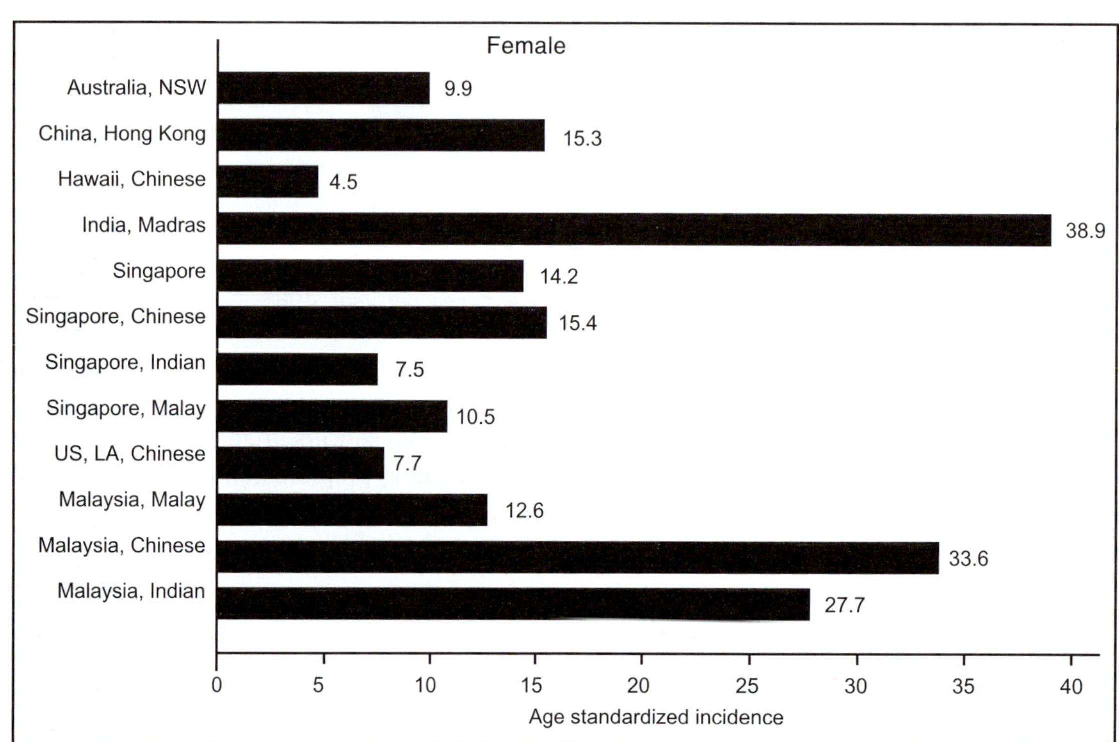

Figure 31.3: Carcinoma Cervix—Age specific cancer incidence per 100,000 population (International comparison) (*Source:* The first report of the National Cancer Registry, Cancer Incidence in Malaysia 2002).

normal physiological process, under the influence of a carcinogenic agent cellular alterations resulting in an atypical transformation zone may occur.

The concept of cervical intraepithelial neoplasia (or CIN) was introduced by Richart[1] to represent a spectrum of intraepithelial abnormalities which were previously called dysplasia and carcinoma-in-situ. The two latter terms imply that carcinoma-in-situ is more serious than dysplasia; one might, therefore, assume they represent 2 different entities resulting in over-treatment of the former and under-treatment of the latter. This is obviously unsatisfactory. The CIN terminology helps to emphasize the concept of a single disease process.

Pathology

The majority of CIN lesions are of squamous origin. The presence of abnormal immature basal cells above the lowermost layer in the epithelium indicates a dysplastic process. As the proliferation of these abnormal cells rises to the surface the grade of the lesion increases. When the abnormality is confined to the lower one-third, it is classified as CIN 1 (which corresponds to mild dysplasia); when the abnormality extends to involve the middle third it is known as CIN 2 (moderate dysplasia) and when greater than two-thirds is involved, the lesion is classified as CIN 3 (severe dysplasia and carcinoma-in-situ).

Microscopically, CIN is characterized by disorganized growth, nuclear abnormalities (such as ↑ nucleus: cytoplasmic ratio, hyperchromasia, nuclear pleomorphism and anisokaryosis) and increased mitosis at any level of the epithelium (*cf* in normal epithelium the increased mitosis is confined to the basal layers). These changes may extend to involve the endocervical glands in 88.6% of CIN 3 lesions.[2]

Etiology of Cervical Cancer

The etiology is multifactoral (Fig. 31.5)—the human papilloma virus (HPV) appears to have a crucial role. This is a sexually transmitted virus; the primary infection with the virus occurs mostly in young adults. The chance of an HPV infection during life is estimated at 80-85%; thus, the prevalence of the infection is high and a large proportion of women and men would be infected by the age of 30 years.[3] The mucosal types of HPV which

have strong affinity for the epithelium of the transformation zone are of 2 types:
- High risk HPV (hrHPV)
- Low risk HPV

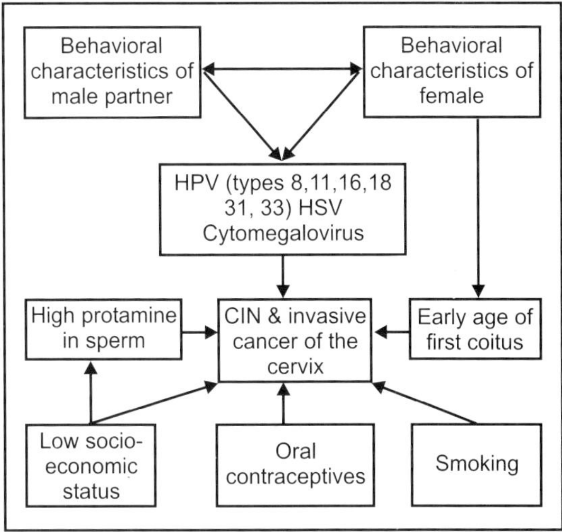

Figure 31.5: Multifactorial etiology of CIN and invasive cancer of the cervix

hrHPV or oncogenic viruses cause 95% of cervical cancer. Eighty percent of hrHPV infections are transient and asymptomatic with mean duration of 6-14 months and with no epithelial abnormalities. Only 20% cause morphological changes in epithelium of the cervix (CIN); only few without intervention will progress to cervical cancer. The only risk factor for progression of a premalignant lesion is persistence of hrHPV infection resulting in development and maintenance of CIN 3 lesions.[4] These hrHPV types include types 6, 11, 16, 18, 31, 33. A Bangkok study reported HPV 16 in 5% normal cervical cytology, 46% in CIN and 61% in cervical cancer. In a Malaysian study HPV-DNA was detected in 95.7% of cervical carcinoma (HPV 16 in 73.9% and HPV 18 in 65.2% of cancer).[5]

The *number of sexual partners* is the most important risk factor for acquisition of hrHPV infection. *Age at first coitus* and *smoking* are not independent risk factors for progressive disease.

Obesity and body fat distribution are associated more strongly with adenocarcinoma than with squamous cell carcinoma, suggesting that *hormonal factors* may play a prominent role in cervical adnocarcinoma.

Most studies show a link between *contraceptive steroids* and cervical cancer and presence of hormone receptors in cervical tissue; the duration of steroid usage is the variable most closely linked to development of cervical neoplasia. The WHO collaborative study[6] (1985) reports relative risk of 1.3-1.8 for users of 5 or > years of pill usage. Figure 31.6 illustrates the possible interaction between steroid hormones, HPV, and p53 in cervical cancer.

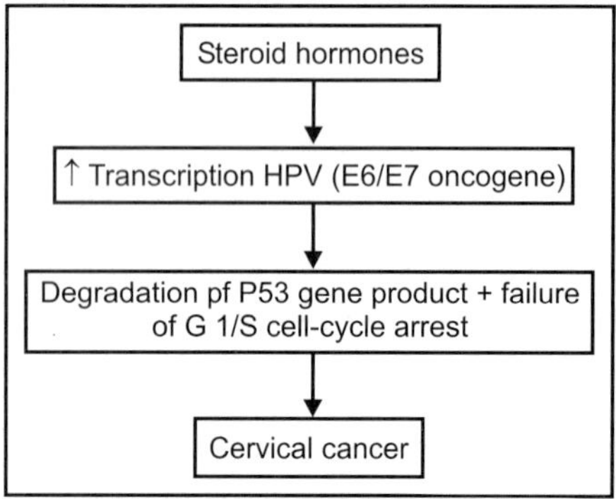

Figure 31.6: Proposed interaction between steroid hormones, HPV, p53 in cervical cancer (Source-Moodley et al, 2003)

Natural History of Cervical Carcinoma

The current understanding of the natural history of the disease is illustrated in Figures 31.7 and 31.8. CIN 3 precedes invasive carcinoma of the cervix in most cases. If CIN 3 is untreated 25% may regress, but majority will develop invasive carcinoma—30% at 10 years, 70% at 12 years and 80% at 30 years. However, it is important to bear in mind that this transit time need not always be slow.

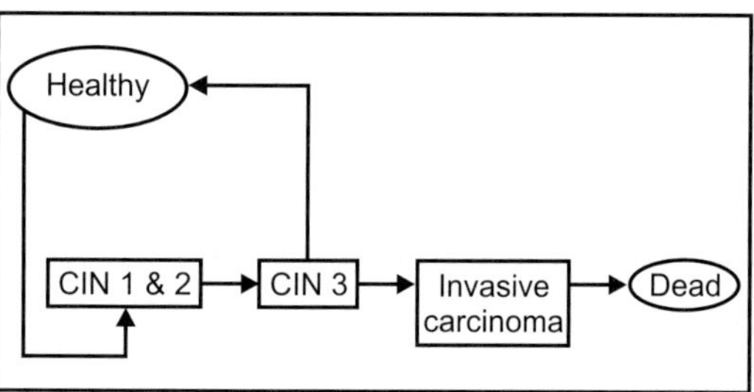

Figure 31.8: Natural history of cervical cancer and its precursor stages as a compartmental model

Management of CIN

An outline of the plan of management of an abnormal smear is given in the chapter on "Gynecological Cancer Screening".

The management can be broadly divided into:
- Ablative techniques
- Excisional techniques

Most patients with CIN lesions can be treated by local ablative techniques; however, certain criteria have to be met:
- the lesion must be seen in its entirety at colposcopy
- colposcopic assessment must be consistent with a CIN lesion; any suggestion of pre-clinical invasion contraindicates local destructive therapy; a cone biopsy is required
- there must be no suspicion colposcopically of abnormal endocervical cells
- close follow-up examination (cytology and colposcopy) is essential particularly in the first year after treatment

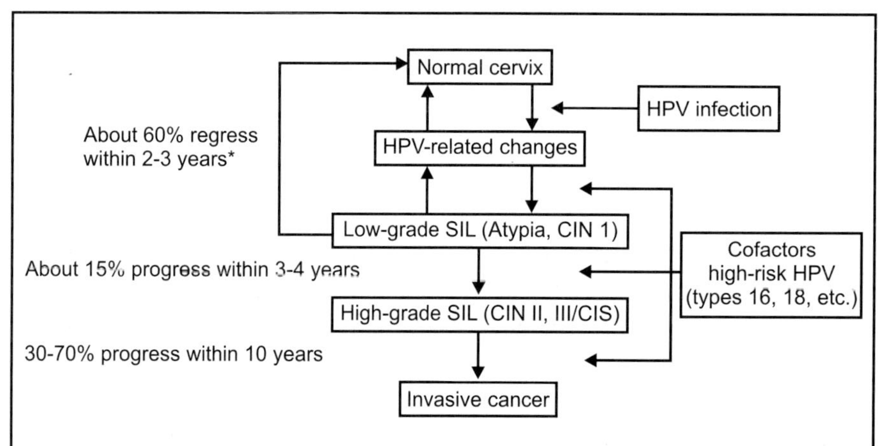

Figure 31.7: Natural history of cervical cancer. Current Understanding

The *ablative techniques* available include:
- radical electrocoagulation diathermy
- cryosurgery
- CO_2 laser ablation

Prior to the procedure, the atypical area is defined by colposcopy and the Schiller iodine staining test. Iodine is not taken up by the glycogen-deficient epithelium which contains CIN lesions. Any local destructive procedure must encompass all the iodine negative (Schiller positive) areas.

Radical Electrocoagulation Diathermy

The procedure usually requires a general anaesthetic and is an extremely effective way of treating all forms of CIN. The author routinely excises the abnormal area(s) initially to provide tissue for further evaluation. The cervix is then dilated to Hegar 9 dilator; this provides adequate exposure of the endocervical canal and discourages postoperative cervical stenosis. The epithelium in the crypts and distal canal is then coagulated by numerous insertions (15 to 20) of the needle electrode to a depth of one cm in the long axis of the cervix, each insertion lasting for at least 1-2 seconds. The ball electrode is then systematically used to fulgurate the epithelial surface until the mucus stops bubbling. A heavy vaginal discharge may persist for about 2 weeks, but other complications are minimal. Up to 98% are cured by this procedure.

Cryosurgery

This can be performed in an outpatient setting without anesthesia. Because of its anatomical configuration and easy accessibility, the cervix is an ideal organ for cryosurgery. A gun-type appliance with interchangeable probe tips of variable shape designed to approximate with the surface area of the atypical epithelium delivers the cryogen (liquid nitrogen, nitrous oxide or carbon dioxide) directly onto the cervix.

Once the probe tip is in place, the refrigerant is circulated until the edge of the iceball extends at least 3-5 mm on to the normal cervix. The tip is defrosted and the cervix examined colposcopically to ensure that all atypical areas are treated. With carbon dioxide a freeze-thaw-freeze technique is recommended.

A watery discharge may last 10-14 days after the procedure.

The primary success rate in treating CIN 3 with cryosurgery is about 95%. The concern is that large lesions with glandular involvement may not be cured by this treatment.

CO$_2$ Laser Ablation

In the 1980s, this was a popular method in the West to treat CIN; the method is performed in the outpatient setting, usually with no anesthesia and if necessary a paracervical block. High cure rates of 95% were reported. However, the high cost of laser equipment and advanced training required are major drawbacks; cryosurgery and radical diathermy coagulation, at a fraction of the cost, give equally good results.

The *excisional methods* available are:
- large loop excision of the transformation zone (LLETZ)
- cold-knife conisation
- laser-excisional conisation
- hysterectomy

Large Loop Excision of the Transformation Zone (LLETZ)

Recently this has become a cost-effective alternative to traditional approaches to therapy of CIN lesions. This can be performed in an outpatient setting using a paracervical block analgesia. Using a diathermy loop connected to a low-voltage output, the whole transformation zone including 10 mm or more of the endocervical canal can be excised; diathermy fulguration of the exposed stroma can help hemostasis.

The resulting thermocoagulation artefact at the margins may interfere with histopathological evaluation. Colposcopic directed biopsies may miss the most significant lesion, especially if taken by the 'average' colposcopist. One of the obvious advantages of LLETZ is in providing more tissue for histological evaluation resulting in increased recognition of those at risk of glandular involvement and early invasive lesions so that appropriate additional therapy can be carried out and management improved; it would have a place in patients for whom local destructive therapy is contraindicated. In a transient population where a high proportion of patients may be lost to follow-up, LLETZ appears reasonable.

Excisional Conisation

This is a combined diagnostic / therapeutic approach. The tissue removed must include the whole transformation zone, including free upper endocervical and lower ectocervical margins. Colposcopy and Schiller's test will help determine how large or small the zone should be. *There is no place today for conisation not preceded by colposcopy and colposcopically directed biopsies.*

The main *indications* for cone biopsy after colposcopic assessment are:

- Inability to visualize the whole transformation zone (upper limit extends into the cervical canal)
- Colposcopic suspicion of occult invasion, even if target biopsies show only CIN3
- Cytology suspicious of adenocarcinoma in situ
- Lesions where cervical cytology indicates a greater possibility of invasive disease than is indicated by colposcopy or the directed biopsy
- Repeated abnormal cytology suggesting neoplasia in the absence of colposcopic abnormality
- Microinvasion on punch biopsy

Cold-knife Conisation

In this technique, the circumferential ectocervical incision is made several millimeters beyond the outer limit of the transformation zone and the cone is then fashioned as dictated by the colposcopic findings. The cone bed is then inspected and bleeding points are diathermized; deep lateral sutures at 3 and 9 o'clock position will help occlude the descending branches of the uterine artery.

The overall complication rate is 23-25%; this includes hemorrhage, pelvic infection and cervical stenosis. Very rarely, a hematocervix/hemotometra may result from severe stenosis of the external os (Fig. 31.9).

Whilst it is important to ensure adequate surgical margins, it is also important not to remove more than is necessary of the endocervical canal to achieve a complete excision of the lesion. This is because of 3 reasons:

- Control of hemorrhage is easier if a small length of endocervical canal is removed

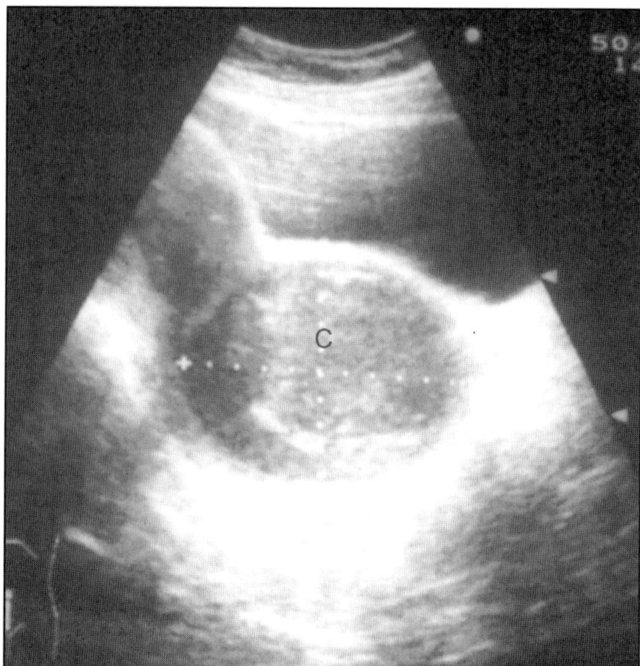

Figure 31.9: Pelvic ultrasound showing "ballooned-out" cervical canal (C) 6 months after cervical cone biopsy; 250 ml of blood was drained after dilatation of the external os

- A slightly reduced length of endocervical canal will not compromise fertility
- Maintenance of internal os is important

The result of a properly planned therapeutic conisation are excellent; long-term follow-up is obligatory. The dilemma arises when the cone biopsy margins are involved by CIN; 50-80% of such patients have been reported to have residual disease at hysterectomy.[7] The author routinely curettes the endocervix and lower part of endometrial cavity immediately after cone biopsy. When 'cone tip' is positive, the findings in the curettage specimens are used to decide whether to follow up the patient, repeat the cone biopsy or perform a hysterectomy.

Laser Excisional Conisation

This requires skill and experience with use of CO_2 laser and excellent clinical judgement. When compared to cold-knife conisation, the intraoperative and immediate postoperative bleeding are reduced. The high cost of the equipment, its maintenance and hazards to the surgeon are disadvantages. LLETZ cone is a simple and cheaper alternative that is now being performed in many clinical units.

Hysterectomy

Routine hysterectomy in the primary treatment of CIN is not justified. The *indications* for the procedure are mainly relative:

- Pre-existing gynecological problems uterine myoma, uterovaginal prolapse, dysfunctional uterine bleeding. Invasive cancer must be adequately excluded prior to hysterectomy
- Resection margins of cone biopsy show evidence of CIN; the alternatives have been discussed earlier
- The lesion extends to vaginal fornix.
  Follow up is essential in all cases.

Adenocarcinoma in situ (AIS)

This is a difficult lesion to diagnose occurring often in association with squamous CIN or at the edge of an invasive adenocarcinoma. The diagnosis is based on the presence of cellular atypia, abnormal mitoses, stratification, papillary projections and outpouchings; the normal architectural pattern of the endocervical crypts is preserved and often only the superficial crypts are involved. Stromal reaction, such as inflammatory infiltrate or edema, are absent, and the adjacent glands should be normal. A punch biopsy alone is insufficient for diagnosis; a cone biopsy, which may be therapeutic, is essential to establish the diagnosis and exclude the possibility of an invasive adenocarcinoma. Like CIN, AIS may be present for several years before invasive carcinoma develops.

Invasive Carcinoma of the Cervix

The most common *symptoms* are:
- Abnormal vaginal bleeding
- Vaginal discharge

Abnormal bleeding occurs in 80-90% of patients; this may be post-coital bleeding, intermenstrual spotting, irregular vaginal bleeding, and post-menopausal bleeding. Some patients may present with only a vaginal discharge—serous or mucoid; some patients may have a foul smelling discharge. Pelvic pain and leg edema are

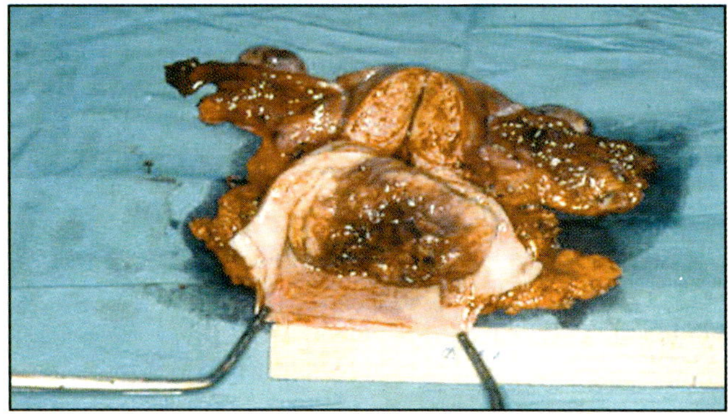

Figure 31.10: Radical hysterectomy specimen showing a large exophytic growth in cervix *(Stage 1B₂ disease)*

usually seen in advanced disease. A minority of patients are completely asymptomatic.

On vaginal speculum examination, the cervix may appear normal in early (microinvasive) cervical cancer, and if the lesion is endocervical. Visible disease takes *two main forms-exophytic* (Fig. 31.10) or *ulcerative*, which often bleeds easily on contact. The tumor may completely replace the cervix which may be distorted. The lesion may extend down the vagina and/or extend laterally into the parametrium; parametrial involvement may result in obstructive uropathy. In order to determine the extent of the disease a rectovaginal examination is essential; this would help determine the degree of cervical expansion and extent of parametrial and uterosacral ligament involvement.

Clinical Staging

This is based on the official staging classification by International Federation of Gynecology and Obstetrics which is based on physical examination and non-invasive tests (Table 31.1 and Fig. 31.11). These tests include biopsies, cystoscopy, sigmoidoscopy, chest radiographs and intravenous urography. Where facilities are available, a CT scan of the chest, abdomen and pelvis will give useful information not detected by above tests and may influence management.

Pathology

Squamous cell carcinoma accounts for 75% of all invasive lesions; there are *2 types*—the much more common and better differentiated large cell carcinoma (non-keratinizing and keratinizing types) and the much

Table 31.1: The International Federation of Gynecology and Obstetrics Staging for Cervical Carcinoma (1994)

Stage 1		**The carcinoma is strictly confined to the cervix (extension to the corpus is disregarded)**
	1a	Invasive carcinoma diagnosed only by microscopy (Pre-clinical carcinoma)
	1a1	Measured stromal invasion of not >3 mm in-depth and horizontal extension of not > 7 mm
	1a2	Measured stromal invasion of >3 mm but not >5 mm in-depth and horizontal extension of not > 7 mm
		(The diagnosis of Stage 1a1 and 1a2 should preferably be made on cone biopsy which includes the entire lesion. Vascular space involvement should not alter the staging but may influence mode of therapy)
	1b	Pre-clinical lesions greater than Stage 1a2 and clinically visible lesions confined to the cervix
	1b1	Clinically visible lesions not > 4 cm
	1b2	Clinically visible lesions > 4 cm
Stage 2		**The carcinoma extends beyond the cervix, but not to the lateral pelvic wall or to the lower third of the vagina**
	2a	No obvious parametrial involvement
	2b	Obvious parametrial involvement present
Stage 3		**The carcinoma extends to the lateral pelvic wall and/or the tumor involves the lower third of vagina. All the cases of hydronephrosis or a non-functioning kidney are included**
	3a	No extension to pelvic wall
	3b	Extension to pelvic wall (as detected by no cancer-free space between the tumor and the pelvic wall on rectovaginal examination) and/or hydronephrosis or non-functioning kidney
Stage 4		**The carcinoma has extended beyond the pelvis or has clinically involved the mucosa of bladder or rectum (Bullous edema does not permit the case to be allotted as Stage 4)**
	4a	Spread of growth to bladder or rectum
	4b	Spread to distant organs

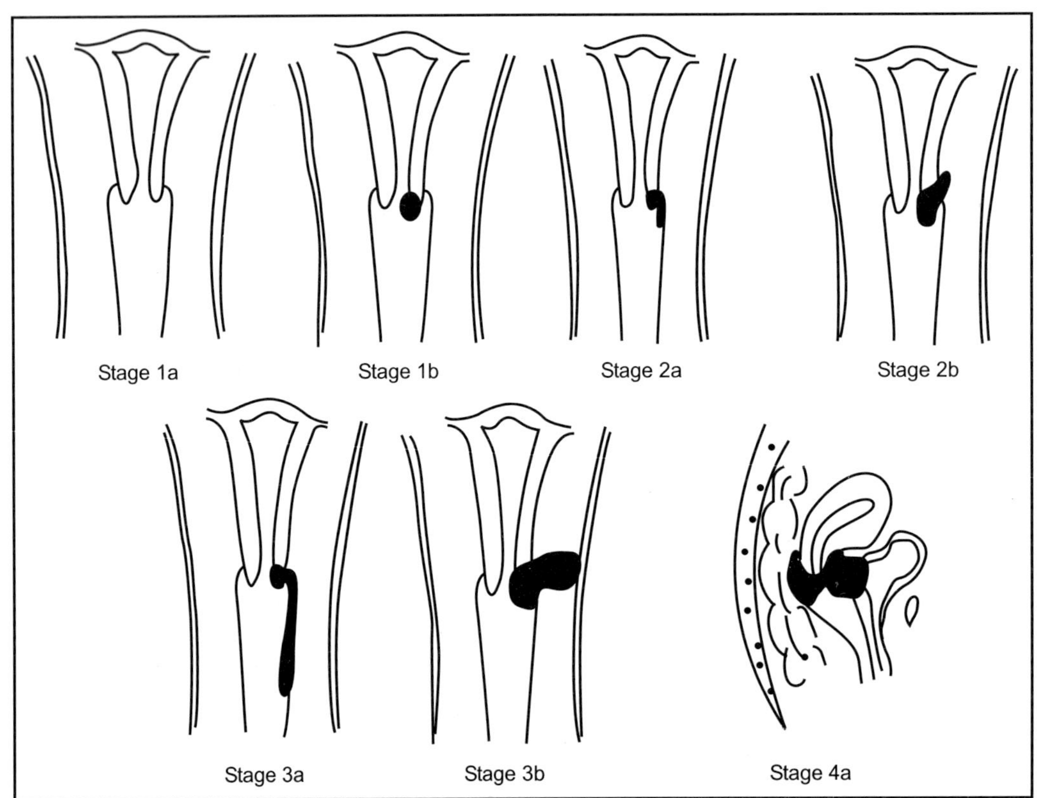

Figure 31.11: Clinical staging of cervical carcinoma (diagrammatic representation)

rarer small cell carcinoma, which is a poorly differentiated lesion.

About 25% of invasive cervical cancers are *adenocarcinoma* or *adenosquamous carcinomas*. The rest involves rarer types such as transitional cell, lymphomas and sarcomas, and melanoma and together these account for fewer than 1% of cases.

Management

Stage 1A (Microinvasive Carcinoma)

There is still controversy over the management of microinvasive cervical cancer. The risk of lymph node metastases depends on the depth of invasion (negligible if < 1 mm, 1% if invasion is 1-3 mm, and 4% if it is 3-5 mm). Hence, if the invasion is < 3 mm, hysterectomy can be avoided—a cone biopsy would suffice. For lesions > 3 mm and in those with lymphovascular permeation an extrafascial hysterectomy and pelvic lymphadenectomy would appear advisable.

Stage 1B and Early 2A

Radical hysterectomy and pelvic lymphadenectomy as well as radical radiotherapy (external pelvic radiation + brachytherapy) are equally effective forms of therapy. The *advantages* of *radical hysterectomy* are, it would allow for:

- Preservation of ovarian function
- Preservation of coital function

Both these important aspects will be compromised if radiotherapy is given. The incidence of ovarian metastases in Stage 1B squamous cell carcinoma is 0-1% allowing for conservation of normal looking ovaries in young women; the conserved ovaries are best transposed (paracaecal on the right and para-colic on the left) thus, protecting the ovaries should pelvic radiation be needed) subsequently. The incidence of ovarian metastases in adenocarcinoma of the cervix is higher (4.3%); in such cases it would not be wise to conserve the ovaries.[8]

Radical hysterectomy and pelvic node dissection (Wertheim's radical hysterectomy) involves removal of the uterus, upper-third of the vagina, parametria and paracolpos and a thorough pelvic lymphadenectomy

(common iliac, external iliac, obturator, internal iliac, gluteal, and presacral nodes) (Fig. 31.12). In older women a bilateral salpingo-oophorectomy is done.

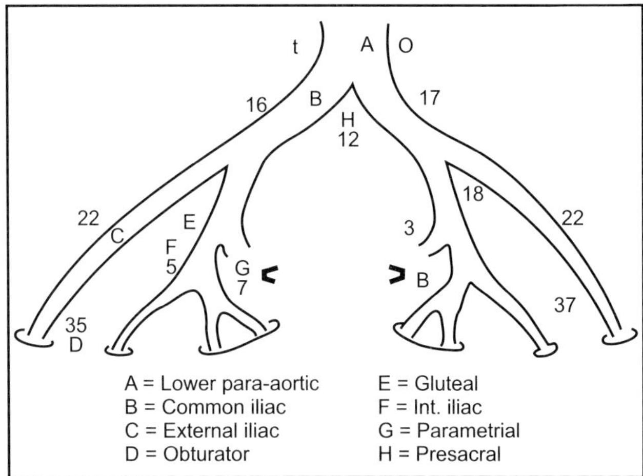

Figure 31.12: Distribution of positive pelvic nodes in 66 patients with stage 1B and early stage 2A carcinoma of the cervix (overall incidence 16.6%)

Complications of radical hysterectomy include:
- Urinary problems
  - Urinary tract infection
  - Bladder atony
  - Urinary fistula (vesico-vaginal, uretero-vaginal)
- Bowel problems
  - Atony of rectum, constipation
- Lymphedema (Fig. 31.13) (in about 1% of cases)

The most serious of these complications is urinary fistula; fortunately this occurs in only 2-3% of patients. The above complications can be minimized with improved surgical technique and appropriate postoperative care; early ambulation and chest physiotherapy are important adjuncts in the prophylaxis against postoperative thromboembolism.

Adjuvant Treatment

The following features seen on histopathological evaluation will adversely affect survival:
- Lymph node metastasis
- Full thickness stromal invasion
- Lympho-vascular tumor permeation
- Microscopic parametrial metastases

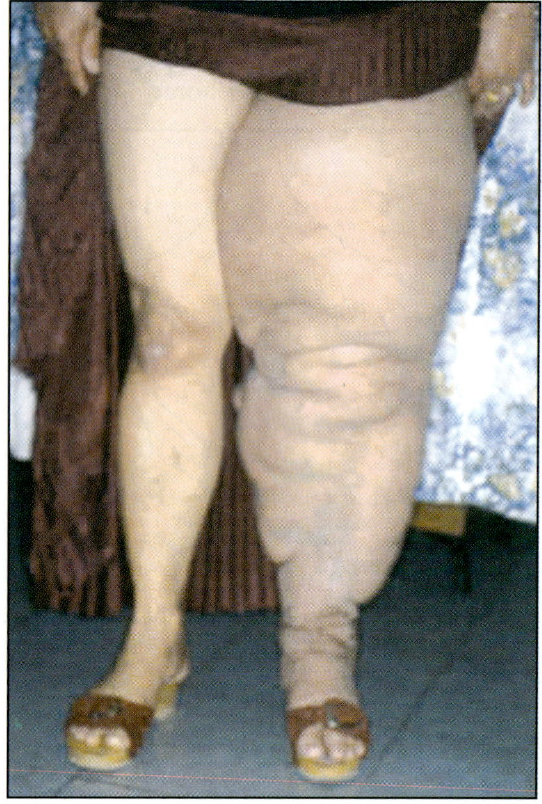

Figure 31.13: Severe lymphoedema. The patient had Wertheim radical hysterectomy and pelvic lymphadenectomy. She developed pelvic recurrence 3 years later and was treated by pelvic irradiation. She remains otherwise well 20 years later

used and for adenocarcinoma and adenosquamous carcinoma better survivals were obtained with cisplatinum, vinblastine and bleomycin (PVB regime). Patients without risk factors have survivals of 98%.[9]

Primary radiation therapy for early stage cervical carcinoma is based primarily on the extent and distribution of the disease; treatment is directed to upper vagina, cervix and parametria, as well as lymph nodes on pelvic wall. Treatment usually begins with external radiation in an attempt to shrink the central tumor; this will help improve the application of subsequent intracavitary caesium therapy.

The *complications* of radiation therapy can be divided into:

- Acute complications (occurring during or immediately after therapy)
  - Perforation of the uterus
  - Sigmoiditis (8%)
  - Hemorrhagic cystitis (3%)
- Chronic complications (occurring as late as 12 to 18 months)
  - Vaginal stenosis (70%)
  - Rectovaginal fistula (1%)
  - Vesicovaginal fistula (1%)
  - Small bowel obstruction (2%).

In order to improve overall survival in these patients, adjuvant treatment is necessary. *Adjuvant pelvic irradiation* in these instances might decrease the incidence of local pelvic recurrences, but the development of distant metastases is not prevented, resulting in no improvement in overall survival. The addition of whole pelvic irradiation to radical surgery also carries a high risk of morbidity and mortality.

Patients with above poor prognostic features can be regarded as having systemic disease requiring systemic measures; in these instances it is fair to assume the presence of micrometastases not only within the pelvis but also at extra-pelvic sites. Using *adjuvant chemotherapy*, we reported 10-year survivals of 86.1% in patients with risk factors; survival in those with squamous cell carcinoma was better if Mitomycin C + 5-fluorouracil (5FU) was

Stage IIa

In patients with extensive involvement of the upper vagina, radiation therapy is the method of choice.

Stage IIb

Most patients with stage IIb lesions will be treated with pelvic radiation (external beam and brachytherapy). For those with bulky disease, currently chemoradiation is advocated, although in some centers neoadjuvant chemotherapy is used to shrink the primary lesion is followed by radical hysterectomy or pelvic irradiation.

Stage IIIa and IIIb

These patients are treated by pelvic irradiation (external beam brachytherapy). In the presence of bulky disease chemoradiation is used.

Stage IVa

Pelvic irradiation is used in most instances. Pelvic exenteration is rarely performed, usually when a recto-vaginal or vesicovaginal fistula is present.

Stage IVb

Pelvic radiation may be used for palliation of bleeding from vagina, bladder or rectum. As distant metastases are present, chemotherapy is often employed; this is only palliative.

The *5-year survivals* for *radiotherapy* are 86.6% for Stage 1, 69.9% for stage II, 42.5% for stage III and 12.3% for stage IV.[10]

More recently, concurrent *chemoradiation* has been used with improved survivals.

Special Situations

Invasive cervical carcinoma found incidentally after simple hysterectomy.

With minimal invasive disease no further treatment is needed. For more severe lesions there are 2 options:
- Immediate postoperative radiotherapy
- Radical excision of the upper vagina and pelvic lymphadenectomy

Positive surgical margins and when residual disease is left behind at radical hysterectomy.

Here, pelvic irradiation is the method of choice.

Cervical Stump Carcinoma

There are 2 options.
- Radical cervicectomy with bilateral lymphadenectomy
- Radiotherapy.

Adhesions and fibrosis from previous surgery make the former difficult, whilst the inability to utilise a uterine source of irradiation may compromise the efficacy of the latter. Thus, in the author's view, subtotal hysterectomy should not be performed in modern gynecological practice.

Bulky Stage 1B2 and Stage 2A Carcinoma of the Cervix

Three options are available:
- Pelvic irradiation (with or without concurrent chemo-therapy) followed by extrafascial hysterectomy
- Radical hysterectomy followed by tailored adjuvant chemotherapy
- Neoadjuvant chemotherapy followed by radical hysterectomy and pelvic lymphadenectomy

Currently, there has been great interest in the third option. A randomised trial will help decide which is the best option.

Fertility Sparing Surgery

Radical hysterectomy remains the mainstay of treatment for stage 1B and early 2A cervical carcinoma. Recently, there has been a great interest in performing conservative (fertility-sparing) surgery in young women with small 1B1 lesions. A laparoscopic / retroperitoneal lymphadenectomy is performed; if frozen section of the nodes show no metastases, a radical trachelectomy, vagino-isthmic anastomosis with a prophylactic cerclage around the isthmus are carried out. The essentials for cure and preservation of fertility are 1 cm upper tumor free margin and 1 cm residual cervical canal. The *contraindications* for the procedure are:
- Presence of L/V permeation
- +ve nodes
- Tumors >2 cm
- Upper endocervical involvement.

Cervical Cancer in Pregnancy

This is rare occurring 1 in 4077 deliveries. About 55% of patients with cervical cancer in pregnancy are asymptomatic. Pregnancy presents an ideal time for cervical screening. The management of an abnormal smear in pregnancy is shown in Figure 31.14. The treatment options available are:
- Radiotherapy
- Radical hysterectomy and pelvic lymphadenectomy.

For stage 1B and early 2A lesions diagnosed before 24 weeks of pregnancy, the pregnancy is disregarded and definitive therapy instituted. Radical hysterectomy and pelvic lymphadenectomy is our preferred choice. The dilemma arises when patients present between 24 to 28 weeks gestation; treatment may be delayed until the fetus has a better chance of survival. When sufficient maturity has been achieved (32-43 weeks) a classical cesarean section is performed, the placenta is left in situ.

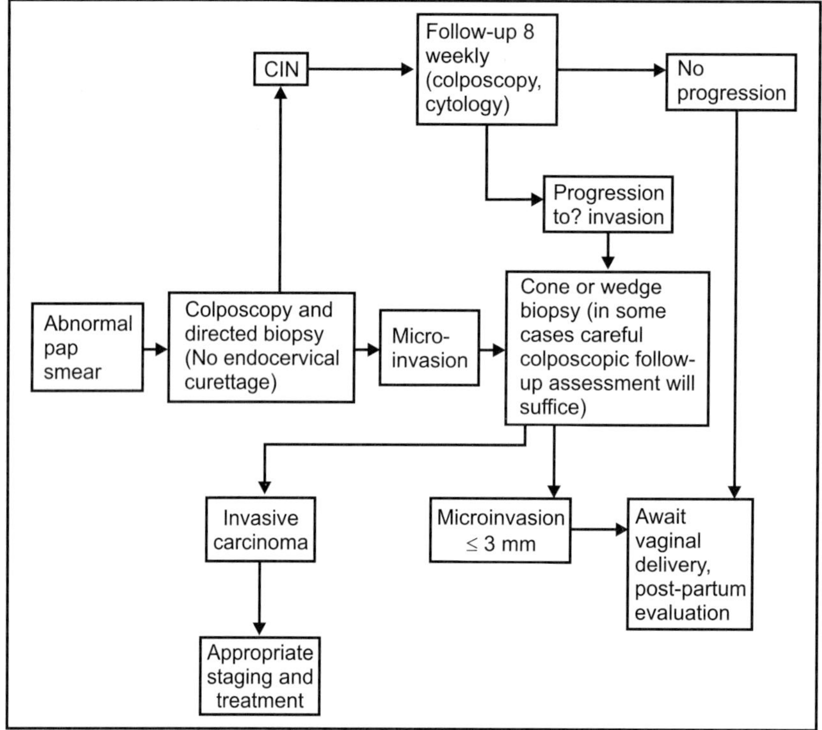

Figure 31.14:   Scheme of evaluation of an abnormal smear in pregnancy

The uterine incision is closed and the radical hysterectomy and pelvic lymphadenectomy is then performed.

For more advanced disease (stage IIB, III and IV) radiotherapy is the treatment of choice. In early pregnancy, external beam radiation results in an abortion; after the uterus is empty brachytherapy completes therapy. Treatment may be delayed in those in the latter part of second or third trimester to achieve fetal viability; the fetus is then delivered by classical cesarean section before radiotherapy. We observed a 5-year survival of 92.8% in our antenatally diagnosed patients, which is similar to the non-pregnant patient; only 25% of those diagnosed and treated in the puerperium survived. Hence, early diagnosis and therapy during pregnancy is important, rather than in the puerperium.[11]

Follow-up

All patients will need long-term follow-up assessments, for reassurance, psychosexual counseling symptomatic relief and early detection of recurrence.

REFERENCES

1. Richart RM. Natural history of cervical intra-epithelial neoplasia. Clin Obstet Gynecol 1967;10: 748-84.
2. Anderson MC, Hartley RB. Cervical cypt involvement by intraepithelial neoplasia. Obstet Gynecol 1980, 55: 546-50.
3. Helmerhorst TJM, Meijer CJLM. Cervical cancer should be considered as a rare complication of oncogenic HPV injection rather than a STD. Int J Gynecol Cancer 2002; 12: 235-36.
4. Nabbenhuis MAE, Walbooners JMM, et al. Relation of human papilloma virus status to cervical lesions and consequences for cervical-cancer screening; a prospective study. Lancet 1999; 354: 20-25.
5. Sivanesaratnam V. Problem of cervical cancer in South- East Asia. Thai J Obstet Gynecol 1999;11: 21-25.
6. WHO Collaborative Study of Neoplasia and Steroid Contraceptives: Invasive cervical cancer and combined oral contraceptives. Br Med J 1985, 290: 961-65.
7. Paterson-Brown S, Chappatte OA, Clark SK et al. The significance of cone biopsy resection margins. Gynecol Oncol 1992;46: 182-85.
8. Sivanesaratnam V, Sen DK, Jayalakshmi P, Ong G. Radical hysterectomy and pelvic lymphadenectomy for early

invasive cancer of the cervix—14-year experience. Int J Gynecol Cancer 1993; 3: 231-38.

9. Sivanesaratnam V. Adjuvant chemotherapy in "high risk" patients after Wertheim hysterectomy—10-year survival. Annals of Academy Medicine S'pore. 1998;27:622-26.

10. Patterson F (Ed). Annual Report on the Results of Treatment in Gynecological Cancer. Int Fed of Gynecology and Obstetrics 1985;19: 216.

11. Sivanesaratnam V, Jayalakshmi P, Loo C. Surgical management of early invasive cancer of the cervix associated with pregnancy. Gynecol Oncol 1993; 48: 68-75.

32.

V Sivanesaratnam
Lim Boon Kiong

Ovarian Cancer

INTRODUCTION

Ovarian cancer is the fourth common cancer among Malaysian women and is a leading cause of death from gynecological cancer. Epithelial ovarian cancer comprise 8 to 85% of all ovarian tumors. The exact etiology is unknown; increasing parity, use of oral contraceptive pills and breastfeeding appear to have a protective effect, whilst low parity/sub-fertility, use of fertility drugs and genetic factors increase the risk.

The overall survival is only 41.6%. The elusive nature of the disease results in 70% of the cases to be in the advanced stage at presentation. A thorough clinical examination and the aid of imaging techniques—ultrasound, CT Scan—will help determine the extent of the disease preoperatively and the subsequent planning of treatment.

Surgery is the main modality of treatment, however, advanced or aggressive the disease. The extent of surgery should be individualized. This would be influenced by age, reproductive status, histological type of tumor, stage of the disease and general medical status.

A second-look laparotomy has little place in the routine management. In patients with persistent or recurrent disease, secondary salvage surgery may be performed in suitable patients. Minimally invasive surgery (laparoscopic surgery) for ovarian masses can do harm if patient selection is not carefully done.

Fertility sparing surgery is possible in patients with germ cell tumors; it is also a viable option for selected patients with stage 1 epithelial ovarian carcinoma after a comprehensive surgical staging.

Chemotherapy has an important role—adjuvant treatment after primary surgery and as neoadjuvant in chemo-debulking of tumors assessed to be inoperable to facilitate subsequent optimal debulking.

Survivals rates are much better when these cases are managed by gynecologic oncologists.

Ovarian carcinoma is the leading cause of death from gynecological cancer in the US. In Malaysia, ovarian carcinoma is the fourth most common cancer among women in Peninsular Malaysia in the year 2002 (after cancers of the breast, cervix uteri and colon) and constituted 5% of total female cancers.[1] It is a leading cause of death from gyanecological cancer because it is difficult to detect before it disseminates; approximately 70% of cases present in advanced stage.

EPIDEMIOLOGY

Malignant neoplasms of the ovaries occur at all ages, including infancy and childhood. Malignant germ cell tumors are most commonly seen in females younger than 20 years, whereas epithelial cancers of the ovary are primarily seen in women older than 50 years. The probability of developing ovarian cancer before the age of 75 is 0.4 to 1.7%. The incidence of epithelial ovarian cancer in women between the age of 40 and 44 is 15 to 16 per 100,000. Epithelial ovarian cancer is infrequent in women below the age of 40, after which the rate increases; in Malaysia the age specific incidence peaks at 60-69 years at 27.0 per 100,000 population.[1] The disease appears to be more common amongst the Chinese (9.9 per 100,000 population) compared to the Malays (8.1 per 100,000 population) and Indians (7.4 per 100,000 population).[1] The lifetime risk of developing ovarian cancer was 1:100 for Chinese, 1:125 for Indians and 1:125 for Malays. It was the third commonest cancer diagnosed in Malay women (after cancers of breast and cervix uteri).

ANATOMY

The ovaries are a pair of solid oval-shaped organs measuring 2-4 cm in diameter; they are situated in the "ovarian fossa" on either side of the pelvis between the bifurcation of the common iliac vessels and medial to bony pelvis. Hence, these are not palpable per abdomen because of this deep location in the pelvis; neither are they easily palpable on pelvic examination, unless they are enlarged. They are connected by a peritoneal fold to the broad ligament, by the infundibulopelvic ligament to the lateral wall of the pelvis and by the ovarian ligament to the cornu of the uterus which continues anterioly as the round ligament.

MODE OF SPREAD

Ovarian cancer spreads mainly by 2 routes:
- Transperitoneal
- Via lymphatics

The viseral and parietal peritoneum, and the omentum are common sites for metastases; subdiaphragmatic and liver surface involvement are also common.

The lymphatic drainage occurs mainly by the ovarian lymphatics to the paraoartic nodes; via accessary external iliac lymphatic channels this may drain into the external iliac, common iliac, hypogastric and lateral sacral nodes and occasionally via the round ligaments into the inguinal nodes.

ETIOLOGICAL FACTORS

The exact etiology of ovarian cancer is unknown but it has been known to have a close association with several factors.

- *Parity*

  The risk of developing ovarian cancer reduces with parity. The relative risk for a nulliparous woman is 1.5 while a woman with parity of more than 3 has a relative risk of 0.73.[2] An associated factor that also reduces the risk is a history of breast feeding, although no consistent relationship has been established between breastfeeding duration and decreased risk.

- *Oral contraceptive pill (OCP)*

  Taking OCP has been associated with the reduction in the risk of developing ovarian cancer. The relative risk of women taking OCP for more than 36 months is 0.4. It has been estimated that oral contraceptives may have prevented over 1,700 cases of ovarian cancer per year in the US.[3] The risk of ovarian cancer is also increased in women with breast cancer and vice versa.[2]

- *Years of ovulation*

  The risk of ovarian cancer increases with number of years of ovulation. Therefore, women with low parity/subfertility, early menarche and late menopause have higher risk of developing ovarian cancer.

- *Hormonal*

  Risk of developing ovarian cancer is said to be increased in patients taking fertility drugs e.g. Clomiphene citrate of more than one year duration. The use of clomiphene for more than 12 ovulatory cycles is associated with a 2 to 4 fold elevated risk. Most of the tumors in this group of patients are borderline malignancy.[4]

- Genetic factors

  Women with genetic risk for ovarian cancer can be divided into two groups:

  - Familial ovarian cancer
  - Hereditary ovarian cancer.

  Hereditary ovarian cancer syndrome is defined as women with at least 2 first-degree relatives with ovarian cancer. Approximately 5% of ovarian cancer has a hereditary basis.[5]

  The lifetime risk for ovarian cancer in the normal population is approximately 1.6%. With one relative affected, the lifetime risk rises to 5%. Lifetime cumulative risk of developing ovarian cancer increases to 7% in patient with at least 2 relatives suffering from ovarian cancer.[5] Approximately 3% of these women have hereditary ovarian cancer syndrome which carry a life-time risk of 25-50% in developing ovarian cancer. At least 2 genes have been identified to be involved in the development of ovarian cancer i.e BRCA1 (location 17q21) and BRCA2 (13q12). BRCA1 is a tumor-suppressor gene that acts as a negative regulator of tumor growth. Mutation of this gene causes dysfunction leading to development of cancer.

  There are two types of hereditary ovarian cancer syndrome that has been identified:

  - Hereditary breast-ovarian cancer syndrome (HBOC) (85-90%). The vast majority is due to mutation of BRCA1 gene with a small proportion due to mutation of BRCA2 gene.
  - Hereditary nonpolyposis colorectal syndrome (HNPCC). This is also an autosomal dominant condition and previously known as Lynch syndrome II. Ovarian cancer occurs in 5-10% of HNPCC. It also increases predisposition to endometrial and stomach cancer.

  In breast-ovarian cancer syndrome, women with either the mother or a sister suffering from breast and/or ovarian cancer has a 50% risk of developing ovarian cancer in her life time. Therefore, women less than 35 years of age with a history of hereditary ovarian cancer syndrome should be monitored with a pelvic examination, ultrasound scan and CA 125 every 6 months. For those above 35 years of age and have completed their family, they should be encouraged to consider prophylactic removal of the ovaries.

Other hereditary factors that has been linked to the occurrence of ovarian cancer are mutation of p53 gene, abnormalities of dominant oncogenes e.g. c-myc, H-ras and Ki-ras.[7]

- *Environmental factors*

  A diet high in meat and animal fat, characteristic of industrialized nations, has been reported in some studies to be associated with an increased risk of ovarian cancer.[2] Some studies disputed the above findings.[8] There have been conflicting reports regarding the association of the use of talcum powder and development of ovarian cancer.[9,10]

- *Others*

  White race and residence in North America and Northern Europe are also at higher risk of developing ovarian cancer.[11] A meta-analysis of 21 studies has shown that there is a small increase (not statistically significant) in overall risk of ovarian cancer in women taking HRT (RR 1.15; CI 1.05-1.27).[12]

The protective effect of factors 1, 2 and 3 which produce periods of *ovulatory rest* support the *incessant ovulation* hypothesis for the etiology of ovarian cancer. According to this hypothesis, ovarian cancer develops from an aberrant repair process of the surface epithelium, which is ruptured and repaired during each ovulatory cycle.[13] The other hypothesis of primary etiology of ovarian cancer is excessive gonado-trophin secretion leading to excessive stimulation of ovary.

SCREENING FOR OVARIAN CANCER

Ovarian cancer is curable when detected at an early stage, but most cases are diagnosed after spread from the ovary has taken place. The typically late diagnosis of ovarian cancer is due to the paucity of symptoms in the early stage as well as the deep location of the ovaries in the pelvis. Screening for ovarian cancer is one way to detect the occurrence of ovarian cancer at the pre-malignant or early stage. This will be discussed in the chapter on "gynecological cancer screening".

PREVENTION OF OVARIAN CANCER

As ovarian cancer cannot be detected early, attention should be directed to its prevention.

- *Oral contraceptive pills*
  Most of what is known about role of oral contraceptive pills in prevention of ovarian cancer is based on epithelial tumor which comprise 80-85% of all ovarian cancers.

  OCP usage reduces the risk of familial and hereditary ovarian cancer. The exact mechanism of risk reduction by OCPs remains to be defined. Decreased ovulation may be its main mechanism but progestational components of OCPs may also exert independent protective effects, including inducing apoptosis on epithelial cells.[14]
- Synthetic *retinoid* (fenretinide) may also protect women from ovarian cancer.[15]
- *Tubal ligation* (RR 0.33) and *hysterectomy* (RR 0.67) may have some protective effect to the occurrence of ovarian cancer.[16] This could be explained by prevention of passage of carcinomagens (e.g. talc) via vagina to the ovaries.
- Prophylactic oophorectomy, generally reduced the risk of ovarian cancer in women. However, this may not be protective to all women especially those with hereditary ovarian cancer syndrome. Follow-up studies have shown that approximately 10% of women in this category developed disseminated intra-abdominal carcinomatosis despite prophylactic oophorectomy.[17] Prophylactic oophorectomy may not be justifiable for women below 50 years without the risk ofovarian cancer.

CLASSIFICATION OF OVARIAN NEOPLASMS

Neoplasm of the ovary can arise from:
- Surface epithelium/serosa
- Ovarian stroma
- Secondary deposit/metastatic

Surface epithelium: During embryonic life, the coelomic cavity forms and is lined by a mesothelial lining of mesodermal origin, parts of which become specialized to form the serosal epithelium covering the gonadal ridge. By process of invagination, this same mesothelial lining gives rise to müllerian duct. Müllerian duct is the origin of fallopian tubes, uterus and vaginal wall. Therefore, it is not surprising that epithelial ovarian carcinoma may show histological features resembling those from these genital organs. Epithelial ovarian tumor which comprise 80 to 85% of all ovarian tumors can be classified into the following types (Table 32.1).

Table 32.1: Classification of epithelial ovarian tumors (80-85%)

1. Serous tumor (resembles fallopian tube)
2. Mucinous tumor (resembles endocervix)
3. Endometrioid tumors
4. Clear cell tumors (resembles endometrial glands during pregnancy rich in glycogen)
5. Transitional-cells or Brenner tumors
6. Mixed epithelial tumors
7. Undifferentiated carcinoma

Ovarian stroma: The second group of ovarian tumors arise from specialized cells in the ovarian stroma. These have been classified into three categories, i.e. germ cell tumors, sex-cord stromal tumors and those of non-specific mesenchymal origin (Table 32.2).

Metastatic ovarian cancer:

Table 32.2: Classifications of Germ-cell, Sex-cord stromal and non-specific mesenchymal tumors

A. *Germ-cell tumors* (10 -15 %)
  a. Dysgerminoma
  b. Yolk-sac tumor (Endodermal sinus tumor)
  c. Embryonal carcinoma
  d. Polyembryoma
  e. Choriocarcinoma
  f. Immature Teratomas
  g. Mixed germ cell tumor
	A. *Non-specific mesenchymal tumors (<1%)*
	  a. Fibroma, haemangioma leiomyoma, lipoma
	  b. Lymphoma
	  c. Sarcoma

B. *Sex-cord stromal tumors* (3-5%)
  1. Granulosa—stromal cell tumors
    a. Granulosa cell tumor
    b. Thecoma
    c. Sclerosing stromal tumor
  2. Sertoli-stromal cell tumors
    a. Sertoli-cell tumor
    b. Leydig-cell tumor
    c. Sertoli-Leydig cell tumor
  3. Gynandroblastoma
  4. Steroid-cell tumors
  5. Unclassified	

DIAGNOSIS

Symptoms and Signs

- *Asymptomatic.*
  Unfortunately ovarian cancer in its early stages does not produce any symptoms or signs that would alert

the clinician to this diagnosis. This explains why approximately two-thirds of all ovarian cancers are already in stage 3 or 4 at diagnosis (Figs 32.1 to 32.3).

- *Gastrointestinal symptoms*
  Most frequent symptoms are those associated with gastrointestinal upset including bloating, abdominal distention and abdominal discomfort.
- *Abdominal mass*
- Respiratory symptoms due to abdominal distention, pleural effusion or metastases.
- Abnormal uterine bleeding due to hormone producing ovarian cancer, such as granulose cell tumors.
- Constitutional symptoms such as loss of apetite, loss of weight, lethargy, etc. are an indication of progressing and advancing disease.
- Acute symptoms are rare; this results from pain due to torsion, rupture, infection or intracystic hemorrhage.

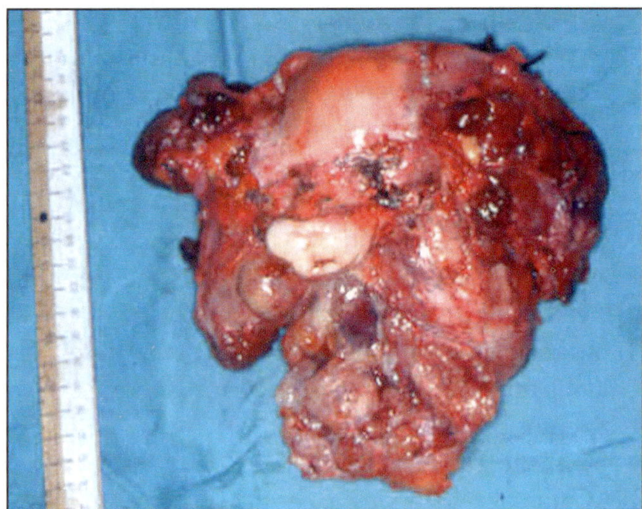

Figure 32.2: The tumor (immature teratoma) has been removed en bloc with the uterus via a retroperitoneal approach; notice that it has eroded through the capsule

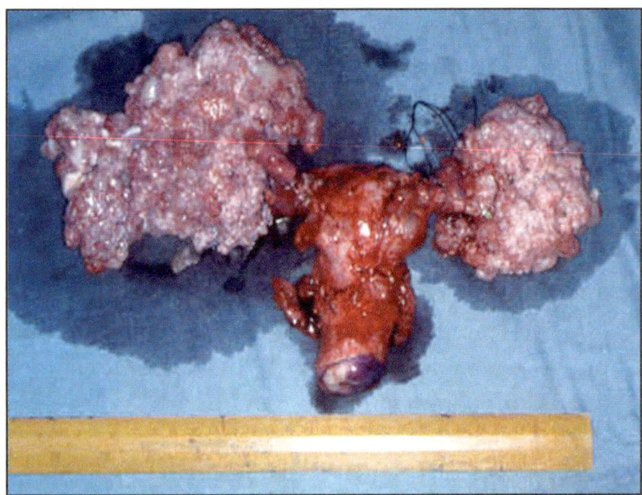

Figure 32.3: Bilateral papillary serous cystadeno-carcinoma of the ovary in a 38-year old patient. Notice the capsule has been completely eroded. There are deposits on the back of the uterus. The patient had ascites, " omental cake" and intraperitoneal deposits

Examination

- *General examination*
  Pallor, loss of weight, palpable left supraclavicular lymph nodes and cachexia are late manifestations.
- *Specific examination*
  Pleural effusion and reduced air entry may indicate lung involvement.

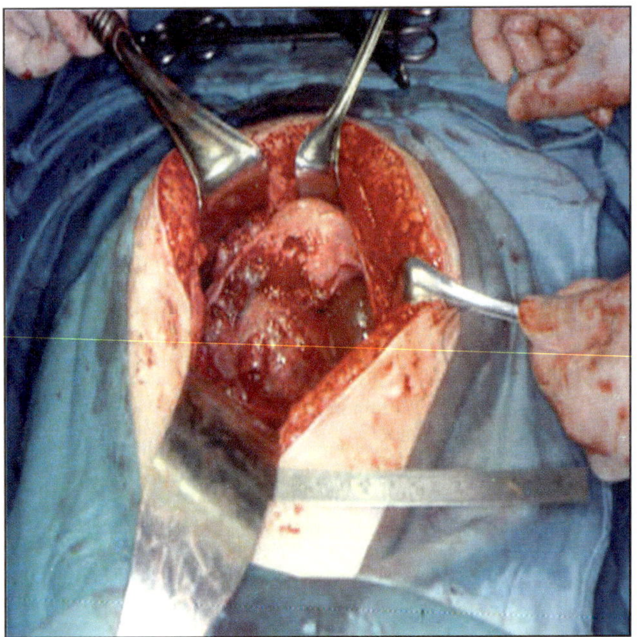

Figure 32.1: Notice the right ovarian tumors (immature teratoma) that has extended anterioly to the right broad ligament; it had infiltrated part of the bladder and was densely adherent to the rectum posterioly. The patient was 28 years of age

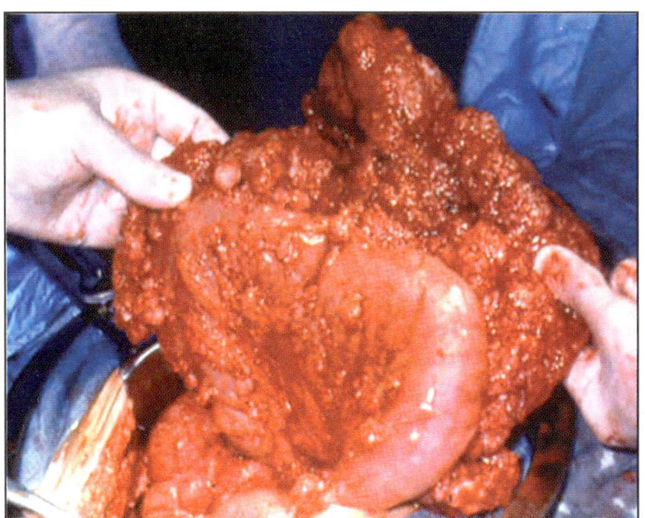

Figure 32.4: "Omental Cake" in a patient with advanced ovarian cancer. Notice the tumor deposits in the omentum and mesocolon

Abdominal distention may be due to ascites (shifting dullness in mild ascites, fluid thrill in gross ascites) or pelvic/abdominal mass. There may also be a palpable abdominal mass (omental cake) (Fig. 32.4) or organomegaly.

Pelvic examination may reveal the presence of an adnexal mass and if the tumor has spread to the bladder and rectum or other surrounding structures, the mass will become fixed/immobile (Figs 32.1 to 32.3). In these instances patients may also present with bowel and urinary symptoms. In addition to a vaginal examination rectal or rectovaginal examination is useful in the evaluation of these masses.

Preoperative Evaluation

Biochemical

Patients could be anemic, hypoproteinemic and suffering from electrolyte deficiencies in advanced stage of ovarian cancer; these need assessment prior to surgery. The tumor markers may be raised. Different type of ovarian cancers produced different tumor markers. As 80% of ovarian cancers are epithelial in origin, CA125 is a common tumor marker to be raised and this should be a routine investigation in a patient with suspected ovarian neoplasm.

Tumor marker is useful in aiding diagnosis but more importantly, it is very useful in assessment of the response to therapy. It can also be used for early detection of recurrence. Overall, approximately 85% of patients with epithelial ovarian cancer have a CA125 level of >35 iu/ml. However, elevated CA125 is found only in 50% of patient with stage 1 disease. In advanced stage >90% will have elevation of CA125.[18-20] CA125 is less often elevated in mucinous, than serous tumors.[21] Other tumor markers are carcinoembryonic antigen(CEA), alpha-fetoprotein(AFP), human chorionic gonadotropin (hCG), inhibin, estrogen and androgen. The CEA level may be elevated in mucinous and Brenner tumor. The AFP level is elevated in endodermal sinus tumor (100%), immature teratoma (62%) and dysgerminoma (12%). The hCG level is invariably elevated in choriocarcinoma. Inhibin and estrogen levels may be elevated in granulosa cell tumor, whilst androgen levels are raised in Sertoli-Leydig cell tumors.

Imaging

Ultrasound is a very useful tool in aiding the diagnosis of ovarian tumors. The ultrasound features of ovarian malignancy are bilaterality, presence of solid areas, papillary projections, ascites, hydronephrosis or liver secondaries. CT scan may be able to identify lymphadenopathy, and detect peritoneal tumor deposits and is useful in the assessment of operability and extent of surgery anticipated pre-operatively. CT scan, however, may not be able to detect lesions smaller than 1 cm size.

Endoscopy

In those with occult blood in stools or significant intestinal symptoms, colonoscopy needs to be done to exclude a primary colonic cancer with ovarian metastases. Similarly, an upper gasto-intestinal endoscopy is important if there are significant gastric symptoms.

Breast Examination

Breast cancer may also metastasise to the ovaries. It is, therefore, important to examine the breasts in all cases; if there are suspicious palpable breast masses bilateral mammograms should be obtained.

STAGES OF OVARIAN CANCER

This is based on the FIGO staging of ovarian cancer:

Stage 1: Tumor limited to the ovaries

1A Tumor limited to one ovary; capsule intact, no tumor on ovarian surface; no malignant cells in ascites or peritoneal washings.

1B Tumor limited to both ovaries; capsule intact. No tumor on ovarian surface; no malignant cells in ascites or peritoneal washings.

1C Tumor limited to one or both ovaries with any of the following: capsule ruptured, tumor on ovarian surface, malignant cells in ascites or peritoneal washings.

Stage 2: Tumor involves one or both ovaries with pelvic extension

2A Extension and/or implants on uterus and/ or tube(s); no malignant cells in ascites or peritoneal washings.

2B Extension to other pelvic tissues; no malignant cells in ascites or peritoneal washings.

2C Pelvic extension (2A or 2B) with malignant cells in ascites or peritoneal washings.

Stage 3: Tumor involves one or both ovaries with microscopically confirmed peritoneal metastasis outside the pelvis and /or regional lymph node metastasis.

3A Microscopic peritoneal metastasis beyond pelvis

3B Macroscopic peritoneal metastasis beyond pelvis 2cm or less in greatest dimension.

3C Peritoneal metastasis beyond pelvis more than 2 cm in greatest dimension and/or regional lymph node metastasis.

Stage 4: Distant metastasis

Liver capsule metastasis is stage 3, while liver parenchymal metastasis is stage 4. Pleural effusion must have positive cytology for stage 4.

TREATMENT OF OVARIAN CARCINOMA

Surgery is the main modality of treatment of ovarian carcinoma, however, advanced or aggressive the tumor is. The extent of surgery is individually tailored, taking into consideration the patient's wishes. As the surgery may include resection of bowel and bowel anastomosis, the preoperative preparation of both small and large bowel is important.

Several *factors* will *influence the extent of surgery* in ovarian carcinoma. These are:

- Age and reproductive status
- Histological type of tumor
- Stage of disease
- General medical status

Staging Laparotomy

The components of a comprehensive surgical staging are:

- A thorough and systematic exploration of the whole peritoneal cavity—this should include examinations of the under-surface of the diaphragam, liver, spleen, stomach and intestines, paraoartic nodes and pelvic structures.
- Cytological/histological sampling of paracolic gutters, subdiaphragmatic and pelvic peritoneal surfaces
- Omentectomy
- Para-oartic and pelvic node sampling

This will help decide whether the disease:

- is confined to one or both ovaries
- has spread locally with metastases confined to pelvis
- is more advanced with intra-abdominal metastases.
- is primary or secondary ovarian carcinoma

From this assessment the extent of surgery needed can be individually tailored. A Pfannenstiel incision (Fig. 32.5) is not adequate to allow this detailed assessment. An adequate upper abdominal exposure is essential for correct staging and optimal tumor excision in patients with ovarian cancer. A vertical incision extending well above the umbilicus is essential. The use of a laparoscopic light source will allow easy visualization of the upper surface of the liver and undersurface of the diaphragm—sites for early metastases.

Surgery for Early Well-encapsulated Epithelial Ovarian Carcinoma

In the young patient where preservation of fertility is desired, a unilateral or bilateral salpingooophorectomy

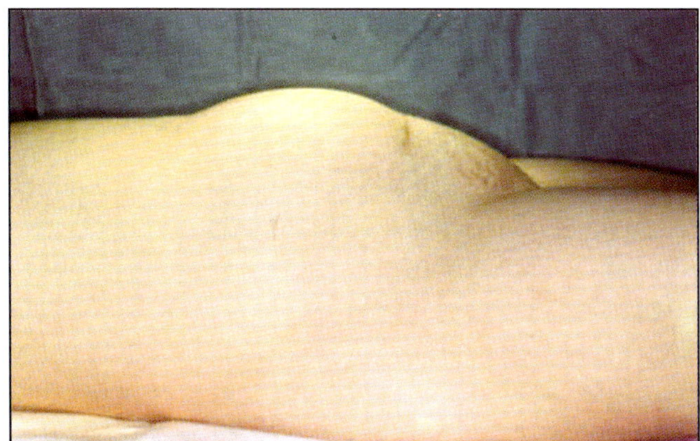

Figure 32.5: The patient has a large suprapubic mass. She was referred after laparotomy via a Pfannenstiel incision showed the tumor to be fixed. This is not an appropriate incision for ovarian cancer surgery. The tumor is illustrated in Figures 32.1 and 32.2 above.

(if there are bilateral tumors present) is performed; ideally these are sent for "frozen section". About a third of these "apparent stage 1 cases" will be understaged if only a unilateral salpingo-oophorectomy is carried out.[26] If the tumor is grade 1 or 2 and the tumor is limited to one or both ovaries without capsular invasion and the peritoneal fluid cytology is negative for malignant cells, *(low risk* cases) the above surgery would suffice; the uterus may be conserved, provided endometrial tumor is excluded. Adjuvant chemotherapy is not necessary.

In the presence of a poorly differentiated carcinoma (grade 3), clear cell carcinoma or positive peritoneal cytology *(high risk* cases) conservative surgery is best avoided and a total hysterectomy, omentectomy with or without pelvic/para-oartic node dissection is performed. Adjuvant chemotherapy in these cases improves survival.

Deliberate puncture and aspiration must be avoided because this is dangerous and can result in iatrogenic tumor spread; malignant ovarian cysts must be removed intact.

In the management of *ovarian germ cell tumors*, the availability of effective chemotherapeutic regimes such as PEB (Cisplatinum, etoposide, bleomycin) and VAC (vincristine, actinomycin D and cyclophosphamide) has made conservative surgery possible even in advanced staged disease in young women.

It must be borne in mind that such conservative surgery is appropriate only in selected young women for the purpose of preserving reproductive function. It is generally *not* recommended when the patient is in the peri- or post-menopausal age.

Surgery for Ovarian Carcinoma with Local Extension (Figs 32.1 and 32.2)

Maximal clearance is only possible via a primary extra-peritoneal approach; a total hysterectomy, omentectomy pelvic/paraoartic lymphadenectomy is performed. This needs competence. Adjuvant chemotherapy improves survival.

Surgery for Ovarian Carcinoma with Disseminated Intraperitoneal Disease

The aim is cytoreductive surgery to achieve no macroscopic residual disease or to residual lesions < 1 cm. To achieve this, the surgery should not increase operative mortality. The initial surgical approach influences survival and, therefore, it should be correctly done. *Optimal debulking* requires judgement and experience in addition to aggressive skills. Thus, advanced ovarian cancers are best not handled surgically by those not familiar with the radical approach to achieve optimal results.

The *benefits* of optimal cytoreduction are:
- improves patient comfort
- improves functional and nutritional status
- improves oxygenation and blood flow resulting in ↑ delivery of cytotoxic drugs to residual tumor
- small volume tumor needs fewer cycles of chemotherapy
- ↓ chance of chemoresistance

The median survival is significantly related to the residual tumor size at conclusion of surgery; the FIGO Annual Report 1998 reported 5 years survival of 56.5% when no microscopic residual disease was achieved, 32.5 % when the residual disease was less that 2 cm and 13.1% when this was > 2 cm. The best results are achieved when these cases are managed by gynecologic oncologists.

Place of Chemotherapy

Chemotherapy plays a very important *adjuvant* role in the treatment for ovarian cancer. Except for a small group of patients with stage 1A, well and moderately differentiated tumors, the rest will require chemotherapy in the postoperative period (adjuvant chemotherapy). The overall 5-year survival in the small group of patients (stage 1A) is greater than 90%, and these patients can be spared the toxicity of chemotherapy.[28]

Surgery alone is rarely, if ever, curative for patients with advanced ovarian cancer. The choice of adjuvant chemotherapy depends on the histological type of cancer, i.e. epithelial or germ cell tumor. The platinum compound remains the most active agent in the treatment of epithelial ovarian cancer. It is also the cornerstone of combination drug regimens. Carboplatin is a second generation platinum compound. It is less nephrotoxic, less neurotoxic and less emetogenic than Cis-platinum.[29] It can be administered in an out patient basis. It's dose limiting toxicity is myelosuppresion, especially thrombocytopenia.

Single agent Carboplatin and combination regimes like Paclitaxel and Carboplatin along with Cis-platinum, Adriamycin (Doxorubicin) and Cyclophosphamide (PAC) are widely used regimes in the treatment of epithelial ovarian cancer. In the most recent randomised trial carried out by the International Collaborative Ovarian Neoplasm (ICON) group, all the 3 regimes were found to be equally effective.[30]

For germ cell tumors, Cis-platinum, Etoposide and Bleomycin (PEB) is the most effective combination.

In selected patients who are poor operative risks with massive, pleural and peritoneal effusions or those who have been assessed pre-operatively to have extensive, fixed pelvic tumors where optimal debulking is unlikely to be achieved, *neoadjuvant chemotherapy* has a role to achieve chemo-debulking and allow optimal surgery to be performed subsequently.

Massive Ovarian Cyst

These tumors are best removed intact. The malignancy rate has been reported to be 27%;[26] thus, siphanage prior to removal is to be avoided because of the risk of spillage of malignant cells. The tumor illustrated in Figure 32.6 was removed intact and weighed 41 kg; it was a mucinous cytadenocarcinma.

"Second Look" Surgery

The role of 'second look' operations remain controversial. In the 1970s this was used to assess patients after adjuvant chemotherapy for complete response both surgically and pathologically. A high complication rate of 63% has been reported previously.[27] A review of the literature shows that 4-53% of patients who had histologically negative second-look procedures subsequently succumbed;[28-32] thus, second-look laparotomy/laparoscopy provides limited prognostic information and has little role outside the scope of experimental treatment protocols.

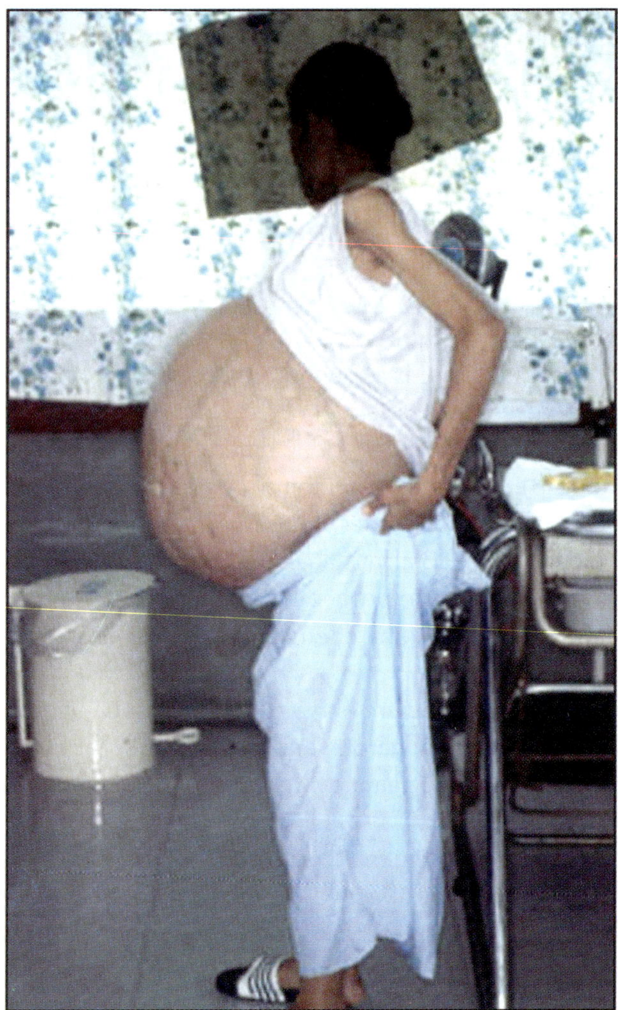

Figure 32.6: Massive ovarian cyst in a 60-year-old lady, it weighed 42 kg and was a mucinous cystadenocarcinoma

Secondary Salvage Surgery

Patients with persistent or recurrent intra-abdominal disease after primary therapy for ovarian cancer are occasionally suitable for surgical excision of their disease. This procedure is referred to as "secondary" cytoreductive surgery. However, the majority of patients with persistent disease will not benefit from such intervention. A suitable patient for this procedure would be one who

* is in good general medical condition
* has no ascites
* has not had cisplatinum combination therapy
* has had a reasonably long interval (>9-12 months) since primary surgery

Optimal debulking should be the aim; only then are patients likely to respond to second-line chemotherapy.

CONCLUSION

Ovarian cancer continues to have an overall poor prognosis compared to other genital cancers; this is primarily due to the advanced stage at presentation. Several advances have transformed the surgical approach to ovarian cancer management in the past 2 decades. For the vast majority of patients considered inoperable in the past, a wide range of surgical procedures are available today; these require experience, fine judgment and aggressiveness on the part of the surgeon. Although surgical cytoreduction is the main modality of therapy today, the importance of adjuvant chemotherapy should not be overlooked. Only a combination of these two modalities will help improve survival in these cases. Individualised management should be the objective to obtain cure in some and palliation in others with advanced disease.

REFERENCES

1. The First Report of the National Cancer Registry. Cancer incidence in Malaysia 2002;148-50.
2. Green MH, Clark JW, Blayney DW.The epidemiology of ovarian cancer. Semin Oncol 1984;11(3):209.
3. Cramer DW, Hutchison GB, Welch WR.Factors affecting the Association of Oral Contraceptives and Ovarian Cancer. N Engl J Med 1982;307:1047.
4. Rossing MA, Daling JR, Weiss NS, et al. Ovarian tunours in a cohort of infertile women. N Engl J Med 1994;331:771.
5. Lynch HT, Bewtra C, Lynch JF. Familial ovarian cancer clinical nuances. Am J Med 1983;81:1073.
6. Schildkraut JM, Thompson WD. Familial ovarian cancer: a population-based case control study. Am J Epidemiology 1988;128:456.
7. Auersperg N, Edelson MI, Mok SC, Johnson SW, Hamilton TC. The biology of ovarian cancer. Semin Oncol 1998;25(3):281.
8. Slattery ML et al .Nutrient intake and ovarian cancer. Am J Epidemiol 1989;130:497.
9. Longo DL , Young RC. Cosmetic talc and ovarian cancer. Lancet 1979;2:349.
10. Piver MS, Baker TR, Jishi MF et al. Familial ovarian cancer. A report of 658 families from the Gilda Radner Familial Ovarian Cancer Registry 1981-1991.Cancer 1993; 1:582.
11. Daly M, Obrams GI. Epidemiology and risk assessment for ovarian cancer. Semin Onco 1998;25:255.
12. Garg PP, Kerlikowske K, Subak L et al. Hormone replacement therapy and the risk of epithelial ovarian cancer: a meta analysis. Obstet Gynecol 1998;92:472.
13. Fathalla, MF. Incessant ovulation—factor in ovarian neoplasia. Lancet 1971;2:163.
14. Rodriguez G. Biologic effect of progestins on the ovarian epithelium: cancer prevention through apoptosis? 1999 (in press).
15. Janerich DT. Can fenretinide protect women against ovarian cancer? J Natl Cancer Inst 1995;87:146.
16. Hankinson SE, Hunter DJ, Colditz GA, et al. Tubal ligation, hysterectomy, and risk of ovarian cancer. A Prospective study. JAMA 1993;270:2813.
17. Tobacman JK, Tucker MA, Kase R, Greene MH, Costa J, Fraumeni JF. Intraabdominal carcinomatosis after prophylactic oophorectomy in ovarian-cancer-prone families. Lancet 1982; 2:795.
18. Bast RC, Klug TL, St John et al. A radioimmunoassay using a monoclonal antibody to monitor the courrsee of epithelial ovarian cancer. N Eng J Med 1983;309:883.
19. Canney PA, Moore M, wilkinsonPM,James RD. Ovarian cancer antigen CA125: A prospective clinical assessment of its role as a tumor marker. Br J Cancer 1984;50:765.
20. Jacobs I, Bast RC. The CA 125 tumor-associated antigen: A review of the literature. Hum Reprod 1989;4:1.
21. Vergote IB, Bormer OP, Abeler VM. Evaluation of serum CA125 levels in the monitoring of ovarian cancer. Am J Obstet Gynecol 1987;157:88.
22. Young RC, Decker DG, Wharton JT. Staging laparotomy in early ovarian cancer. JAMA 1983; 250:3072.
23. Young RC, Walton LA, Ellenberg SS. Adjuvant therapy in stage I and II epithelial ovarian cancer. Results of two prospective randomized trials. N Engl J Med 1990; 322:1021.
24. Canetta R, Bragman K, Smaldone L. Carboplatin: current status and future prospects. Cancer Treat Rev 1988; 15:17.
25. The International Collaborative Ovarian Neoplasm Group. Paclitaxel plus carboplatin versus standard chemotherapy with either single agent carboplatin or cyclophosphamide, doxorubicin and cisplatin in women with ovarian cancer: the ICON 3 randomised trial. The Lancet 2002; 360:505.

26. Dottors DJ, Katz VL, Curvie J. Massive ovarian cyst. A comprehensive surgical approach. Obst Gynecol Surv 1988; 43: 191.

27. Chambers S, Chambers JT, Kohorn ET. Evaluation of the role of second-look surgery in ovarian cancer. Obstet Gynecol 1988; 72: 404.

28. Greco F, Julin CG, Richardson R et al. Advanced ovarian cancer: Brief intensive combination chemotherapy and second look operations. Obstet Gynecol 1981;58: 199.

29. Jones S, Khoo IS, Whitaker S. Evaluation of ovarian cancer by second look laparotomy after treatment. Anst NZJ Surgery 1981;51: 30

30. Luseley DM, Chan KK, Fielding JWL et al. Second-look laparotomy in the management of epithelial ovarian carcinoma: an evaluation of fifty cases. Obstet Gynecol 1984;64: 421.

31. Ho G, Beller U, Speyer JL, Columbo N et al. A reassessment of the role of second-look laparotomy in advanced ovarian cancer. J of Oncol 1988;5: 1316.

32. Copeland IJ, Gershenson DM. Ovarian cancer recurrences in patient with no marcoscopic tumor at second-look laparotomy. Obstet Gynecol 1988;68: 873.

33.

Sapna Ahuja
Sambit Mukhopadhyay
Sabaratnam Arulkumaran

Uterine Malignancy

PART Three

Gynecologic Oncology

INTRODUCTION

Endometrial cancer constitutes 25-30% of all gynecological malignancies. It is the commonest gynecological cancer in the United States. Nearly 25% of those affected die of the disease. Survival is about 75% for those with adenocarcinoma but is only about 50% for those with rarer types of histology like clear cell and papillary serous carcinoma.

EPIDEMIOLOGY AND RISK FACTORS

The incidence of the disease varies between country to country and between different racial groups, being 7 times higher in the white North Americans when compared to their Chinese counterparts.

The median age of patients with endometrial cancer is 61 years. 75% of endometrial cancers occur in postmenopausal women, 3-8% occur in women under 45 years of age and 25% occur in premenopausal women.

Risk factors for endometrial cancer: most risk ractors for endometrial cancer seem to act by unopposed or excessive stimulation of the endometrium with estrogen.

- Obesity and disorders of insulin metabolism are recognized risk factors. There is increased conversion of androgens to estrogen in adipose tissues specifically oestrone. Obese women also have reduced levels of sex hormone binding globulin leading to increased levels of free estrogen available.
- Nulliparity, late menopause, early menarche.
- Polycystic ovarian syndrome.
- Functioning ovarian tumors like granulosa-theca cell tumors are associated with endometrial cancer in 10% of cases and with endometrial hyperplasia in 50% of cases.
- Exogenous estrogen can lead to a 7-10 fold increase in the incidence of endometrial cancer. Giving progestogen for 12-14 days each month can reduce this risk.
- Personal history or family history of breast or colon carcinoma. The Lynch 2 syndrome predisposes women to hereditary non-polyposis colonic cancer, endometrial cancer and ovarian cancer.
- Tamoxifen therapy: tamoxifen is given to women with breast cancer and this predisposes them to endometrial polyps, endometrial hyperplasia and less commonly cancers and sarcomas of the uterus. Breast cancer per se is associated with two-fold increase in endometrial cancer.

Factors decreasing the risk of endometrial cancer include the following:

- Oral contraception decreases the risk of endometrial cancer by about 50% specially if taken for 10 years or more and this effect lasts even 20 years after discontinuation.
- Progestogens.
- Early menopause may decrease the risk of endometrial cancer.

PATHOLOGY

Endometrial Hyperplasia

In simple hyperplasia there is an increased stromal and glandular component but the stromal/glandular ratio is normal. This usually regresses spontaneously in 80% of cases. One percent of cases can progress to endometrial cancer.

Crowding of glandular elements occurs in complex hyperplasia. If nuclear and cytological abnormalities exist, then it is classified as atypical hyperplasia. Complex and atypical hyperplasia can progress to endometrial cancer in 3% and 23% of cases respectively. The risk of malignant change depends on the degree of nuclear/cytological atypia rather than architectural atypia.

HISTOLOGY

Endometrial cancer commonly arises from the endometrial glandular cells and endometrial stromal sarcoma arises from the stroma. The malignant mixed mullerian tumor is derived from both the glandular and stromal components and is very uncommon.

The various subtypes of endometrial cancer are:

- The endometrioid carcinoma or adenocarcinoma: 75% of endometrial cancers are of this type and the prognosis is quite good. Atypical hyperplasia and well differentiated adenocarcinoma may coexist.
- Adenoacanthoma and adenosquamous cancers: about 25% of adenocarcinomas have areas of squamous metaplasia. If the squamous component is benign then it is called an adenoacanthoma. When the squamous component is cytologically malignant then it is called an adenosquamous cancer and the prognosis for this is much worse than that of adenocarcinomas. This happens as these cancers have a poorer grade and are more likely to invade the myometrium and lymphovascular space.

- Serous papillary cancers: they account for <10% of all endometrial cancers. They mostly occur in older women and are more likely to have myometrial invasion, lymphovascular invasion and extrauterine spread. The 5-year survival rate is around 50%.
- Clear cell cancers: These cancers account for < 5% of endometrial cancers and have a 5-year survival rate of < 35%. They are not related to intrauterine exposure to diethylstilbestrol.

SPREAD OF THE DISEASE

Spread occurs by invading the myometrium and deeper invasion is associated with lymphatic and vascular involvement. The endometrium can also be involved by contiguous spread. Direct spread occurs to the para-aortic nodes and less likely to the supraclavicular and inguinal nodes. Cervical involvement occurs due to lymphatic and stromal spread and less commonly due to surface extension. Spread to the ovaries can occur in metastatic disease or a primary cancer may coexist. Transperitoneal spread occurs either via the myometrium or through the fallopian tubes.

PROGNOSTIC FACTORS

Most prognostic factors are interrelated. The purpose of identifying prognostic factors is to identify a group of patients who require adjuvant therapy. The low risk group consists of patients with well differentiated, grade 1 tumors, with no myometrial invasion and intraperitoneal disease. The risk of nodal involvement in these cases is 0%. The high risk group comprises those patients with myometrial invasion and/or intraperitoneal disease. These women have a 15-60% chance of nodal disease.

The various factors taken into consideration are:

- Lymph node involvement
- Lymphovascular space involvement
- Histological subtype
- Positive peritoneal cytology
- Myometrial invasion
- Steroid receptor status

- CA125 level
- Stage of the disease
- Degree of differentiation
- Ploidy status
- Tumor size
- Age
- Morphometric assessment

The most important of the above factors are the presense or absence of positive peritoneal cytology, tumor grade, depth of myometrial penetration, lymph node involvement and the presense or absense of extrauterine disease.

CLINICAL FEATURES

Abnormal vaginal bleeding is the commonest presenting symptom with endometrial cancer and the majority (75-80%) of patients are postmenopausal. Premenopausal and perimenopausal women with heavy and irregular bleeding are also at risk of having endometrial cancer. A postmenopausal woman not on hormone replacement therapy with vaginal bleeding has a 10% chance of having an endometrial cancer.

Abnormal vaginal discharge may be associated with pyometra (pus in uterine cavity) and deserves further investigation. Pyometra in a postmenopausal woman is associated with endometrial cancer in 50% of cases.

Pain may be a presenting symptom in pyometra and advanced metastatic disease. Pain in advanced disease is usually due to neuronal involvement or compression of nerves from metastatic disease.

DIAGNOSIS

Endometrial sampling is the mainstay of diagnosis of endometral cancer.

Endometrial sampling may be done in an outpatient setting using a pipelle sampler (or similar device). The accuracy of such sampling is 90%, with a failure rate of 8-20%.

An ultrasound scan measuring endometrial thickness in postmenopausal women with abnormal bleeding also helps to identify patients at risk of endometrial cancer. Endometrial cancer is very unlikely if the endometrial thickness is less than 4 mm.

Hysteroscopy and curettage may be carried out either as an outpatient or as an inpatient under general anesthetic.

Dilatation and curettage will only sample about 60% of the endometrium and is likely to miss 10% of endometrial lesions.

Once the diagnosis of endometrial cancer is confirmed, a chest X-ray, blood biochemistry and urinalysis should be carried out. Magnetic resonance imaging should be considered if extra-uterine spread is suspected particularly in poorly differentiated lesions.

STAGING

Endometrial cancer is staged surgically. The FIGO staging of endometrial cancer is as follows:

Ia	tumor limited to the endometrium
Ib	invasion of inner half of the myometrium
Ic	invasion of outer half of the myometrium
IIa	endocervical glandular involvement
IIb	endocervical stromal involvement
IIIa	tumor invasion of serosa and/or adnexae and/or positive peritoneal cytology
IIIb	vaginal metastasis
IIIc	metastasis to pelvic and/or paraaortic nodes
IVa	tumor invasion of bladder and/or bowel mucosa
IVb	distant metastasis including intra-abdominal disease and/or inguinal nodes

In addition each stage can be divided into G1, G2, G3 based on the tumor grade.

Screening

Several screening methods have been evaluated to screen asymptomatic women for endometrial cancer. No method has been found to reduce the morbidity or the mortality from endometrial cancer. The methods evaluated include endometrial biopsy, vaginal ultrasound, progestogen challenge test, papinicolaou smear of the cervix, vaginal pool smear, etc.

MANAGEMENT

Surgery

Exploratory laparotomy with total abdominal hysterectomy and bilateral salpingo-oophorectomy (TAH+BSO) is the operation of choice and surgical staging should include:

- aspiration of peritoneal fluid or peritoneal washings
- palpation and inspection of all peritoneal structures
- palpation/biopsy of the pelvic and paraaortic nodes

Cervical involvement necessitates parametrial resection and lymphadenectomy.

TAH+BSO is sufficient if the histology is a well differentiated adenocarcinoma, there is minimal myometrial invasion on imaging and if the tumor is superficial on sectioning the uterus. Pelvic and para-aortic lymphadenectomy may be indicated in poorly differentiated lesions, histology other than pure adenocarcinoma and deeper myometrial invasion.

The role of lymphadenectomy may be defined by the results of the ongoing ASTEC study (A Study in the Treatment of Endometrial Cancer).

Stage 2 disease requires an exploratory laparotomy as for stage 1. Parametrial excision (radical hysterectomy) has been recommended but all these patients would receive postoperative radiotherapy.

Debulking surgery should be carried out in FIGO stage 3 and 4 disease. This may help to reduce the incidence of bladder/bowel symptoms, vaginal discharge and pelvic pain.

Radiotherapy

The incidence of vaginal vault and pelvic recurrences are reduced after adjuvant radiotherapy but survival is not affected. This can be given as teletherapy or brachytherapy or a combination of both. Adjuvant radiotherapy is given to high risk patients.

Radiotherapy can be used as a primary mode of treatment in patients who are medically unfit for surgery, and also to give symptomatic relief in case of pelvic recurrences.

Cytotoxic Therapy

Both single agent and combination therapy can be used in case of recurrences. Combination regimens give higher response rates. Drugs like cisplatin, carboplatin and doxorubicin give response rates of >20%. Combination therapy produces slightly higher response rates of about 35%. However, responses are usually partial and shortlived. High risk patients like those with serous papillary tumors are usually considered for adjuvant chemotherapy.

Hormonal Therapy

Response rates to progestogens are quite low and may be less than 25%. Since side effects are minimal they are used at some stage of management and can be continued indefinitely if a response is achieved. If the tumor is progestogen receptor positive then a response is more likely.

Table 33.1: Surgical FIGO stage distribution and 5-year survival

Stage	% of cases	% 5-year survival
I	81.3	82.9
II	11.2	70.8
III	5.9	39.2
IV	1.7	27.3
All stages		78.1

Hormone Replacement Therapy (HRT)

Retrospective studies suggest that there are no adverse effects if HRT is given after treatment of the cancer. Consensus is that it can be offered to younger women with a good prognosis. Whether additional progestogens must be added is still unanswered.

Recurrent Disease

Clinical examination is the mainstay of follow-up. Some use vault cytology but there is no data to attest its value. In 50% of cases recurrence is local and one third of patients have distant metastasis. Recurrence occurs in one-third of patients in a year and in three quarters of patients in 3 years. Treatment depends on the site of recurrence and previous treatment given to the patient.

Conclusion

Surgery is the mainstay of management of endometrial cancer. Though the FIGO classification requires lymphadenectomy and histology this is unlikely to be routinely undertaken for low and medium risk patients. Adjuvant radiotherapy reduces the risk of vault recurrence but survival is not affected. The response rate of chemotherapy is generally poor.

Uterine Sarcomas

Uterine sarcomas can be the following three types. Myometrial cells can give rise to leiomyosarcomas (LMS), endometrial stroma gives rise to endometrial stromal sarcomas (ESS), and both cell types can give rise to malignant mixed mesodermal sarcomas (MMMT). As the mixed mesodermal tumor consists of both epithelial and stromal elements it is also called carcinosarcoma. Sarcomas account for only 3% of uterine malignancies and less than 1% of gynecological cancers.

Leiomyosarcomas

One percent of leiomyomas actually have a leiomyosarcoma at hysterectomy. About one-third of uterine sarcomas are leiomyosarcomas. The mean age of presentation is about 52 years.

Five percent of patients have a history of pelvic irradiation. Presenting symptoms can be postmenopausal bleeding, irregular vaginal bleeding, vaginal discharge, abdominal or pelvic pain, weight loss or abnormal cytology. A leiomyosarcoma must be excluded in a rapidly growing uterine mass or fibroid uterus.

Macroscopically a leiomyosarcoma looks similar to a leiomyoma but may be more pale or yellow and usually has areas of hemorrhage and necrosis. They are more likely to be single and measure more than 10 cm in size. Microscopically the three main criteria for diagnosis are hypercellularity, nuclear atypia and frequent mitotic figures more than or equal to 10 per high power field.

The treatment of choice is total abdominal hysterectomy with bilateral salpingo-oopherectomy. A full staging laparotomy should be performed on patients where the diagnosis is known preoperatively including pelvic washings as is done in all cases of ovarian cancer. The role of adjuvant radiotherapy or chemotherapy is unclear.

Endometrial Stromal Tumors

An endometrial stromal nodule is a benign tumor composed of endometrial stroma and located in the myometrium. An endometrial stromal sarcoma can arise from endometrial stroma, adenomyosis and rarely from pelvic endometriosis. It can be low grade or high grade. Endometrial sarcomas account for about 15% of all uterine sarcomas. More than 50% of tumors occur in premenopausal women and occasionally they occur in young girls. Clinical presentation is usually with abnormal vaginal bleeding, discharge or pain.

Macroscopically the tumor may be polypoidal or infiltrating in nature. Miscoscopically there is evidence of nuclear atypia and mitotic figures but the margins are usually well defined. In a low-grade tumor the characteristic feature is the infiltrating margin of the tumor. Mitotic figures are usually less than 10 per high power field in a low-grade tumor and more than 10 per high power field in the high-grade tumor.

Treatment consists of total abdominal hysterectomy and bilateral salpingo-oopherectomy (TAH+BSO). Adjuvant pelvic radiotherapy may be used to improve local control. Progestins or chemotherapy may be used in recurrent disease.

Malignant Mixed Müllerian Tumor

This tumor consists of both epithelial and mesenchymal elements. The benign end of the spectrum is an adenofibroma and at the malignant end is the carcinosarcoma or the mixed mullerian tumor.

Patients usually present at the age of 65 years with abdominal or pelvic pain, abnormal vaginal bleeding or a pelvic mass. As disease spread occurs early, presentation may be due to symptoms of extra-uterine disease (gastrointestinal or urological symptoms). A considerable number of patients have a prior history of pelvic irradiation which may have been given more than 15 years ago.

Macroscopically the tumor may fill the endometrial cavity and protrude through the cervical os. Microscopically the epithelial component may be an endometroid or a squamous cell carcinoma. The stromal component may be homologous or heterologous. The homologous forms consist of endometrial stromal sarcoma or fibrosarcoma and heterologous forms consist of rhabdomyosarcoma, osteosarcoma or chondrosarcoma. Tumor spread is similar to a poorly differentiated endometrial carcinoma and management should be in the same manner.

A staging laparotomy with TAH+BSO should be carried out. Radiotherapy is said to reduce local pelvic recurrence in those with poor prognostic factors. Chemotherapy using various combination regimes including adriamycin, ifosfamide and doxyrubicin are under investigation.

CONCLUSION

The advanced uterine sarcomas have a poor 2-year survival of less than 50%. The five year survival is 20-40%. Presently trials are trying to find out the optimal adjuvant treatment following surgical excision of the tumor.

REFERENCES

1. Michael A Quinn, Malcolm C Anderson, Carmel AE Coulter, W Patrick Soutter. Malignant disease of the uterus. In Text Book of Gynecology, 2nd edn. Robert W. Shaw, W. Patrick Soutter, Stuart L. Stanton, Churchill Livingstone; 585-605.
2. BD Rufford, FG Lawton. Endometrial cancer. Current Obstetrics and Gynecology 2001;11(5): 290-295.
3. AJ Papadopoulos, A Kenney. Solid malignant uterine tumors. Current Obstetrics and Gynecology October 2001; 11(5): 296-301.
4. Frank Lawton. Management of endometrial cancer. The Obstetrician and Gynecologist 2003; 5: 79-83.

34.

V Sivanesaratnam

Vulvar Cancer

INTRODUCTION

Malignancies in the vulva are uncommon and comprise 3-4% of genital tract malignancies. Internationally, the incidence of vulvar cancer varies, the highest rates being seen in Portuguese South America and in Portugal; the lowest rates are seen in Asian countries.[1] Asian women who have migrated to Australia continue to be at significantly lower risk for this malignancy.[2] The true incidence in Malaysia is not known. The University of Malaya Medical Centre is a major referral center for gynecological malignancies. Of the 3,125 gynecological malignancies managed during a 12-year period, vulvar malignancies comprised 2.8% (Table 34.1); thus, this malignancy is rare in Malaysia.

Table 34.1: Gynecological malignancies managed at the University of Malaya Medical Centre, KL 1991-2002

Malignancy	Number	%
Carcinoma cervix	1,466	47.0
Carcinoma of ovary	960	30.7
GTD	284	9.1
Carcinoma endometrium	269	8.6
Carcinoma vulva	88	2.8
Carcinoma of vagina	16	0.5
Others	42	1.3
Total	3,125	100.00

It is essentially a disease of the elderly with a mean age of 56 years in Malaysian women. Over the past 2 decades a subset of women younger than 50 years with squamous cell carcinoma has emerged.[3]

Ninety percent of the malignancies seen are squamous cell carcinomas; melanomas, adenocarcinoma, basal-cell carcinoma and sarcomas are far less commonly seen.

Etiology

Most vulvar cancers occur in postmenopausal women; more recently there is a trend towards a younger age at presentation. No specific etiological factor has been identified for vulvar cancer. Recent studies suggest 2 different *etiological types* of vulvar cancer:

- *One occurring in younger women:* This is related to human papilloma virus (HPV) and smoking, and commonly associated with vulvar intraepithelial neoplasia (VIN)

- *The other occurring in older women:* This is the more common type and is unrelated to smoking or human papilloma virus infection, and concurrent VIN is uncommon

Other diseases associated with vulvar cancer include lymphogranuloma venereum and granuloma inguinale. A positive serology for syphilis is present in 5% of vulvar cancers; these patients tend to have more poorly differentiated tumors. Vulvar cancer has also been associated with immunosuppression and a history of cervical neoplasia.

Squamous Cell Carcinoma

This accounts for 90% of vulvar cancers.

Clinical Presentation

The most common symptom is long standing vulvar pruritus and a recognizable lesion which is usually raised, fleshy, ulcerated or warty in appearance (Figs 34.1 and 34.2).

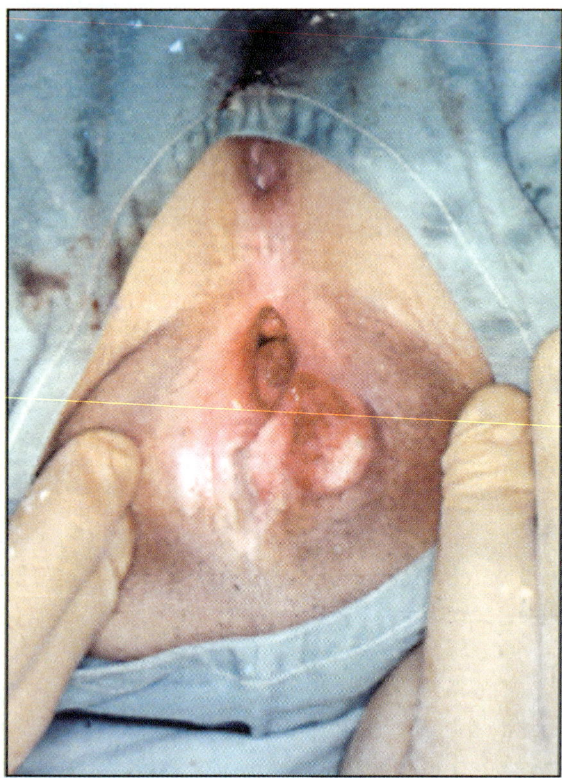

Figure 34.1: The 2 cm lesion arises on the left labium majus; note the typical irregular surface and superficial ulceration of a squamous cell carcinoma

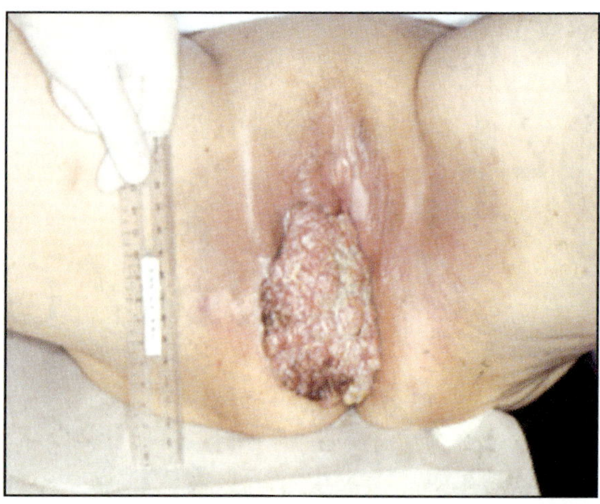

Figure 34.2: This patient ignored her symptoms and an obvious tumor in the lower vulva for more than 1 year. Such a late presentation is not unusual amongst Asian patients

Other symptoms include vulvar pain, bleeding, dysuria and discharge. In many parts of Asia-Oceania at the time of diagnosis, squamous cell carcinoma of the vulva is often large and exophytic and fungating (Figs 34.2 and 34.3) because of delay in treatment. Such late presentations are often due to:

- Fear of cancer
- Cultural taboos
- Ignorance
- Lack of appropriate facilities

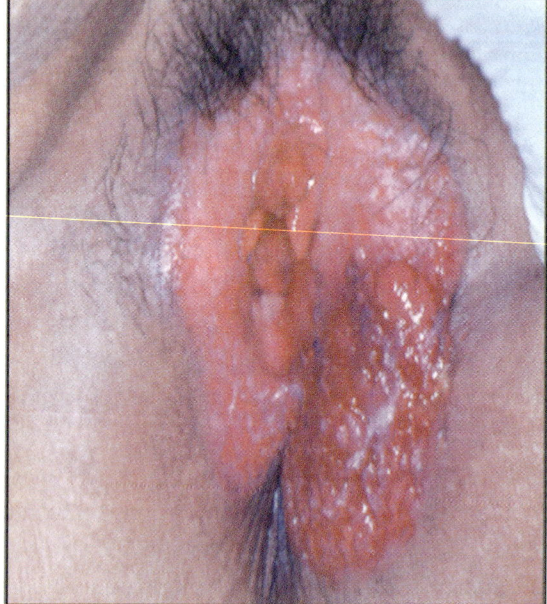

Figure 34.3: Squamous cell carcinoma of vulva involving both labia majora, anus and medial aspect of the upper thigh

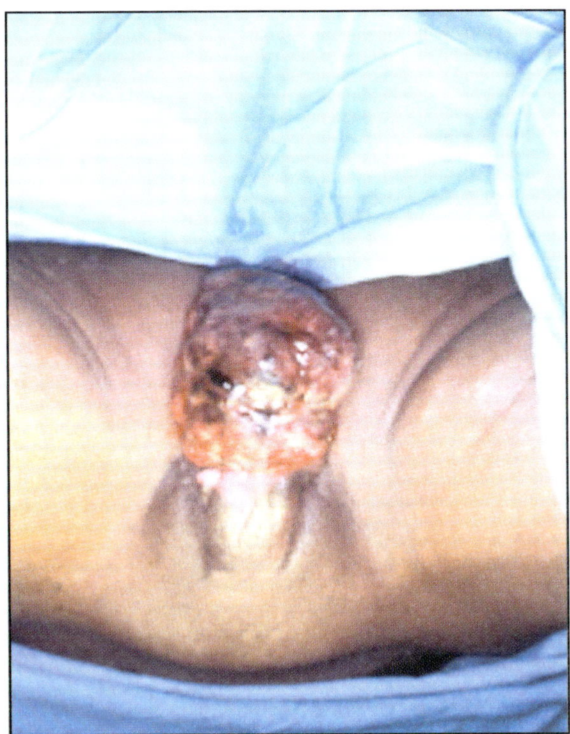

Figure 34.4A: A large clitoral squamous cell carcinoma—
This is relatively uncommon (see Fig. 34.4(B))

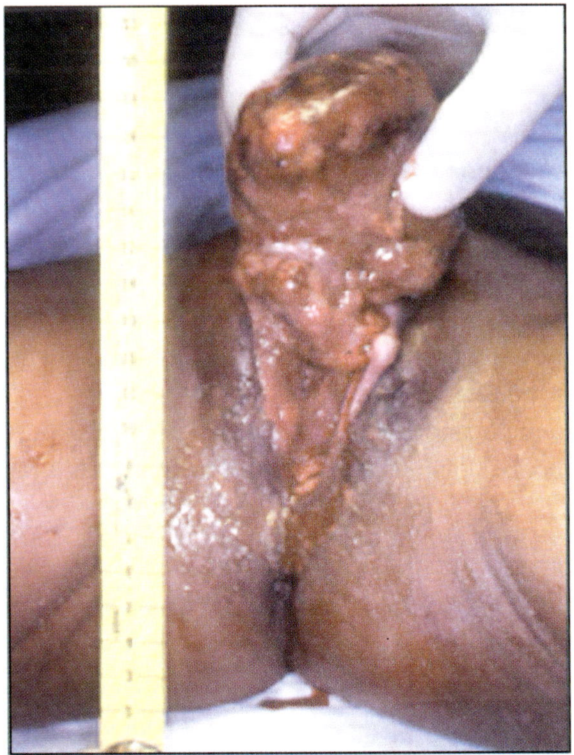

Figure 34.4B: Large clitoral squamous cell carcinoma
(see Fig. 34.4(A))

Many seek traditional treatment first, thus delaying definitive therapy. In contrast to the exophytic type, some tumors may grow as endophytic masses with ulceration.

Most of the lesions occur in the labia majora, favoring the medial aspect (Fig. 34.1); primary involvement of the labia minora is seen in less than 30% of patients. Primary clitoral (Fig. 34.4) and periurethral sites are less common.

In approximately 5% of cases the lesions are multifocal (Fig. 34.5)

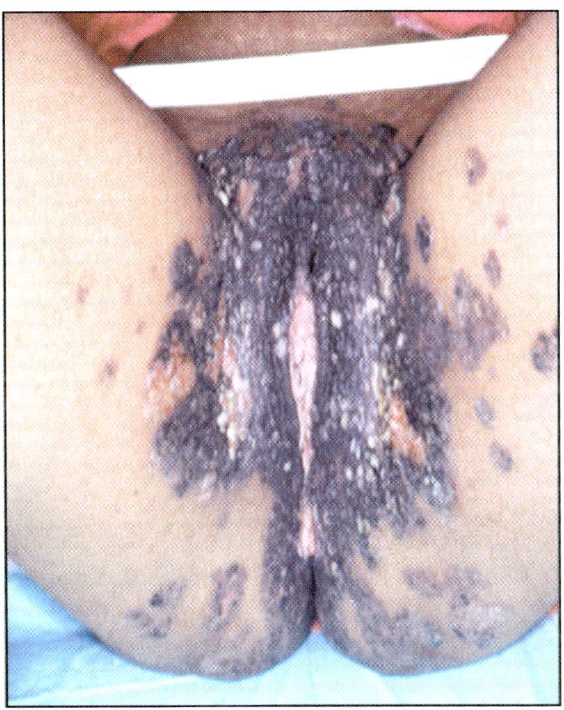

Figure 34.5: Extensive squamous cell carcinoma of the vulva. Note the multifocal lesions extending to the medial aspects of both thighs and buttocks. Such an occurrence is extremely rare

The *clinical examination* should include a thorough examination of the vulva, vestibule, introitus, perineum and anus. Because neoplasms of the lower female genital tract are often multicentric, the vagina and cervix should be evaluated; a complete pelvic examination including cervical cytology is essential. The groins should be carefully palpated for lymph node involvement.

Diagnosis

This requires a wedge biopsy which can be carried out as an office procedure under local anesthesia; this should include surrounding normal skin and underlying connective tissue. For small lesions, an excisional biopsy is preferred.

In those with a large primary tumor, a computed tomography (CT) is useful to determine extent of spread of disease. Where there is involvement of the vestibule a cystoscopic evaluation is useful to determine extent of urethral and bladder involvement. If the anus is involved a procto-sigmoidoscopy is useful.

Pattern of Spread

There are three modalities of spread:
- Direct extension to adjacent organs such as urethra, vagina and anus (Fig. 34.3)
- Lymphatic embolization to regional lymph nodes
- Hematogenous spread to distant sites (lungs, liver, bone)

The predominant method of spread is by lymphatic embolization. As demonstrated by Perry-Jones,[4] the lymplatics of the vulva course superiorly to the area of the mons pubis and then turn to drain in the ipsilateral superficial inguinal nodes located between the Camper's fascia and fascia lata; lymphatics from here perforate through the cribriform fascia to the deep inguinal (femoral) nodes. The latter number 1 to 4; the Cloquet node (Rosenmuller) which is the most cephalad of the femoral nodes, is absent in 50% of cases. These nodes are situated medial to the femoral vein within the fossa ovalis, there are no nodes distal to the lower margin of the fossa ovalis. Thus, there is no need to remove the fascia lata lateral to the femoral vessels; this reduces risk of injury to the femoral nerve. From the inguino-femoral nodes the lymphatics drain into the pelvic nodes, and in particular the external iliac nodes. The lymphatics from laterally situated lesions drain to the ipsilateral nodes; the vulvar lymphatic channels do not cross labio-crural folds on to the medial aspects of the thigh, and drainage to the contralateral groin is rare.

Lymphatics from the clitoris and anterior aspect of vulva and perineum drain to both groins. Direct lymphatic pathways from the clitoris and Bartholin's glands to the pelvic nodes have also been observed. This pattern of spread is illustrated in Figure 34.6.

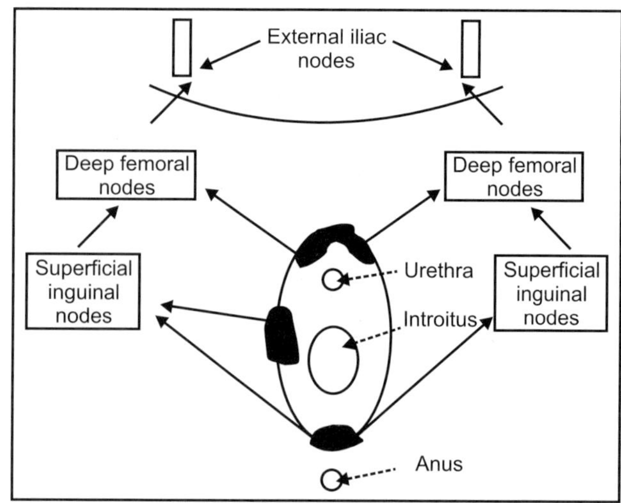

Figure 34.6: Schematic representation of potential lymphatic spread from vulvar cancer (Modified from Stanley Way)

An Australian study using bipedal lymphangiograms[5] demonstrated no nodes medial to the pubic tubercle and no nodes in outer 15-20% of a line drawn from the anterior aspect of the anterior-superior iliac spine to the pubic tubercle. Occasional lymphatics from the leg traverse this outer area to join axillary lymphatics; thus, limiting the lateral extent of groin incision will help reduce postoperative lymphedema.

Lymph Node Metastases

The incidence of groin lymph node metastasis is approximately 30%; this is related to the size of the tumor and stage of the disease. The incidence of pelvic lymph node involvement is approximately 5-6%, such patients usually have 3 or more positive inguinal nodes. The occurrence of pelvic node metastases without groin node metastases is extremely rare.

Hematogenous spread occurs late in the disease; the absence of lymphatic metastases in such patients is rarely seen.

Staging

This is now based on a surgical-pathological staging (Table 34.2).

Management

The surgical approach to vulvar cancer has continued to change over the past 4-5 decades. In 1912, Basset

Table 34.2: FIGO Staging for vulvar cancer

Stage	Surgico-pathological findings
0	Vulvar intraepithelial neoplasia (VIN)
I	Tumor confined to vulva or perineum or both, 2 cm or < in greatest diameter (no nodal metastases)
1a	Stromal invasion 1.0 mm or less
1b	Stromal invasion > 1.0 mm
II	Tumor confined to vulva or perineum or both. More than 2 cm in greatest diameter (no nodal metastases)
III	Tumor of any size with one or both of the following (a) adjacent spread to the lower urethra, vagina and anus (b) unilateral lymph node metastases
IV a	Tumor involving the upper urethra, bladder mucosa, rectal mucosa, or pelvic bones or bilateral groin node metastases
IV b	Any distant metastases including pelvic lymph nodes

proposed *en bloc* resection of the vulvar tumor and inguino-femoral nodes; the lines of excision were inadequate resulting in poor survival. Tausig[6] and Way[7] advocated a more radical surgical excision which included the entire vulva and mons and extended laterally over and including the inguinal nodes and inferiorly extending to the urogenital diaphragm. This had been extremely successful from a curative point of view, with overall survival rates of 65%. However, the postoperative morbidity was extremely high; there was extensive wound infection and dehiscence, resulting in greatly delayed healing; there were also psychological and psychosexual sequelae. Monaghan[8] using this traditional vulvectomy reported 5-year survivals of 94.3% in node negative patients and 62.5% in node positive patients.

Since mid-1970/early 1980 such a radical approach which was associated with significant morbidity was questioned and prompted a reappraisal, as these lesions were now being detected early and, therefore, considerably smaller than those seen so commonly in the first half of the 20th century. Currently more than 50% of these lesions seen in the West are in Stage 1 disease at the time of diagnosis. Furthermore, the disease is now being diagnosed more frequently in the young, some of whom are in the twenties. The extensive radical procedures performed in the past have helped define the patterns of local lymphatic spread, incidence of nodal metastases and pathological features of the primary tumor; these accumulated data have helped in predicting the risk of nodal metastases allowing for customization of extent of surgery based on:

- Lesion size
- Location
- Depth of invasion
- Clinical suspicion of lymph node metastasis

For instance, for small T1 squamous cell carcinoma there are no positive nodes if the depth of invasion is < 1mm; the incidence of nodal metastases increases as the depth of invasion increases, 7.7% for depth of 1.1-2 mm to 34.2% for depths > 5 mm.[9] The incidence of lymph node metastases according to clinical stage[9] are:

Stage I	10.7%
Stage II	26.2%
Stage III	64.2%
Stage IV	88.9%

Management of Early Vulvar Cancer

The management of early vulvar lesions should be individualized with emphasis on carrying out the most conservative procedure that will achieve cure for the patient.

Thus, for small lesions (< 2 cm) that are laterally situated with < 1 mm depth of invasion a wide radical excision (with 10 mm clear margins) would suffice; there is no need to perform a lymphadenectomy, thus sparing the patient the potential morbidity.

For laterally situated lesions with depth of invasion exceeding 1mm or lesions > 2 cm in size, a wide radical excision may be performed with an ipsilateral inguino-femoral lymphadenectomy; if a metastatic deposit is noted, the contra-lateral lymphadenectomy should also be performed (see Fig. 34.6). In the presence of an otherwise normal-looking vulva, such vulvar-sparing surgery is a safe surgical option regardless of the depth of invasion. Conserve the clitoris where possible.

For mid-line lesions (Figs 34.4 and 34.6) the resection should include bilateral inguino-femoral lymphadenectomy. Metastases to the femoral nodes can occur without involvement of the superficial inguinal nodes. Thus, if groin node dissection is indicated a thorough inguino-femoral lymphadenectomy is mandatory. It is also important to bear in mind that patients who develop recurrent disease in an undissected or incompletely dissected groin have a very high mortality (92%).

Incision

Recently there has been a shift to the *triple incision* technique (separate groin incision for lymphadenectomy) to reduce postoperative morbidity (Fig. 34.7). The advantages are:
- Primary closure is easily achieved
- Primary healing occurs in > 65% or cases
- Mean hospital stay is markedly reduced

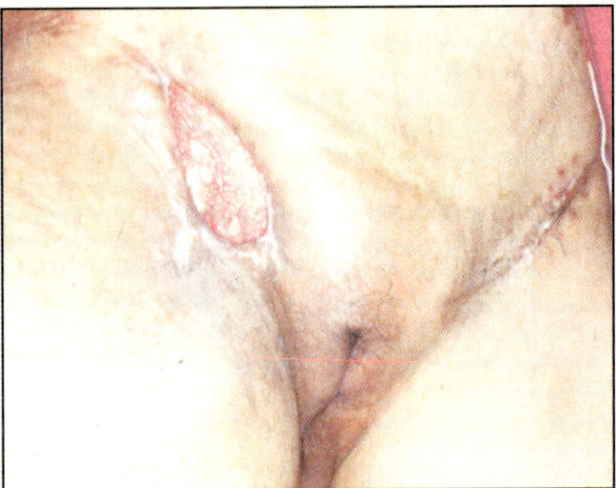

Figure 34.7: Wide radical excision of a 2 cm lesion over the perineum and bilateral groin node dissection had been done. Note superficial breakdown of wound in right groin. The normal vulvar appearance is preserved

Whilst such a conservative approach is generally safe, *skin bridge metastases* has been reported; this results from 2 possible mechanisms:
- Transit metastatic emboli
- Retrograde permeation of lymphatics

Thus, separate groin incisions are probably not advisable when more than microscopic lymph node metastases are present.

Modified Twombley-Ulfelder Technique

As stated earlier, unlike in the West, a majority of our patients present with large bulky tumors. We have used the modified Twombley-Ulfelder technique which helps preserve sufficient skin to achieve primary skin closure (Figs 34.8 to 34.11).

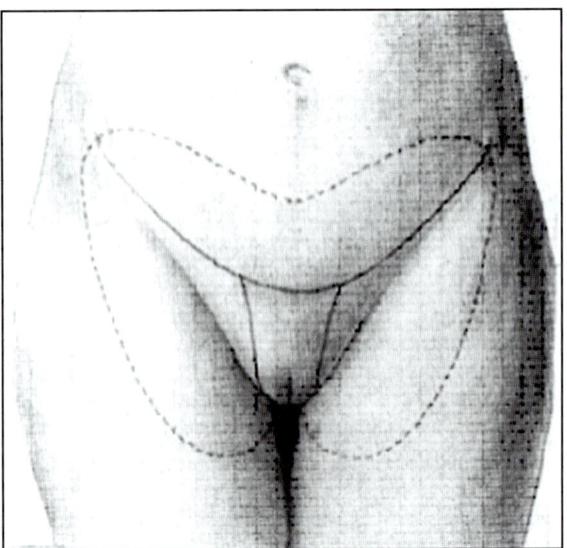

Figure 34.8: Skin incision for radical vulvectomy. The dotted lines indicate the limits of the superficial groin dissection (adopted from Twombley GH, Cancer)

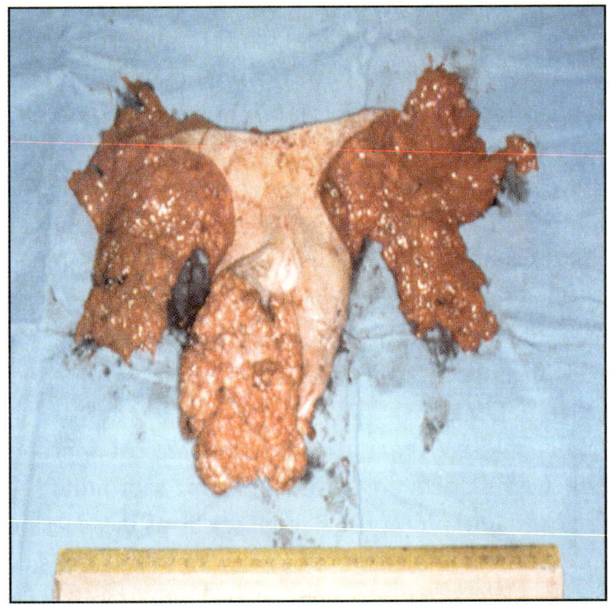

Figure 34.9: Radical vulvectomy specimen (using the technique above) from patient shown in Figure 34.2

Special Situations

- *Lesion in close proximity to the urethra:* Here, the distal 1cm of urethra can be resected; this does not compromise urethral continence.
- *Lesion close to or involving the clitoris:* Here, anterior vulvar irradiation is an option; it will sterilize the tumor without interfering with clitoral sensitivity.

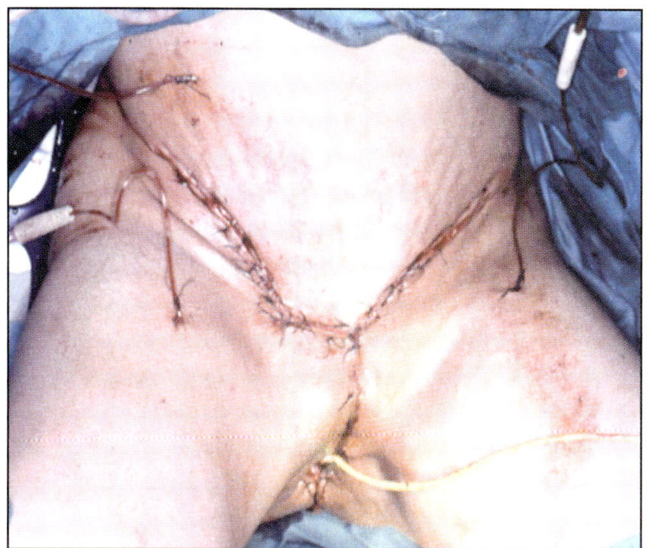

Figure 34.10: Primary skin closure is easily obtained

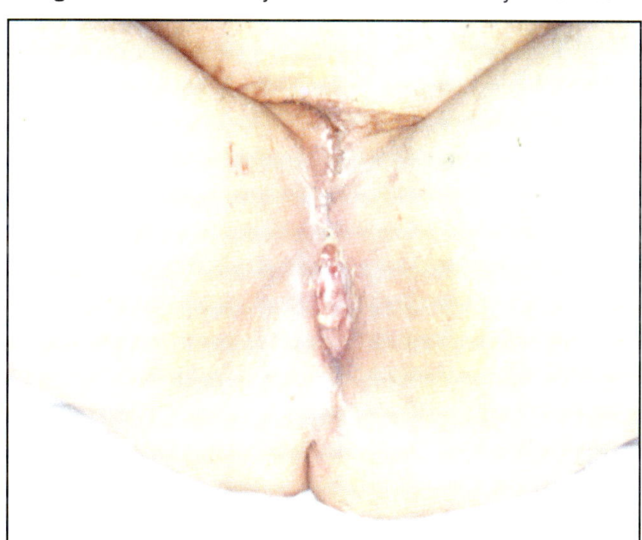

Figure 34.11: Appearance of the operation site 6 months later. Satisfactory wound healing is obtained

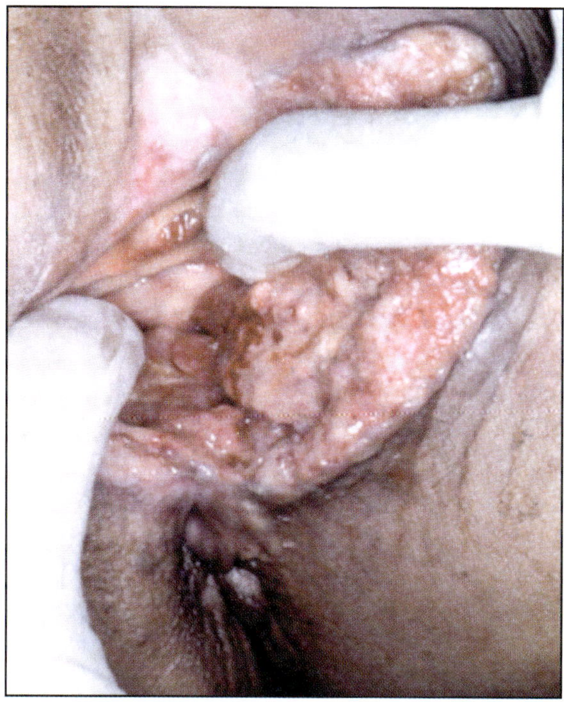

Figure 34.12: Note the large vulval growth extending downwards to involve the anus. A radical vulvectomy (with "en bloc" groin node dissection and posterior exenteration was done (see Figs 34.13 and 34.14)

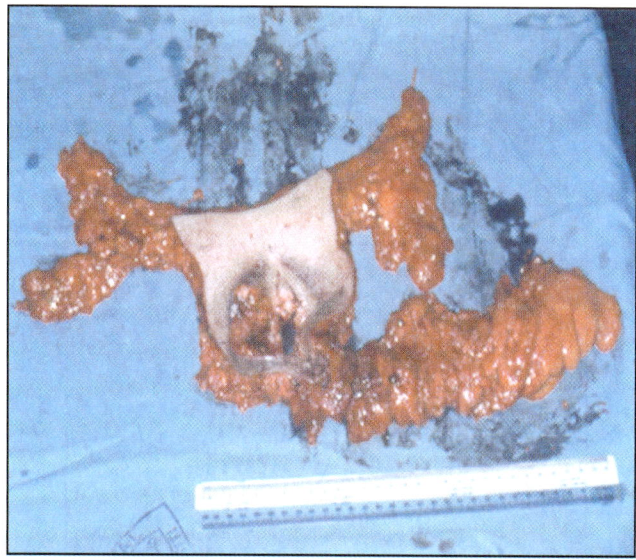

Figure 34.13: Radical vulvectomy specimen *en bloc* with groin nodes and rectum and anus

- *Proximity of the lesions to the anus:* When the lesion is extensive and involves the anus as shown in Figure 34.12, a more radical procedure is necessary

  An alternative approach in the management of such lesions is *irradiation* to the vulva which would help preserve the vulval contour as well as the anus (Figs 34.3 and 34.15).

- *Carcinoma of the vulva in pregnancy:* This is extremely rare. The first case of squamous cell carcinoma of the vulva in Malaysia and possibly the second in Asia was reported by us.[10] Treatment is individualized; radical excision with or without ipsilateral or bilateral inguinal lymphadenectomy is carried out as in the non-pregnant patient until 36 weeks, beyond which the definitive therapy is

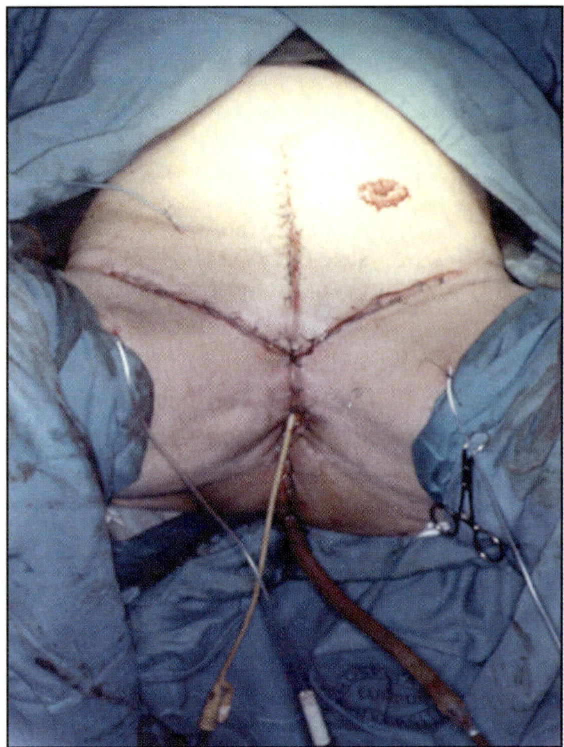

Figure 34.14: Primary skin closure has been achieved. Note the colostomy in the left iliac fossa

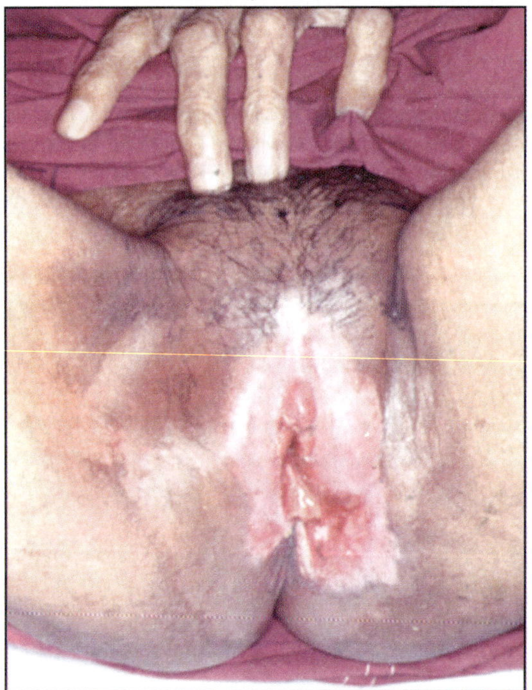

Figure 34.15: Please refer to Figure 34.3. Surgical excision of the lesion which had extended to the medial aspect of the thigh would have required reconstructive surgery to close the large raw area. Note the satisfactory response after radiotherapy and preservation of vulvar appearance 6 months after

deferred into the puerperium. These tumors can be aggressive and grow rapidly during pregnancy as observed by us (Fig. 34.16).

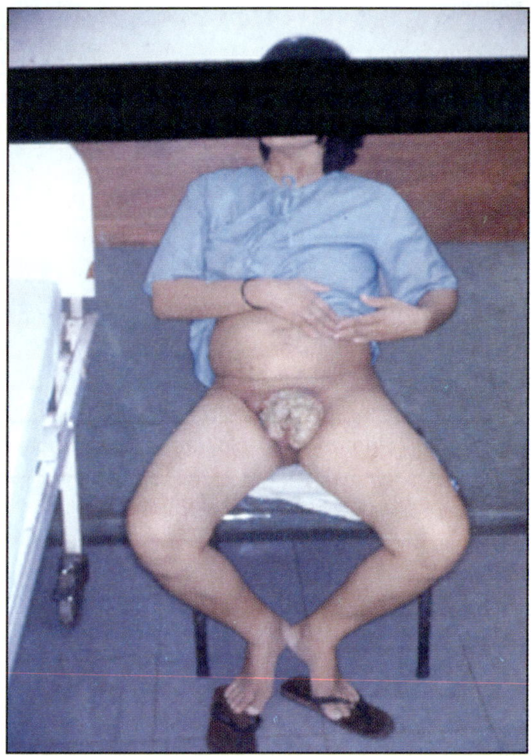

Figure 34.16: Carcinoma of the vulva in pregnancy. The 28-year-old patient was referred soon after a term vaginal delivery. Notice the large exophytic growth and groin node enlargement. Radical vulvectomy and bilateral inguino-femoral lymphadenectomy was performed; there was metastases to 17 nodes. She succumbed 6 months later

Lymphatic Mapping

Recently there has been a great interest in locating the sentinel node using intraoperative mapping with lymphoscintigraphy. Selective sentinel node biopsy in early vulvar cancer is done using this technique; if this was negative for metastases it would spare the patient the morbidity associated with lymphadenectomy. Whilst this is reliable in a majority of cases, occasional false negative sentinel nodes have been reported.

Other Vulvar Malignancies

Malignant Melanoma of Vulva

This is rare in Malaysia; in the West this is the second most common type of vulvar cancer, occurring predominantly in postmenopausal white women and involving the labia minora or clitoris. Diagnosis is based on an excisional biopsy (for small lesions) for histological diagnosis. The overall prognosis is poor with 5 year-survival of 30%; hence, the surgical approach now is towards vulvar conservation with radical excision of the primary tumor.

Verrucous Carcinoma

This is a variant of squamous cell carcinoma. This cauliflower tumor may be difficult to distinguish from condylomata acuminata or squamous papilloma. It is a locally aggressive tumor that pushes into, rather than invades, the underlying structures; metastasis to regional nodes is rare. Treatment is radical excision; radiation therapy is contraindicated as it may induce anaplastic transformation.

Basal Cell Carcinoma

This locally invasive, non-metastatic tumor is rare; it usually presents as a 'rodent' ulcer and involves the labium majus. Treatment is wide local excision.

Bartholin's Gland Carcinoma

Primary carcinoma of *Bartholin's* gland accounts for 5% of all vulvar cancers. The histological types noted are adenocarcinomas, squamous cell carcinomas and rarely transitional cell carcinomas. Current therapy consists of hemivulvectomy, ipsilateral inguino-femoral lymphadenectomy; pelvic lymphadenectomy is performed for those with positive groin nodes.

Vulvar Sarcomas

These constitute 1 to 2% of vulvar cancers; leiomyosarcomas are the most common. Wide local excision is the recommended initial treatment. Recurrences are likely with lesions > 5 cm diameter with infiltrating margins.

Transitional Cell Carcinoma

This may be a primary tumor of the vulva, arising from the Bartholin's glands. Rarely, it may be an extension of a primary tumor in bladder or urethra on to the vulva (Figs 34.17 to 34.19).

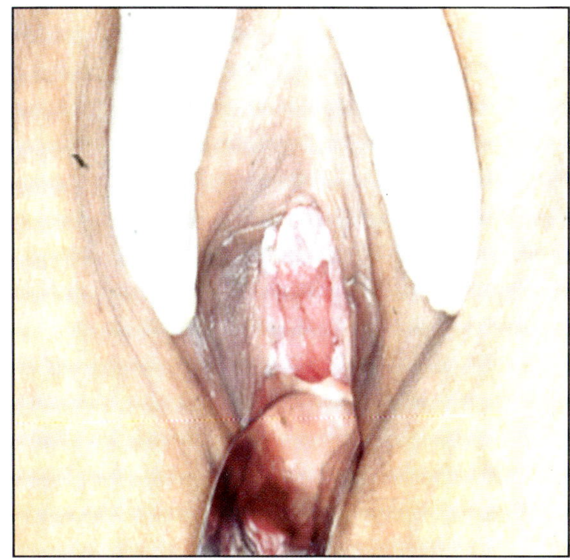

Figure 34.17: Transitional cell carcinoma of bladder extending to involve the clitoris, vestibule and labia minora. An anterior exenteration, radical vulvectomy and bilateral inguino-femoral node dissection and ileal conduit were done (Fig. 34.18). The posterior vaginal wall was preserved and swung forward to create a vaginal lumen (Fig. 34.19)

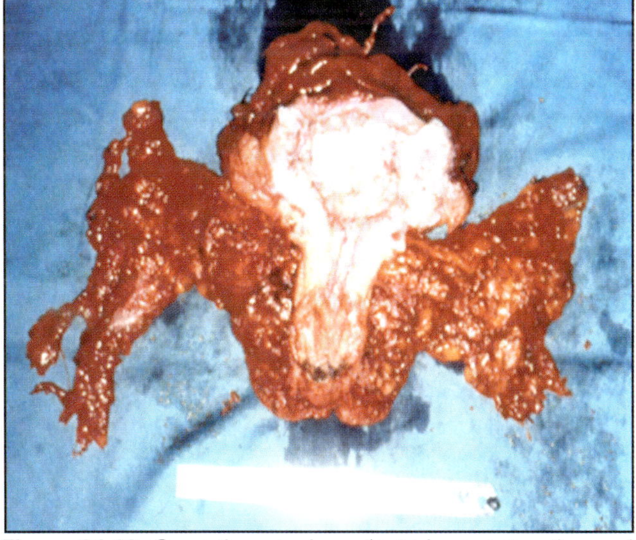

Figure 34.18: Operative specimen (anterior exenteration and radical vulvectomy) of above showing transitional cell carcinoma of bladder extending down to the urethra

Summary

Recent advances in the surgical approach to vulvar malignancies suggest the following:

- More limited resection of primary lesion for unifocal tumors and, otherwise, normal vulva

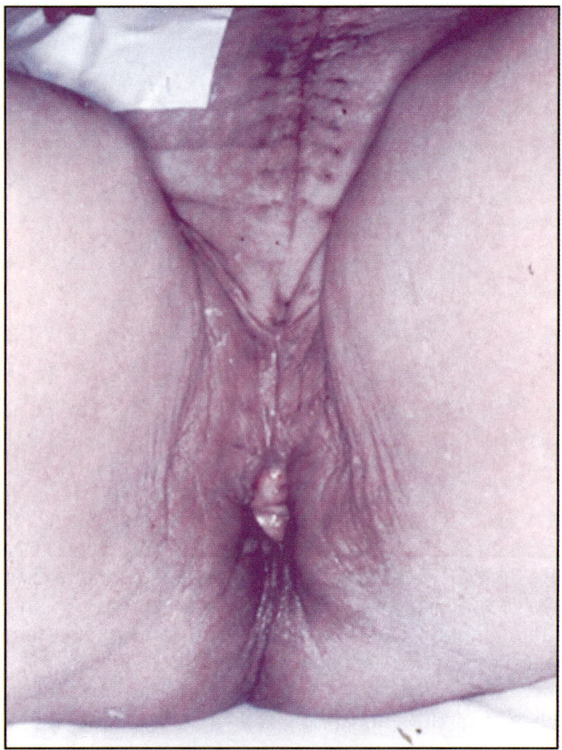

Figure 34.19: The above patient 6 months after surgery. There is satisfactory healing with a functioning ileal conduit and satisfactory vaginal lumen

- Omission of groin node dissection for T_1 tumors and < 1mm stromal invasion
- Elimination of routine pelvic lymphadenectomy
- Use of separate groin incisions for inguino-femoral lymphadenectomy

- Omission of contralateral groin node dissection for lateral T_1 lesions/negative ipsilateral nodes
- Use of postoperative radiation to groin recurrence in those with multiple positive groin nodes
- Care should be individualized.

REFERENCES

1. Parkin M, Muir CS, Wheelan SL et al. Cancer incidence in five Continents. Vol VI. Lyon International Agency for Research on Cancer, 1993.
2. Giles GG, Farrugia H, Silver B, Staples MP. Cancer in Victoria, Melbourne: Anti-Cancer Council of Victoria, 1992.
3. Jones RW, Bananyai J, Sables S. Trends in squamous cell carcinoma of the vulva: the influence of vulvar intra-epithelial neoplasia. Obstet Gynecol 1997; 90: 448-52.
4. Parry-Jones E. Lymphatics of the vulva. J Obstet Gynecol Br Empire 1963; 70: 751.
5. Nicklin JL, Hacker NF, Heintze SW. An anatomical study of inguinal node topography and clinical implications for the surgical management of vulvar cancer. Int. J Gynecol Cancer 1995;5:128-33.
6. Chu J, Tamimi H, Figge D. Femoral node metastases with negative inguinal nodes in early vulvar cancer. Am J Obstet Gynecol 1981;140:337-39.
7. Taussig F. Carcinoma of the vulva: an analysis of 155 cases. Am J Obstet Gynecol 1940; 40: 764.
8. Way S. Carcinoma of vulva. Am J Obstet Gynecol 1960; 79: 692.
9. Hacker NF. Vulvar cancer. In Practical Gynecologic Oncology (2nd ed) Ed. Berek JS and Hacker NF. Williams and Wilkinson, Sydney 1994.
10. Sivanesaratnam V, Pathmanathan R. Carcinoma of the vulva in pregnancy, a rare occurrence. Asia-Oceania J Obstet Gynecol 1990; 16: 207-10.

35.

V Sivanesaratnam

Gestational Trophoblastic Neoplasia

INTRODUCTION

Gestational trophoblastic neoplasia (GTN) encompasses a spectrum of clinical and histological entities and comprise a group of neoplastic disorders arising from trophoblastic tissue of the placenta (Tables 35.1 and 35.2).

Table 35.1: Gestational trophoblastic neoplasia—clinical entities

- Gestational trophoblastic disease
- Gestational trophoblastic tumor (clinical evidence of either choriocarcinoma/invasive mole)
- Metastatic gestational tophoblastic tumor (clinical evidence of invasive mole/choriocarcinoma beyond the body of uterus)
- Non-metastasising gestational trophoblastic tumor

Table 35.2: Gestational trophoblastic neoplasia—histological entities

- Hydatidiform mole
- Invasive mole (chorioadenoma destruens)
- Gestational choriocarcinoma
- Placental site tumor

GTN is a common gynecological problem in Malaysia and other South-East Asian countries (Table 35.3). Due to the lack of a Tumor Register in many of these countries, the true incidence is unknown.

Table 35.3: Incidence of hydatidiform mole in Asia[1]

Center	Author	Year	Rate per 1000	Type of denominator
Singapore	Teoh et al	1971	1.2	Deliveries
Japan	Takeuchi	1982	1.96	Pregnancies
Indonesia	Farid Aziz	1984	12.9	Pregnancies
Malaysia	Sivanesaratnam	1991	2.8	Deliveries
Philippines	Panililo	1987	7.0	Deliveries

HYDATIDIFORM MOLE

Hydatidiform mole is more prevalent in Indonesia and Philippines (Table 35.3). In Malaysia the incidence was reported as 2.8 per 1000 deliveries; a significantly higher incidence among the Chinese was observed (5.52 per 1000 deliveries, $p < 0.001$)[2] (Table 35.4).

Table 35.4: Hydatidiform mole—Racial incidence (University Hospital, Kuala Lumpur 1978-1987)

Race	No. with molar pregnancy	Total deliveries	Incidence per 1000 deliveries
Malay	91	34,344	2.66
Chinese	51	9,247	5.52*
Indian	12	13,497	0.89
Others	5	344	14.70
Total	159	57,430	2.78

* $p < 0.001$

On the basis of gross morphology, histopathology and karyotype (Table 35.5) hydatidiform mole may be categorised into:

- Complete hydatidiform mole
- Partial hydatidiform mole

A complete mole is a hydatidiform mole without an embryo or fetus. Macroscopically, it is characterized by clusters of "grape-like" vesicles of varying sizes (Fig. 35.1).

Table 35.5 shows the histological differences between complete and partial moles. These features are often subject to inter- and intra-observer variations.

Clinical Features

The classical clinical features include:
- vaginal bleeding
- anemia

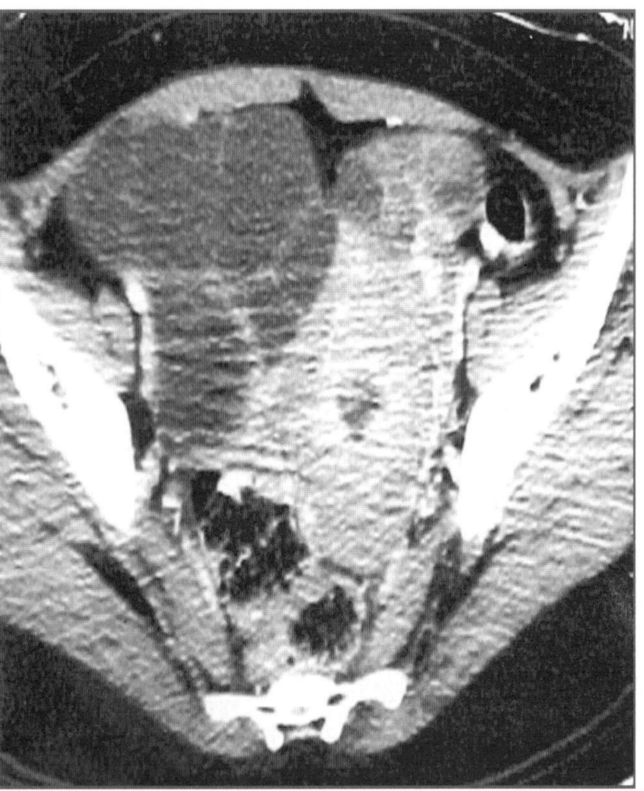

Figure 35.1: Notice the clusters of "grape-like" vesicles within the uterine cavity. The patient had a hysterectomy performed (Today, hysterectomy is seldom performed for hydatidiform mole)

- excessive uterine enlargement
- hyperemesis gravidarum
- hyperthyroidism
- toxaemia of pregnancy
- theca-luteal cysts

Vaginal bleeding is the most common presenting symptom, occurring in 97% of cases. This occurs in the early second trimester of pregnancy and is often

Table 35.5: Differences between complete and partial mole

Features	Complete mole	Partial mole
Fetal or embryonic tissue	absent	present
Hydatidiform swelling and cavitation of villi	diffuse	focal
Circumferential trophoblastic proliferation with or without atypia	diffuse	focal
Scalloping of chorionic villi	absent	marked
Stromal trophoblastic inclusions	absent	marked
Fetal stromal vessels	absent	absent
Karyotype	46xx; 46xy (entirely paternal origin)	69xxy; 69xyy (triploid—extra haploid set paternal origin)

intermittent and prolonged (*cf.* ectopic tubal pregnancy where a similar pattern occurs but in the early first trimester). Molar tissue may separate from the decidua and disrupt maternal vessels; this results in large volume of retained blood within the uterine cavity causing the *excessive uterine enlargement* seen in about 70% of patients and *anemia* in 50% of patients.

Pre-eclampsia is observed in about 25% of patients. The diagnosis of hydatidiform mole should be considered whenever pre-eclampsia develops before 20 weeks gestation. *Hyperemesis gravidarum* occurs in 25% of patients, particularly in those with excessive uterine enlargement and markedly elevated hCG levels.

Hyperthyroidism occurs in about 5% of patients; tachycardia, warm skin and tremor may be present. The diagnosis is confirmed by detection of elevated levels of free thyroxine (T_4) and triiodothyronine (T_3). These clinical and biochemical features rapidly revert to normal soon after uterine evacuation, confirming the features are *transient*. The therapy, therefore, need not be prolonged.

Theca-luteal cysts (>6 cm) are present in about 50% of patients with complete mole. These are thin-walled multiloculated cysts that are often bilateral (Fig. 35.2).

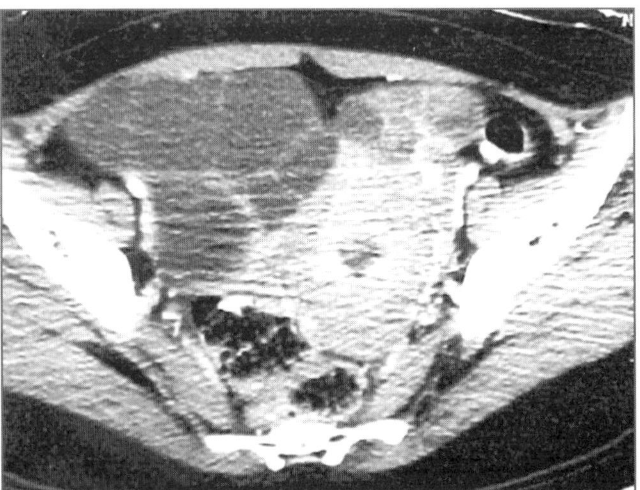

Figure 35.2: Notice the typical large thin-walled multiloculated cysts. The patient had uterine evacuation for complete mole 1 week earlier

Their formation is related to the high level of circulating hCG. Because the uterus is often excessively large, these cysts may not be easily palpable.

Spontaneous regression occurs after molar evacuation within 8 to 10 weeks. Continued persistence of these cysts would indicate persistence of trophoblastic mole.

Diagnosis of Molar Pregnancy

The diagnosis of a *complete mole* is nearly always made by ultrasonography; the chorionic villi of complete hydatidiform moles proliferate diffusely with hydropic swelling and produce a characteristic vesicular sonographic pattern or "snow-storm" pattern. The increasing use of high resolution ultrasound has led to the earlier diagnosis of molar pregnancy when the patient is asymptomatic; in the first trimester the typical appearance of the complete mole has been reported as a complex, echogenic, intrauterine mass containing many small cystic spaces.

Management of Molar Pregnancy

Once the diagnosis of hydatidiform mole is confirmed (by ultrasound) the uterine cavity must be emptied; *suction curettage* is the preferred method. An oxytocin infusion (20 units in 500ml saline) is commenced soon after induction to aid in the uterine evacuation and minimise the risk of uterine perforation. The aim in the management is to prevent malignant sequelae; thus, complete evacuation of the uterus is essential. In 25% of our cases, complete evacuation was not achieved at the first attempt.[2] A routine ultrasound examination one week later should be performed. If residual molar tissue is still present a second evacuation needs to be done; the uterus is now smaller and firmer and can be curetted without fear of perforation. The danger of repeated curettage is the development of Asherman's syndrome; fertility in these patients can be restored by lysis of intra-uterine adhesions.[3]

Acute respiratory distress occurring in 27% of cases during or after evacuation of uteri larger than 16 weeks has been reported.[4] This is caused by a combination of factors—trophoblastic embolization, pre-eclampsia, anaemia, fluid overload and hyperthyroidism.[4] With cardiovascular and respiratory support in intensive care, response is usual within 72 hours.

In the situation of a *twin pregnancy*, where there is one viable fetus and the other pregnancy is molar, if the mother wishes, the pregnancy should be allowed to proceed after appropriate counselling. Whilst the probability of achieving a viable pregnancy is 40%, there are risks of complications such as pulmonary embolism and pre-eclampsia. No increased risk of developing GTN after such twin pregnancy has been reported.[5]

Follow-up

The patients should be seen weekly. At these visits a pelvic examination looking for vaginal nodules, and regression in size of uterus and theca-luteal cysts are noted and the serum hCG levels assessed. These weekly visits are continued till the hCG levels return to normal (< 2mlU/ml), after which the patient is seen 2 weekly for the next 3 months and monthly for the next 9 months.

Contraception after Molar Pregnancy

The potential for persistent trophoblastic proliferation after initial evacuation of a hydatidiform mole is well recognized. The failure to note a progressive decline in the serum hCG after molar evacuation is generally indicative of trophoblastic malignancy.

In the UK, the use of combined oral contraceptives pill (OC) in such patients before hCG levels returned to normal resulted in a 2–fold increase of post-molar tumor requiring chemotherapy.[6] However, it can be used safely after the hCG levels have returned to normal;[7] we prefer to advise the use of barrier method of contraception till the hCG levels return to normal. It must, however, be noted that OC_s do not postpone the occurrence of choriocarcinoma; thus, women on OC in the post-molar period run the same risk of developing choriocarcinoma as their counterparts not on OC. Close follow-up is, therefore, essential.

Partial Hydatidiform Mole (phm) (Fig. 35.3)

As a result of lack of awareness and the lack of detailed routine histopathological evaluation of the placenta and products of conception evacuated at abortion, resulting in under-reporting, the true incidence of PHM is unknown. In our own institution we reported[8] that 30% of all molar pregnancies were, in fact, PHM. The

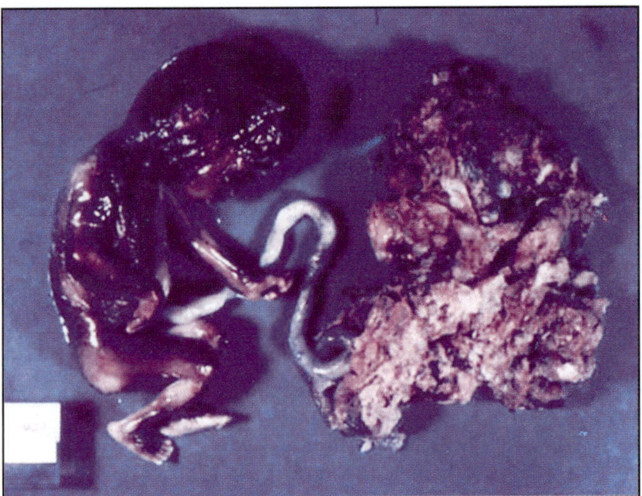

Figure 35.3: Partial mole-note the macerated fetus and vesicles in the placenta

histopathological differences from a complete mole are shown in Table 35.5.

Whilst the ultrasound features of a complete mole are reliable, the *ultrasound diagnosis of a partial mole* is more complex. The finding of cystic spaces in the placenta and a ratio of transverse to antero-posterior diameter of the gestation sac > 1.5 is required for the reliable diagnosis of partial molar pregnancy.[9]

The clinical features characteristic of complete mole are usually absent in PHM. However, one of our patients at 19 weeks gestation had a 24 weeks' enlarged uterus.[1] The hCG levels have been said to be not higher than in normal pregnancies; yet in one of our cases the urinary pregnancy test was positive at a dilution of 1: 4096.

Until as recently as 1988, various authors have claimed that no choriocarcinoma has been associated with PHM.[10, 11] This is in spite of the first documented case by us in early 1981[12] of malignant evolution with fatal outcome in a patient with PHM. The partial mole is, thus, part of a spectrum of GTN and not an entity by itself and is potentially malignant. It, therefore, requires close follow-up as for complete moles.

Invasive Mole

The diagnosis of an invasive mole cannot be made on evacuation of the uterus alone; the exact incidence is not known. At a time when hysterectomy was considered proper for molar pregnancy, Acosta-Sison[13] reported 18 histologically proven cases in a series of 210—an incidence of 8.6%.

Recent advances in treatment and the current practice of uterine conservation in a majority of cases of molar pregnancy mean that a pathological diagnosis of an invasive mole cannot be made; abdominal or transvaginal scans are not always helpful in detecting myometrial invasion. Deep myometrial invasion can result in uterine perforation and massive intraperitoneal hemorrhage. The gross appearance of hemorrhage and necrosis in the uterine wall can be confused with choriocarcinoma. Detailed histopathological evaluation showing persistence of villous structures confirm an invasive mole as was shown in one of our patients.[14]

Although invasive mole is generally less malignant than choriocarcinoma, 3.4% of documented cases of invasive mole have subsequently died from histologically varified chriocarcinoma.[15] Thus, chemotherapy should not be witheld in the presence of metastases, or failure of hCG regression and persistence of theca-luteal cysts as we have observed.[14]

PROPHYLAXIS AGAINST CHORIOCARCINOMA

Selective Preventive Chemotherapy

It is well known that embolization of trophoblasts occurs during uterine contraction, stimulation by oxytocics and during evacuation of the uterus. The role of chemotherapy at the time of molar evacuation remains controversial.[16] However, we have shown that such prophylaxis is not justified as it does not significantly reduce the malignancy rate;[17] this study showed that the neoplasia takes longer to be detected.

The disadvantage of routine chemotherapy is that a large number of patients (80-90%) who are unlikely to develop persistent GTN, will be unnecessarily exposed to the toxic effects of these drugs. '*Selective preventive chemotherapy*' has been practised by us for the past 25 years.[17] This is used in patients identified at risk of developing GTN/Choriocarcinoma, i.e.

- Those with a very slow decline in hCG levels
- Those with an initial fall but subsequent rise in hCG levels
- Those in whom an initial fall is followed by a plateau

These patients will receive the "low risk" regime chemotherapy[18] (Methotrexate 50 gm i.v on day 1, 3, 5, 7, 9 with oral folinic acid 12 mg 24-30 hours after each dose of methotrexate; course repeated after 7-10 day). The justifications for such an approach are:

- a long period of observation without treatment often results in many seeking non-effective traditional native treatment, so that we may see them only when the disease is already well advanced.
- the 'low risk' chemotherapy regime above has minimal toxicity; the risk is definitely less than that of metastatic GTN.
- the theoretical risk of development of tumor resistance is obviated by the administration of full course of chemotherapy in all instances until biochemical remission is achieved.
- normal reproductive function and normal offspring have been shown in long-term follow–up studies after chemotherapy.[19]

Follow-up of patients receiving 'selection preventive chemotherapy' for more than 10 years showed none developed choriocarcinoma, indicating the value of such therapy.

Role of Prophylactic Hysterectomy

In 1966 Tow[20] advocated prophylactic hysterectomy in patients with molar pregnancy at 40 years or more, or in those para 3 or more, as the rate of subsequent malignancy in such patients was significantly increased 3½ times. Hence, it is not unusual to see this practice adopted in many developing countries of Asia.

The subsequent development of widespread metastasis to brain and lungs observed as late as 9 years[18] and the need for close follow-up of patients with radioimmunoassay even after hysterectomy, means that 'prophylactic hysterectomy' is less justified today.

PLACENTAL SITE TUMOR (PST)

This very rare tumor is now recognized as a variant of gestational trophoblastic neoplasia, and can follow any type of pregnancy. It is composed of only one type of trophoblastic cell (cytotrophoblast); as syncytial cell which are the source of hCG are absent, the hCG production in PST is variable or absent. Curettage is needed to confirm the diagnosis. The clinical course is variable; the only case we have seen in the past 25 years presented with nephrotic syndrome.[18]

Hysterectomy and multi-agent chemotherapy play a major role in the clinical management of this tumor.[21,22]

CHORIOCARCINOMA

The risk of choriocarcinoma is 1000-fold higher after hydatidiform mole than after an abortion or normal pregnancy. Choriocarcinoma is, thus, more prevalent in the countries of South-East Asia. An incidence of gestational trophoblastic tumor/choriocarcinoma of 1.59 per 1000 deliveries was reported in our centre.[1] As shown in Table 35.6, choriocarcinoma is also more commonly seen among the Chinese (4.59 per 1000 deliveries) compared to Malays and Indians.

Table 35.6: Gestational trophoblastic tumor/choriocarcinoma (University Hospital, 1981-1990)—Racial distribution)

Race	No of cases	Total delivery	Incidence per 1000 deliveries
Malay	40	37, 380	1.07
Chinese	44	9, 581	4.58*
Indian	13	14, 210	0.91
Others	1	510	1.96
Total	98	61, 681	1.59

p < 0.001

The most common sites of disease are the uterus and lungs (Table 35.7).

Table 35.7: Choriocarcinoma–sites of disease (n= 98, University Hospital Kuala Lumpur 1981-1990)

Genital	Number	Extragenital	Number
Uterus	36	Lungs	78
Vagina	8	Brain	14
Paravaginal	8	Liver	11
Cervix (Fig. 35.9)	3	Porta-hepatis	2
Fallopian tube	2	Kidney	1
Stomach	1		
Spleen	1		
Para-aortic nodes	1		

In view of the various sites of disease, choriocarcinoma may present with
- genital tract manifestations
- extragenital tract manifestations

Genital Tract Manifestations

The most common site is the uterus. There is enlargement of the uterus to a varying degree. The symptomas include:

Amenorrhea

The occurrence of amenorrhea after molar evacuation may indicate choriocarcinoma. An ultrasound assessment of the uterus would exclude an intrauterine pregnancy as the cause of the amenorrhea.

Vaginal Bleeding

This could be intermittent and prolonged. If such bleeding occurs after evacuation of a mole, abortion or normal delivery, possibility of uterine choriocarcinoma should be borne in mind (Fig. 35.4).

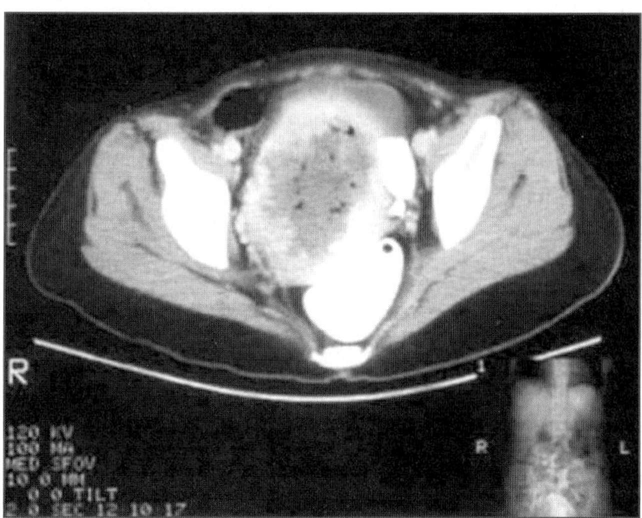

Figure 35.4: CT scan of pelvis showing appearances of uterine choriocarcinoma

Intraperitoneal Hemorrhage

Choriocarcinoma is invasive; thus, the uterine wall can be perforated by tumor resulting in intraperitoneal hemorrhage. The presence of prior amenorrhea can make distinction from a ruptured ectopic pregnancy difficult; the diagnosis is often discovered only at surgery.

Vaginal Metastasis

The commonest location is at the introitus, suburethral in position (Fig. 35.5). The differential diagnosis of a bluish nodule at this location include endometriosis, and melanoma.

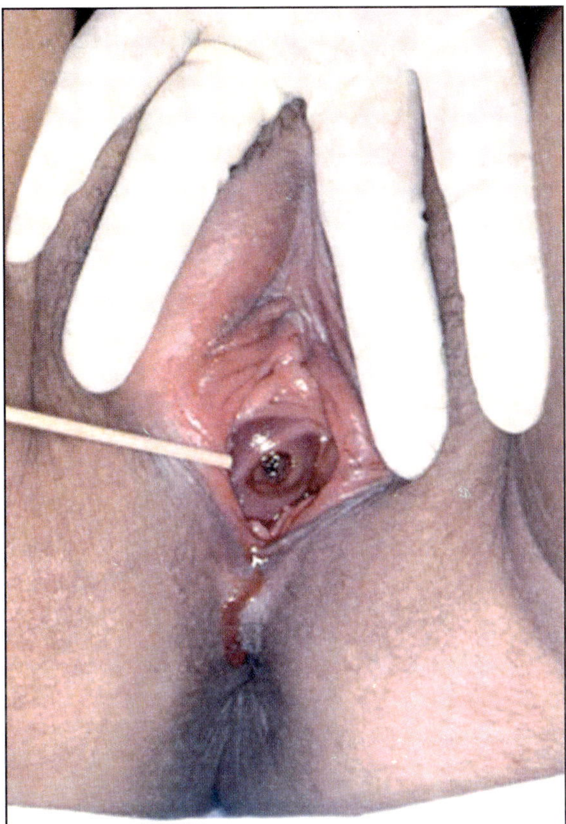

Fig. 35.5: Typical location of vaginal metastasis of choriocarcinoma (an endometriotic nodule or melanoma at this site will also have a similar appearance)

Extragenital Manifestations

The *lungs* are the commonest sites for extragenital metastasis. 'Canon-ball' lesion, either single or multiple, on chest radiograph or CT scan are typical (Fig. 35.7). Miliary lesions, are also sometimes seen; the association of hemoptysis in such patients may be mistaken for miliary TB. If the lesion is pleural based, hemo-thorax could occur causing respiratory difficulty.

The *brain* is the next most common site for extra-genital metastases (Fig. 35.8). Depending on the location the patient may have varied neurological symptoms and signs and may be mistaken for a primary brain tumor, cerebrovascular accident or even psychosis.

Secondaries can also occur in the *liver*. If the liver involvement is extensive, or if lesions occur in the bile

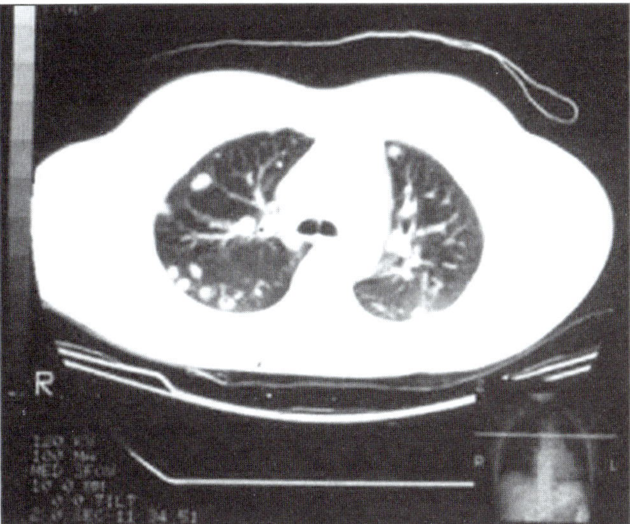

Figure 35.6: CT scan of thorax showing typical rounded metastatic lesions in the lungs in a patient with choriocarcinoma

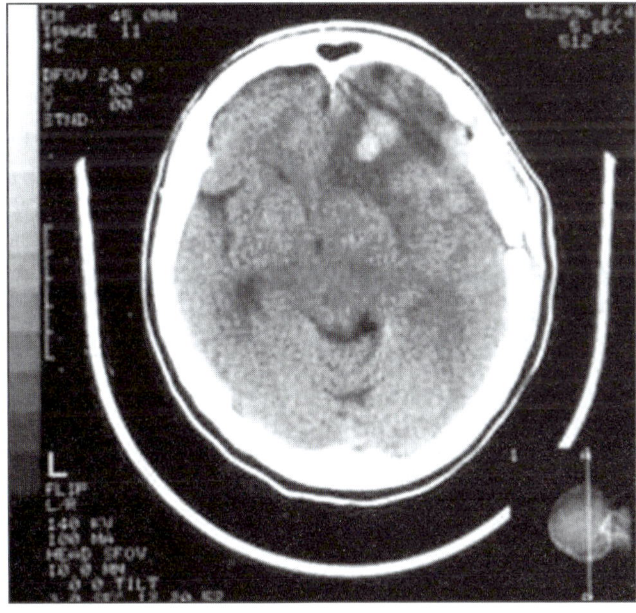

Figure 35.7: Choriocarcinoma with brain metastases. Note the rather hyperdence lesion with surrounding edema in the right frontal lobe. She also had severe jaundice (see Figure 35.8)

duct or porta-hepatis, jaundice may be the mode of presentation (Fig. 35.8).

Other sites for metastases include the *upper gastrointestinal tract* (presentating as hematemesis), *lower gastrointestinal tract* (presenting as malena), and *kidneys* (presenting as hematuria).

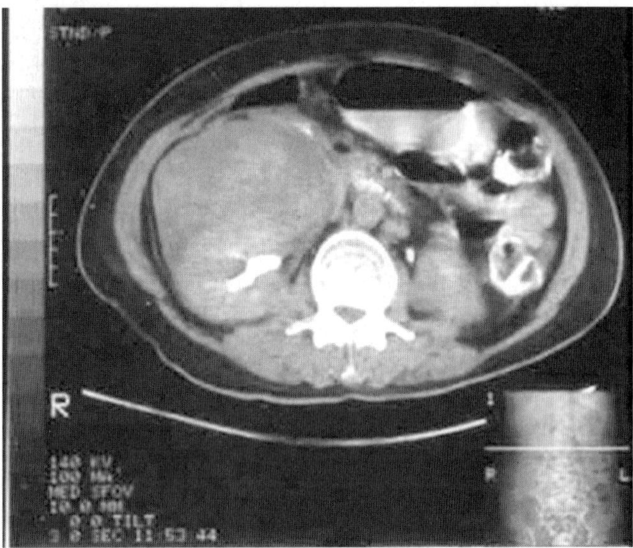

Figure 35.8: Choriocarcinoma. Note the large tumor mass in the region of portahepatis. She was intensely jaundiced and had brain and lung metastates (Figures 35.6 and 35.7). She responded to chemotherapy

Choriocarcinoma is, thus, one of the great mimics of other diseases. A high index of suspicion is crucial for early diagnosis. Clinicians must, therefore, keep in mind the possibility of choriocarcinoma in all women in the reproductive age group. A test for hCG should be a reflex response to any such presentation.

Management of Choriocarcinoma

The strategies in therapy include:
- chemotherapy
- interventional surgery in localized resistant disease
- radiotherapy

Chemotherapy

This remains the main modality of treatment. The severity of the disease has been graded according to various prognostic factors. The WHO prognostic scoring system (1983)[23] and revised FIGO staging system (1992)[24] are shown below.

For purposes of assigning appropriate chemotherapy we have categorized our patients into low, medium and high risk groups (Table 35.10)[18]

As decribed earlier, those in the 'low-risk' group receive "*selective preventive chemotherapy*". Patients in the 'medium-risk' group, receive methotrexate and

Table 35.8: WHO prognostic scoring system (1983)[23]

	Score			
Prognostic factors	0	1	2	4
Age (year)	=39	> 39	-	-
Antecedent pregnancy	Hydatidiform Mole	Abortion	Term	-
Interval (months)	<4	4 -6	7-12	> 12
hCG IU/l	$<10^3$	10^3-10^4	10^4-10^5	$>10^5$
Blood Groups (female + male.	- A x 0	0 x A AB	B	
Largest tumor Including uterine (cm)	-	3-5	5	
Sites of metastases Liver	-	Spleen, kidney	GI tract,	Brain
No. of metastases	-	1-4	4-8	>8
Prior chemotherapy	-	-	single drug	2 or more drugs

Table 35.9: Revised FIGO staging system 1992[24]

Stage
1   Disease confined to the uterus
2   Disease extends outside uterus but is limited to the genital structures (adnexa, vagina, broad ligament)
3   Disease extends to the lungs with or without known genital tract involment
4   Disease at other metastatic sites
Sub-stage
A   No risk factors
B   One risk factor
C   Two risk factors
Risk factors
1   hCG > 100,000 U/l
2   Duration to diagnosis > 6 months

Table 35.10: Choriocarcinoma—'risk' groups, University Hospital, Kuala Lumpur classification[18]

Low risk
- Persistent trophoblastic disease after molar evacuation (no radiological evidence of disease)

Medium risk
- Lesions in the uterus (uterine size < 8 weeks)
- Vaginal nodule
- < 3 lung nodules (each < 2 cm size)

High risk
- > 3 lung nodules
- metastases to brain, liver or kidneys
- uterine tumor (uterine size > 8 weeks)
- Paravaginal masses
- Failed chemotherapy

actinomycin D with folinic acid. Those in the 'high-risk' group receive the modified CHAMOCA or EMA–PE regimes. For the severely jaundiced patient we have found cisplatinum/etoposide/bleomycin combination safe and effective. For details of these regimes please refer to our publication.[18] We reported survivals of 98% in patients in the 'medium-risk' group and 61.7% in 'high-risk' group. Survival according to FIGO staging were 100%, 80%, 78.6% and 68.2%. for stage 1, 2, 3 and 4 respectively.[18]

The reasons for the *poor survival* in our *high-risk* cases are *multifactoral*:

- Multiorgan involvement
- Large bulky disease at time of presentation
- Late referrals
- Previous failed chemotherapy
- Poor patient compliance in some instances

We also observed significantly lower survival (50%) when the interval between the antecedent pregnancy (mole) and the development of GTN exceeded 24 months.[1]

Chemotherapy administered optimally is generally very effective therapy for choriocarcinoma, as shown by the remarkable response noted in Figures 35.10 and 35.11.

Side Effects of Chemotherapy

Apart from nausea and vomiting, the *severe side effects* include *severe mucositis* (Fig. 35.11) and extravasation of drugs causing skin necrosis (Fig. 35.12). Patient compliance will be enhanced if these side effects are minimized.

Another uncommon side-effect following chemotherapy is 'transient menopause' characterised by amenorrhea, and elevated FSH and LH levels; with the use of cyclical oral contraceptives return of normal ovulatory cycles is the norm.[1]

Cerebral Metastases

Patients with central nervous system metastases have one of the worst prognosis, with variable survival rates. The use of chemotherapy (with intrathecal MTX) as the main modality, with craniotomy and excision of metastasis or whole brain irradiation in a few, resulted in an overall survival rate of 84.6%.[1]

Role of Surgery

As chemotherapy is effective as primary treatment, surgery has only a limited role. Solitary nodules in the lungs not responding to chemotherapy can be excised at thoracotomy. Similarly, hysterectomy need not be

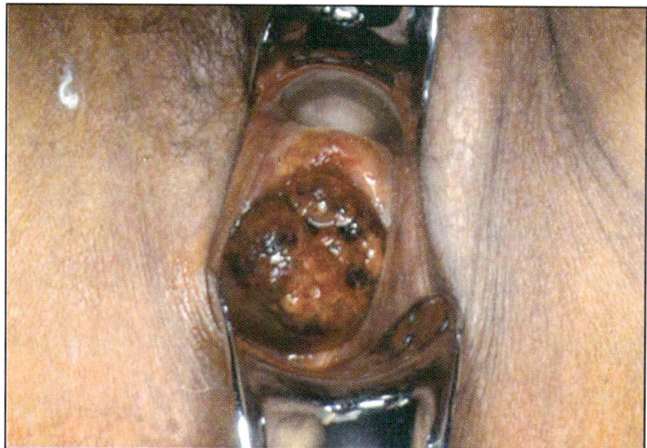

Figure 35.9: Note the large hemorrhagic / blackish tumor in the cervix. The patient also had liver, lung and brain metastases

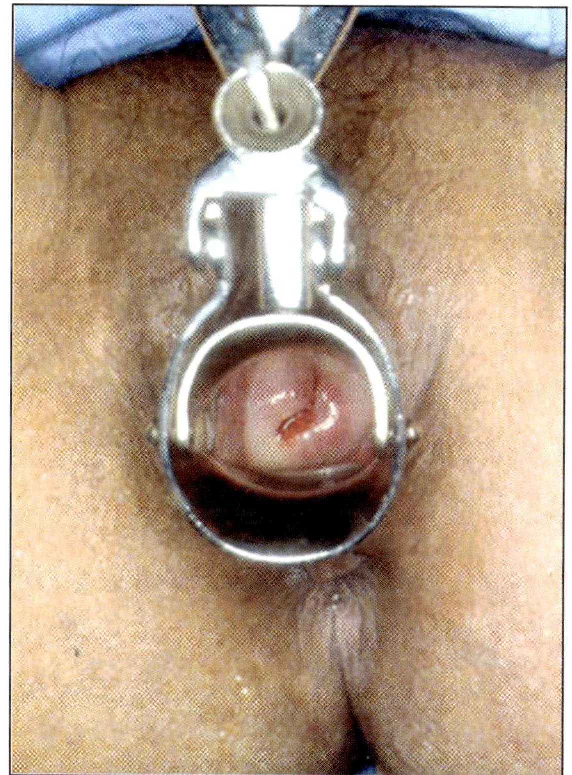

Figure 35.10: Normal appearance of the cervix after successful treatment with combination chemotherapy

performed routinely; it is only indicated for resistant disease or severe hemorrhage (Fig. 35.13)

Future Pregnancies

Women after molar evacuation should be advised not to conceive until their hCG levels have been normal

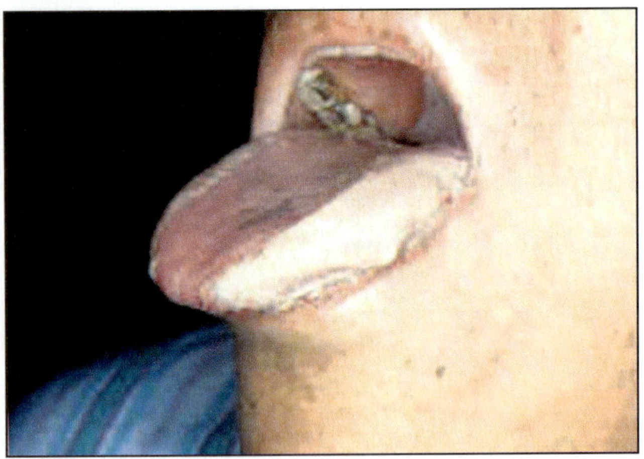

Figure 35.11: Note the severe oral mucositis after high dose MTX. This could be prevented with appropriate doses of folinic acid

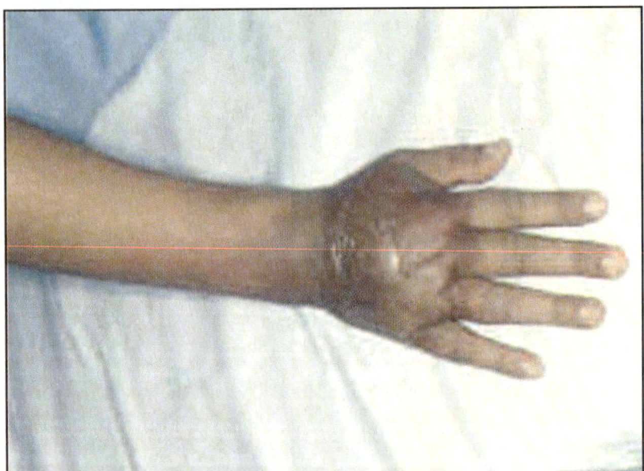

Figure 35.12: Extravasation of drug causing skin necrosis. This is preventable

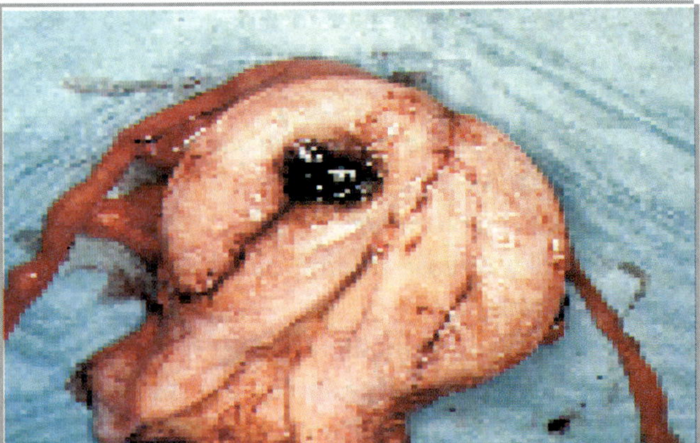

Figure 35.13: Hysterectomy specimen for resistant choriocarcinoma. Note the blackish lesion in wall of uterus; Biochemical response was achieved soon after.

diagnosis, the extent of the disease and where optimal care during chemotherapy is available.

for 6 months. Those who have had chemotherapy are advised not to conceive for one year after completion of treatment.

Pregnancies can occur after treatment of gestational trophoblastic tumors; in one large study[19] 86% succeeded in having at least one live birth. Successful pregnancies are even possible in patients with ceberal metastases.[1,25, 26]

CONCLUSION

Gestational trophoblastic neoplasia are highly curable. Best results will not be achieved unless these cases are referred promptly to specialized centers where appropriate facilities are available to determine the correct

REFERENCES

1. Sivanesaratnam V. Gestational trophoblastic disease in Malaysia and the Pacific Basin. Contemp Rev Obstet Gynecol 1995;7:179-84.
2. Sivanesaratnam V. The President's Lecture: Gestational trophoblastic disease—the Malaysian experience. Proceedings of the 3rd Malaysian Congress of Obstetrics and gynecology, Kuala Lumpur 1991.
3. Sivanesaratnam V. Asherman's syndrome successfully treated by the insertion of a multiload copper 250 device. J Obstet. Gynecol 1986;7:22-23.
4. Twiggs LB, Morrow DP, Schlaerth JB. Acute pulmonary complications of hydatidiform mole. Am J Obstet Gynecol 1979;135:189-94.
5. Sabire NJ, Foskett M, Paradinas FJ, et al. Outcome of twin pregnancies with complete hydatidiform mole and healthy co-twin. Lancet 2002; 359: 2165-66.
6. Stone M, Dent J, Kardona A, et al. Relationship of oral contraception to development of trophoblastic tumor after evacuation of hydatidiform mole. Br J Obstet Gynecol 1976; 83:913-16.
7. Newlands ES. Presentation and management of persistent gestational trophoblastic disease and gestational trophoblastic tumors in the UK. In: Hancock BW, Newlands ES, Berkowitz RS, Cole IA. Eds. Gestational Trophoblastic Disease London: Chapman and Hall 1997;143-56.
8. Cheah PL, Looi LM, Sivanesaratnam V. Hydatidiform molar pregnancy in Malaysian women, a histopathological study from the University Hospital, Kuala Lumpur. Malaysian Journal of Pathology 1993; 15: 59-63.
9. Fine C, Bundy AL, Berkowitz R et al. Sonographic diagnosis of patient hydatidiform mole. Obstet Gynecol 1989;73: 414-18.

10. Szulman AE. Trophoblastic disease: clinical pathology of hydatidiform mole. Obstet Gyne Clinics of North America 1988; 15: 443-56.

11. Bagshawe KD. Trophoblastic neoplasia—current results and therapeutic issues. In Magreth 1 (ed) New directions in Cancer Treatment. London: Springer 1988;514.

12. Looi LM, Sivanesaratnam V. Malignant evolution with fatal outcome in a patient with partial hydatidiform node. Aust NZJ Obstet Gynecol 1981;21:51-52.

13. Acosta-Sison H. Indications for immediate hysterectomy with currettage in cases of hydatidiform mole. Am J Obstet Gynecol 1961;81:715-17.

14. Goh JYL, Sivanearatnam V, Peh SC. Perforating invasive mole with subsequent metastases. Sing J Obstet Gynecol 1987;18:151-53.

15. Obir WB. The pathology of choriocarcinoma. Annals of the New York Academy of Sciences 1971;172:299-426.

16. Goldstein DP. Prevention of gestational trophoblastic disease by use of actinomycin D in molar pregnancies. Obstet Gynecol 1974; 43: 475-79.

17. Sivanesaratnam V, Ng KH. Prophylaxis against choriocarcinoma. Med J Malaysia 1977; 3: 219-31.

18. Sivanesaratnam V. Management of gestational trophoblastic disease in developing countries. Best Practice & Research Clinical Obstetric and Gynecology 2003;17: 925-42.

19. Rustin GJ, Booth M, Dent J et al. Pregnancy after cytotoxic chemotherapy for gestational trophoblastic tumors. Br Med J 1984; 288: 183-206.

20. Tow WSH. The influence of the primary treatment of hydatidiform mole and its subsequent course. J Obstet Gynecol Br Cwlth 1966; 77: 544-52.

21. Newlands ES, Bower M, Fisher RA, Paradinas FJ. Management of placental site trophoblastic tumors. J Reprod Med 1998; 43: 53-59.

22. Feltmate CM, Genest DR, Wise L et al. Placental site trophoblastic tumor: 17-year experience at New England Trophoblastic Disease Centre. Gynecol Oncol 2001; 82: 415-19.

23. World Health Organisation. Gestational Trophoblastic Disease Who Technical Report series 692. Geneva: WHO, 1983.

24. FIGO Oncology Committee Report. International Journal of Gynecology and Obstetrics 1992;39: 149-50.

25. Sen Dk, Sivanesaratnam V, Chuah CY et al. Cerebal metastases from choriocarcinoma. Acta Obstet Gynecol Scand 1987;66:425-28

26. Sivanesaratnam V, Sen DK. Normal pregnancy after successful treatment of choriocarcoma with cerebral metastases. J Reprod Med 1988; 33: 402-03.

Sapna Ahuja
Sambit Mukhopadhyay
Sabaratnam Arulkumaran

36.

Radiotherapy and Chemotherapy in Gynecological Malignancies

Radiotherapy and chemotherapy are used to treat gynecological cancers. In this chapter the basic principles of radiotherapy and chemotherapy are highlighted. This is followed by a brief description of the role of radiotherapy and chemotherapy in the treatment of individual gynecological malignancies.

RADIOTHERAPY

The use of ionising radiation is called radiotherapy. Ionising radiation plays a major role in the treatment of malignant diseases including gynecological cancers. Its role in the treatment of cervical cancer is well established.

Radiation Physics

Ionising radiation broadly consists of *electromagnetic* and *particulate* radiation. X-rays and gamma rays are types of electromagnetic radiation. Particulate radiation includes electrons (negative charges), protons (positive charges), neutrons (no charge) and negative iT mesons. The nuclei of the atoms of radioactive elements are unstable. They undergo spontaneous transformation, changing to isotopes of other elements and during this process emit alpha, beta and gamma radiation. Radioisotopes like radium are found naturally but others are now produced artificially.

The half-life is the time taken for the radioisotope to decay to half its original activity. The rate of decay of each isotope is characteristic for that element. The half-lives of some radioactive elements are:

Radium-226	1620 years
Radiocesium-137	37 years
Radiocobalt-60	5 years
Radiogold-198	2.7 days

Alpha rays consist of a stream of fast moving particles but have very little penetrating power (each resembles the nucleus of a helium atom).

Beta rays consist of a stream of fast moving particles but the penetrating power varies and is usually less than 1 cm. Most have a negative charge (electrons) but some have a positive charge (positrons).

X-rays and gamma rays are identical types of radiation, characterized by a short wavelength and high frequency. Both consist of photons or packets of energy, which are absorbed by tissue and have the power to break chemical bonds and lead to biological change and cell death.

The linear accelerator is a machine, which is used to produce X-rays. Part of the energy of electrons, which are accelerated to very high kinetic energies, is converted to X-rays.

When radioactive isotopes like cobalt-60 decay to reach a stable form they emit gamma rays. These rays have great penetrating power being able to pass through the body and even through 3 mm metal screens of lead.

The Gray

The dose of radiation energy received by tissues is expressed, as Gray. One Gray is the equivalent of 1J/kg. Earlier radiation was measured in rads; one Gray is the equivalent of 100 rads.

Radiobiology

Radiobiology is the study of the effects of ionising radiation on living matter. The principal target in the cell is the DNA. Cell death is the loss of clonogenic capacity or loss of the ability of the cell to divide. Damage to the DNA will lead to altered cell metabolism and reproduction. Cells in mitosis are vulnerable and malignant cells are more susceptible to a dose of radiation than normal cells. Anaplastic tumors tend to be more responsive than well-differentiated tumors. Cells like those of the gonads are more sensitive compared to other tissues. Recovery of normal tissues is greater than malignant tissues as long as the dose of radiation is not too large and is given over a period of time.

In all tumors there are areas, which are hypoxic, and these areas are relatively protected from radiation. Hypoxic conditions require three times the dose required to treat under fully oxygenated conditions. The ratio of these doses is the oxygen enhancement ratio. Hyperbaric oxygen chamber increases the sensitivity of radiotherapy by increasing the oxygen concentration in the tumors.

Radiotherapy Techniques

Teletherapy is external irradiation where the tumor is at a distance from the source of ionising radiation. External radiation is given by either mega-voltage or super-voltage equipment. Rays are directed through the skin to deeper structures from an external source, and hence, the skin reaction is avoided. The aim is to deliver a homogenous dose to the tumor volume while giving a low dose to the surrounding normal tissues and therefore, accurate localisation of the tumor is essential. The overall dose will be influenced by the age and general condition of the patient.

Brachytherapy is either *intracavitary* or *interstitial* irradiation where the source is a short distance from the tumor. The dose of radiation in brachytherapy is determined by the inverse square law, which states that the dose of radiation at a given point is inversely proportional to the square of the distance from the source. There is a rapid fall off of the radiation dose around the source and less damage to normal tissues. The advantage of this technique is that a high dose of radiation can be achieved over a small area and sensitive tissues within the pelvis particularly the bladder and bowel can be spared excessive doses. Radium-226 was used in the past but it has a long half-life and emits a toxic gas-radon and therefore, an isotope like caesium-137, which has a shorter half-life, has replaced this.

The intravaginal and intrauterine devices are examples of *intracavitary* therapy used in gynecological cancers. Though there are large varieties of applicators, their basic design is the same and they usually consist of a hollow stem that holds the radioactive source.

In the *Manchester technique* a single uterine tube (tandem) containing the caesium-137 is inserted into the uterine cavity and smaller tubes containing the caesium-137 in plastic vaginal ovoids (colpostats) are inserted into the lateral vaginal fornices. However, this direct insertion technique has been replaced by the *after loading technique* in most centers. Here the applicators are positioned without hazard to the operator, the accuracy of the placement is identified with X-rays and only then the radioactive source is inserted. Remote after loading systems are preferred to the manual system to avoid radiation risk to the theater staff. With this system the radioactive source is stored in the patient's room in a lead lined safe and is connected to the intravaginal and intrauterine tubes using hollow tubes.

Interstitial brachytherapy involves the direct insertion of radioactive sources like needles, wires or seeds into the tumor. An example is the treatment of vaginal carcinoma. The isotopes commonly used for this procedure are Iridium-192, Caesium-137, Iodine-125.

Instillation of radioisotopes in solution—early ovarian cancers have been treated using isotopes like gold or phosphorus linked to carrier colloids, giving high dose radiation to a depth of 4-6 mm. Postsurgical adhesions limit the free flow of the radioactive solution and some tumor sites receive a low dosage and an over dosage may be delivered to other sites. The role of this technique requires further research and is not presently established.

Radiation Damage

Tolerance of normal tissues limits the dose of radiation. Large single fractions cause more damage than multiple small fractions. Early reactions occur immediately after the course of radiotherapy and usually recover quickly. Late reactions are usually permanent and slowly progressive and can occur from an year after the treatment. They are commonly due to loss of blood supply and fibrosis. Rapidly proliferating tissues are more susceptible and result in early reactions involving the skin, bowel and bone marrow. Slowly dividing tissues like the kidney show late reactions.

Early Reactions

Skin reactions include erythema, dryness of the skin and moist desquamation.

Gastrointestinal side effects are not uncommon and include anorexia, nausea, vomiting and diarrhea. More serious problems include enteritis, proctitis and colitis. Treatment is supportive with the use of analgesics, antiemetics, antidiarrheal agents and intravenous fluids.

Bone marrow cells are susceptible to radiotherapy. White cell counts and platelets fall early but anemia sets in later due to the long life span of the red cells. Blood and platelet transfusions may be required.

Involvement of the bladder mucosa can lead to cystitis.

Late Complications

Gastrointestinal side effects include bleeding, stenosis, malabsorption and rarely rectovaginal fistulae. Special diets and nutritional support may be required. Damage to the blood supply of the liver and kidneys can lead to cirrhosis and loss of renal function.

Hemorrhagic cystitis and telangiectasis of the bladder are common, but vesicovaginal fistulae and ureteric damage are rare.

Vaginal stenosis and atrophic changes in the vulva may occur. Even small doses of radiation can cause ovarian failure. The endometrium is quite resistant to radiotherapy and may persist after treatment for cancer cervix.

Safety Precautions

Medical and other personnel coming in contact with radioactive material should take the required training and be acquainted with proper precautions specially with relation to those who are pregnant. Warning signs must be displayed in appropriate areas. Staff involved should wear film badges and the walls of treatment rooms should be reinforced with lead or brick.

Radiotherapy in Gynecological Malignancies

Cervical Cancer

Cervical cancer is sensitive to radiotherapy. Stages Ib and IIa can be treated by surgery (radical hysterectomy with lymphadnectomy) or radiotherapy. Small volume stage Ib in a younger patient is managed by surgery. Bulky stage Ia and IIb disease, more advanced disease and older patients with poor surgical risk factors, regardless of the size of the tumor are managed by radiotherapy. The 5-year survival rates are comparable to surgical treatment being 85-90% for stage Ib and 70-75% for stage IIa. The treatment of choice for stages IIb to IV is radiotherapy and the 5-year survival rates for stages IIb, III and IV are 50-60%, 30-35% and <10% respectively. The radiothereupeutic techniques employed for the treatment of cervical cancer are intracavitary and external beam radiation. Early stage disease can be managed by intracavitary therapy alone but more advanced disease requires the addition of external beam therapy. As the disease becomes more advanced the balance between external and intra-cavitary therapy alters. Curative doses of radiation are usually directed to the pelvic tumor with its local extensions and to the regional lymph nodes.

Brachytherapy: Two hypothetical points within the pelvis are referred to with respect to the dose of radiation received within the pelvis and in relation to the tumor. Point A is 2 cm lateral to the uterine canal and 2 cm above the cervical os. This lies in the paracervical region close to the uterine artery and ureter. Point B is 5 cm lateral to the central uterine canal and 2 cm above the cervical os. The dose to point B is usually one third the dose to point A due to the rapid fall-off in dose with intracavitary radiation.

Radiopaque intrauterine and vaginal applicators are inserted under general anesthesia and the radioactive sources are inserted using the after-loading technique as already described.

In the Manchester system, 6600-7600 cGy are given to point A in two treatments each lasting 70 hours and at an interval of 4-7 days. The Amersham system is currently used and is a modification of this technique. The Stockholm and the Paris techniques are not used anymore.

Teletherapy or external radiation is given before intracavitary irradiation to reduce the size of the tumor mass so that intracavitary therapy is more effective. The field of treatment extends from the junction of L4-L5 to the lower border of the obturator foramen and the lateral margins lie 1 cm outside the bony margins of the pelvis. Vaginal involvement requires the lower margin to be shifted to the introitus.

It is a common practice to add the doses from brachytherapy and teletherapy and give the dose prescription with reference to point A and point B. Usually the summated dose to point A is 7500-8500 cGy and to point B is 4500-6500 cGy. The dose to the bladder and the rectum is limited to <6000 cGy.

Endometrial Cancer

- In stage I disease radiotherapy is usually given as an adjunct to surgery in those with adverse prognostic factors which include invasion of >50% of the myometrium, a high grade tumor or a large tumor. This will consist of either brachytherapy to the vault or teletherapy or a combination of both. Post-operative adjuvant vault radiation will reduce the incidence of vaginal and pelvic recurrence but does not affect survival.

  Brachytherapy alone is given in a dose of 60 Gy to the surface of the vagina. If teletherapy is added then this is reduced to 30 Gy.

- If the patient is unfit for surgery then radiation can be used as the only modality of treatment though it is more effective when given as an adjuvant to surgery than when given alone.

- In stage II, III and IV treatment has to be individualized and a combination of radiotherapy and surgery can be used. In stage II if the cervical involvement is microscopic then treatment is as for stage I disease and if there is macroscopic cervical involvement then treatment is with radiotherapy as for cervical cancer.

- Radiotherapy also plays a curative role in those with isolated pelvic or vaginal and pelvic recurrences.

- In those with non-resectable intrapelvic or metastatic disease radiotherapy plays a role in palliative management.

- Survival rates are 80-85% for stage I disease, 55-60% for stage II disease, 35-40% for stage III disease and <10% for stage IV disease.

Ovarian Cancer

Chemotherapy has replaced radiotherapy in the management of early ovarian cancer. At present there is no role for radiotherapy in the management of advanced ovarian cancer. Therapy with intraperitoneal radioactive phosphorus has not shown to be effective but intraperitoneal radioactive antibody therapy is under research.

Cancer of the Vulva

Surgery is the mainstay of treatment, but radiotherapy has a proven role in the treatment of groin node disease after inguinofemoral lymphadenectomy. Those who have large tumors extending to or involving the urethra, vagina or anus benefit from preoperative radiotherapy alone or with combined chemotherapy to facilitate surgery and reduce morbidity. Postoperative radiotherapy should be considered if the disease free margin is less than 8 mm. Women with more than microscopic disease in one groin node need post radiotherapy. Radiotherapy can act as a useful adjunct but not a substitute to surgery.

Concurrent radiotherapy and chemotherapy are in experimental stages.

Cancer of the Vagina

Stage I-IIa can be treated entirely with radiotherapy using interstitial therapy with Iridium-192. The groin nodes are included if the tumor involves the lower half of the vagina. Vaginal stenosis is more likely when more advanced tumors are treated. Advanced cases require the addition of teletherapy.

Trophoblastic Tumors

The role of radiotherapy in the treatment of trophoblastic diseases lies in the palliative management of advanced disease. External irradiation may be used for brain metastasis and to control vaginal bleeding not responding to any other modality of treatment.

CHEMOTHERAPY

The effects of mustard gas on the bone marrow cells were first noticed during the World War 1 and it was since then that cytotoxic chemotherapy was developed.

Cellular Biology

Every dividing cell goes through the following phases
- G1 phase—diploid DNA, phase of variable length
- S phase—synthesis of DNA occurs, and DNA content is doubled

- G2 phase—tetraploid DNA content
- G0 Phase—in this phase cells are not actively dividing

After the pre-mitotic phase the cell starts the mitotic phase, and cell division begins.

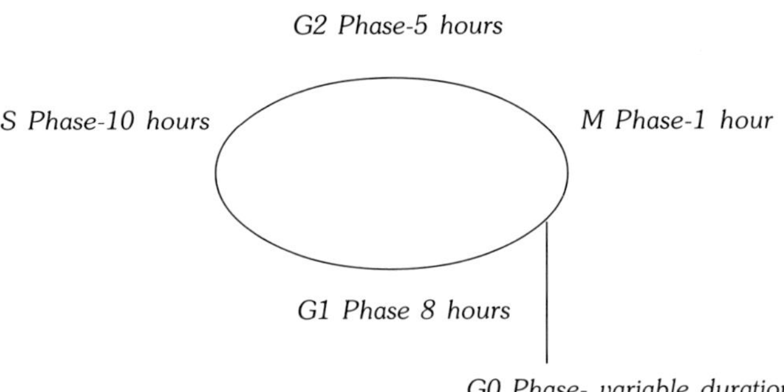

Basic Principles of Chemotherapy

- A constant proportion of cells are killed and not a given number—this is known as *fractional cell kill hypothesis.* Therefore, chemotherapeutic agents work more effectively on smaller tumors. In ovarian cancers debulking of the tumor thus decreasing the number of cells and removal of the hypoxic areas of the tumor makes the tumor more susceptible to chemotherapy.
- Drugs used in chemotherapy kill rapidly dividing cells and they are not tumor specific, hence gut and marrow cells are very susceptible to the toxic effects of chemotherapy.

Classification

Classification can be according to biological activity or according to the action on the cell cycle.

specific agents
1. Cell Cycle
   non-specific agents

Cell cycle specific agents are:
G1 Phase Actinomycin D
G2 Phase Bleomycin
S Phase Methotrexate, 5 fluorouracil and hydroxyurea
M Phase Vinblastine and vincristine
Cell cycle non-specific agents are the alkylating agents.

Table 36.1: Modalities of therapeutic regimens

Group	Drugs	Uses	Side effects
Alkylating agents-cross link strands of DNA by forming covalent bonds between alkylating and nitrogen groups preventing cell division that leads to cell death	Cyclophosphamide Chlorambucil Mephalan Treosulphan Ifosphamide	Ovarian cancers, breast cancer and soft tissue sarcomas	Vomiting, myelotoxicity; cyclophosphamide and ifosphamide-fatal encephalopathy
Platinum agents-action is similar to that of alkylating agents	Cisplatin	Ovarian, germ cell and cervical cancer	Nausea, vomiting, severe nephrotoxicity (measure clearance before every course), peripheral neuropathy and myelotoxocity limited to anemia
	Carboplatin	Ovarian and germ cell cancer	Severe myelotoxicity especially thrombocytopenia; minimal vomiting, nephrotoxicity and neurotoxicity
Antimetabolites-these drugs resemble metabolites required for the synthesis of nucleic acids and proteins			
Folic acid antagonist- inhibits the enzyme dihydrofolate reductase	Methotrexate	Breast and ovarian cancer	Oral ulceration, hepatotoxicity, myelosuppression
*Pyrimidine analogue-*blocks thymidine synthesis and the incorporation of uracil into DNA	5-Fluorouracil	Breast and ovarian cancer	Myelosuppression, nausea, vomiting and alopecia
Vinca alkaloids-spindle poisons which cause metaphase arrest by interfering with microtubular assembly	Vincristine	Germ cell cancers, cervical cancers and sarcomas	Peripheral and autonomic neuropathy, cranial nerve palsies and alopecia
	Vinblastine	Choriocarcinoma and germ cell cancers	Myelosuppression, alopecia, nausea and vomiting
Antitumor antibiotics- Interfere with tumor cell replication			
Forms irreversible complexes with DNA	actinomycin D	Germ cell ovarian tumors, soft tissue sarcoma and choriocarcinoma	Nausea and vomiting, skin necrosis, mucosal ulceration
	Doxorubicin	Ovarian, breast and endometrial cancer	Myelosuppression, alopecia cardiotoxicity and necrotic ulcers if infused s/c
Breaks up DNA chains, and interferes with DNA replication	Bleomycin	Cervical cancer, germ cell tumors of the ovary and malignant effusions	Pulmonary fibrosis, febrile reactions, hyperpigmentation
Miscellaneous			
Taxols-cytotoxic action causing polymerisation of the microtubules	Paclitaxel Docetaxel	Breast and ovarian cancers	Myelosuppression, alopecia, cardiac arrhythmias and

Contd...

Contd...

Etoposide		Ovarian germ cell tumors and choriocarcinoma
Hormones	Glucocorticoids	Used as antiemetics in terminal care
	Tamoxifen	Breast and endometrial cancer
Biological agents	Vaccines, antibodies, activated lymphocytes and cytokines	A role has yet to be defined for these in gynecological cancers

2. Biological classification
   - Alkylating agents
   - Platinum agents
   - Antimetabolites
   - Vinca alkaloids-derived from the *periwinkle plant-Vinca Rosea*
   - Antitumor antibiotics
   - Miscellaneous-taxols, etoposide, hormones and biological agents.

Single Agent vs Combination Chemotherapy

Combination chemotherapy can be curative and more beneficial than single agents in germ cell tumors but similar benefit is not seen in epithelial ovarian cancers. The theoretical advantages of combination chemotherapy are:
- Drugs with different mechanisms of action can be combined to give a synergistic effect
- Drug resistance is less likely to develop
- Two drugs with different spectrum of side effects can be combined to avoid cumulative toxic effects

Sequential Therapy

This approach is useful in treating germ cell tumors and trophoblastic disease but not epithelial tumors. Different drugs are given in turn as this allows for a shorter treatment time, and severely myelotoxic drugs can be alternated with those with no effect on the marrow. Drug resistance is also less likely to develop.

Duration of Chemotherapy

Prolonged therapy with chemothereupeutic agents can cause toxicity. Leukemias and secondary cancers have been known to develop. There is evidence that 5 courses are as good as 8 in the treatment of advanced ovarian cancers. In practice it is usually given for 6 to 12 months. Sometimes tumor markers influence the dose and duration of chemotherapy.

Chemotherapy in Gynecological Malignancies

Cervical Cancer

Chemotherapy can play a role in causing tumor regression but radiotherapy and surgery are the only modalities of treatment that can cure cervical cancer. Significant response rates are seen with cisplatin, methotrexate and bleomycin when used as single agents. Combination chemotherapy with cisplatin also gives good response rates.

The combination of 'neoadjuvant' chemotherapy and radiotherapy has not proved to improve survival. Further research is required to assess the role of chemotherapy with surgery.

Endometrial Cancer

Cytotoxic agents play a small role in the management of advanced disease which has failed to respond to hormonal therapy. Adriamycin, cisplatin, cyclophosphamide and hexamethylmelamine are useful single agents. Combination therapy has nothing to add to single agent therapy.

Ovarian Cancer

The standard treatment of ovarian cancer is cytoreductive surgery aiming to leave a tumor mass of no more than 1 cm in diameter. This maximises the effect of subsequent cytotoxic chemotherapy. Surgery alone is sufficient for the treatment of early cancers of epithelial origin but chemotherapy plays a role in the management of all other ovarian cancers. Chemotherapy is given to prolong remission and median survival postoperatively, and as palliation for advanced and recurrent disease. Chemotherapy is commenced within 6 weeks of surgery and 5 to 6 cycles are given at an interval of 3 to 4 weeks each.

The platinum drugs are now the most effective and widely used drugs either alone or in combination. Carboplatin is as effective as cisplatin but causes minimal nephrotoxicity and less incidence of nausea and vomiting. Leucopinea and thrombocytopinea are the dose limiting toxicities of carboplatin. Newer drugs like paclitaxel, docetaxol and gemcitabine have shown promising results.

Combination regimens using cisplatin when compared with single agent therapy have shown improvement in clinical response but no improvement in survival. Interim results comparing single agent carboplatin with combination therapy CAP (cyclophosphamide, doxorubicin, cisplatin) have shown no survival difference between the two.

Paclitaxel has been used to treat platinum resistant cases as second line drug therapy. Initial trials have shown response rates of 22%.

Combinations using paclitaxel with cisplatin have shown better survival rates compared to conventional combination therapy in ovarian cancers. Further results using the above combination are awaited from the ongoing European trial.

Presently intraperitoneal therapy using cisplatin can only be considered in research settings and has been found to be of limited benefit so far.

Ovarian cancers tend to present in fairly advanced stage and despite platinum therapy the overall survival rate(25-30%) for metastatic disease has not changed significantly. A 5 year survival figure of 60-70% for stage I and 10% for stage III-IV is quoted in the literature.

Cancer of the Vulva and Vagina

Concurrent chemoradiotherapy for the treatment of vulval carcinoma remains an experimental procedure.

There is no role for the treatment of vaginal cancer with chemotherapy.

Trophoblastic Disease

The term gestational trophoblastic disease (GTD) describes a patient who has had either a complete or a partial mole and has persistently raised hCG concentrations. After evacuation of a hydatiform mole prophylactic treatment should be started with actinomycin D for 5 days at a dose of 12 mcg/kg if

- there is a high level of hCG more than 4 weeks after evacuation (serum hCG >20 000U/L, urine hCG >30 000U/L)
- there is a rising titre of hCG at any time after evacuation
- there is histological evidence of choriocarcinoma or there is evidence of metastasis at anytime

The term gestational trophoblastic tumors (GTT) include invasive mole, placental site trophoblastic tumor and choriocarcinoma. Methotrexate, actinomycin D and etoposide are the drugs with greatest activity in gestational trophoblastic tumors, but other drugs shown to be of value are 6-mercaptopurine, vincristine, cyclophosphamide, cisplatin and hydroxyurea.

A prognostic scoring system has been adopted by the World Health Organization, for the treatment of patients with gestational trophoblastic tumors. Patients are classified as low, medium and high risk based on the prognostic factors which include age, antecedent pregnancy, hCG level, blood group, size of the tumor, site and number of metastasis and interval since previous pregnancy. Low risk patients receive primary single-agent chemotherapy and high risk patients receive primary intensive combination chemotherapy (low risk= <4, medium risk=5-7, high risk=>8)

Methotrexate followed by folinic acid is the standard treatment followed in patients with low risk disease. This regimen is given over 8 days and is repeated every 14 days until hCG levels are undetectable for 6 weeks. Multidrug regimens are used in high risk disease. The MAC 111 regimen is used at Boston and the EMA/CO (EMA is etoposide, methotrexate and actinomycin D; CO is cyclophosphamide and vincristine) regimen is used at Charing Cross Hospital. The long term survival for high risk patients has been shown to be 86% with a maximum follow up of 16 years.

CONCLUSIONS

Radiotherapy is the mainstay of treatment in advanced cervical cancer and cancer of the vagina. Chemotherapy is curative in case of germ call tumors of the ovary and trophoblastic tumors. A multidisciplinary team approach plays an important role in the management of gynecological malignancies with involvement of doctors, radiographers, engineers, physicists, pharmacists and healthcare providers.

REFERENCES

1. Joanna Lambert, Clare C. Vernon. The principles of radiotherapy and chemotherapy. In: Robert E Shaw, W Patrick Soutter, Stuart L Stanton (Eds): Gynecology (2nd edn), Edinburgh: Churchill Livingstone, 1997; 505-520.
2. Robert C Young, Gillian M Thomas. General principles of Cancer Therapy. In: Jonathan S Berek (Ed). Novak's Gynecology (12th edn), USA: Williams and Wilkins, 1996; 1015-57.
3. Tim Chard, Richard Lilford. Pharmacology. In Basic Sciences for Obstetrics and Gynecology (5th edn), London: Springer, 1998; 181-183.
4. Professor ES. Newlands. Trophoblastic disease. RCOG PACE review 96/10.
5. Gordon M Stirrat. Conditions of the lower genital tract. In:Aids to Obstetrics and Gynecology for MRCOG 4th edn, Edinburgh: Churchill Livingstone, 1997; 250-277.

37. Palliative Care

O Tamizian
Sabaratnam Arulkumaran

INTRODUCTION

Palliative care should not be viewed as synonymous to terminal care. Although cure is no longer the aim of treatment, the patient may still enjoy a fruitful and rewarding life. The patient needs to lead a life as normal as possible with effective relief from pain and distressing symptoms, coupled with consistent and effective response to changes in wellbeing. Focusing on the quality of life and what it means for individual women and their families is paramount. In order to elicit the detail of problems, fears and anxieties it is essential to develop excellent communication skills. Patients need sensitive, clear and repeated explanations of the diagnosis and its implications along with the potential effects of any treatments (curative or palliative) on activities of daily living and well being. Breaking the news of a diagnosis of cancer is one of the doctor's first responsibilities and as such, the manner in which it is performed influences the course of the doctor–patient relationship.

SYMPTOM MANAGEMENT

The principles involved in symptom management are based around thorough evaluation and assessment of the problem, to identify the best course of action. Symptoms need to be appreciated in the context of the beliefs of the individual, their understanding of the situation, their coping mechanism and expectations. Understanding the pathophysiology of a specific problem enables appropriate management plans to be initiated. Combining treatment both for the cause and the symptom is generally the best approach. Any intervention should be evaluated with respect to its appropriateness regarding improvement in quality of life prior to implementation and any actual benefit confirmed after the implementation.

Pain Control

Pain is a physical as well as an emotional experience, therefore, consideration should be given to the physical, emotional, social and spiritual aspects of suffering. This in turn will enable more rapid relief of pain with less use of medication and hence, fewer side effects. Appropriate management of pain control requires determination of cause or mechanism of underlying pain in order to direct appropriate treatment against it. The basic principles involved in the assessment of pain need to be revisited and detailed information about the site, radiation, duration, nature, relieving and exacerbating features need to be obtained.

It is important to determine whether the pain is cancer related and if so its characteristics. In the assessment of pain, it is essential to incorporate how the pain is limiting the patient's activities, what the patient thinks the pain may be due to, as well as, review what analgesia has been tried and with what success and adverse effects. Clearly a fine balance needs to be struck regarding the need for investigations to determine cause of pain in the very ill patient, and investigations only performed if they will significantly alter management and benefit the patient. Successful management of pain will need some sort of 'contract' or 'agreement' between the patient and physician as to achievable goals and potential side effects or changes in lifestyle the patient may have to make as a result of treatment. Ensuring a full night's sleep undisturbed by pain should be an initial aim. During the daytime a balance needs to be struck of keeping the patient comfortable, whilst ensuring she can engage in social activities and carry out arrangements for her life.

The importance of regular administration of analgesia in maintaining adequate pain relief cannot be sufficiently emphasized. Regular analgesia is required to prevent recurrence of pain. Analgesia prescribed should be in appropriate doses and dose intervals determined by the pharmacokinetics of the medication. The preferred route of administration is the oral route, being least disruptive and giving the patient maximal control. Anticipation and measures to prevent or ameliorate adverse effects may improve acceptability and tolerance.

The two broad classifications of analgesic drugs non-opioids and opioids, have differing mechanisms of action. Non-opioid analgesics such as Paracetamol and non-steroidals (NSAIDs) reduce inflammation and prostaglandin synthesis, thereby reducing painful stimuli. Opioids on the other hand are thought to act both peripherally and centrally through inhibition of nociceptive transmission at spinal cord, brainstem and possibly at peripheral nerve level. Visceral/soft tissue pain can be controlled in the majority of settings using the WHO analgesic ladder with a combination of non - opioids with or without adjuvants, progressing to opioids and adding non-opioids with or without adjuvants in more severe pain. In bone pain, NSAIDs are the first line, but opioids are also helpful. Bone pain secondary to metastatic disease often responds to radiotherapy either in a single high dose fraction or in series of low dose fractions. In certain circumstances bone metastases may lead to pathological fractures and therefore orthopedic assistance to plate and support such bones may be helpful in maintaining function of the limb.

Opioid Analgesia

When patients are being commenced on strong opioids, it is advisable to achieve pain control initially with a four hourly dose such as 10 mg although a smaller dose may be advisable in renal failure, hepatic impairment or the very frail. The regular dose needs to be supplemented with equivalent doses administered on an 'as required' basis. The regular dose needs to be readjusted on a daily basis including increasing the 'as required' dose for breakthrough pain. Once pain control has been achieved it is then possible to convert the 4 hourly dose to a once or twice daily long acting agent or an alternative route such as a transdermal patch but at all times having a fast short acting opioid available for breakthrough pain. When converting between strong opioids or different routes of administration, great care should be taken using conversion tables or seeking advice from a specialist pharmacist.

Neuropathic Pain

Pain originating from damage to the nervous system may be difficult to manage with conventional opioid or non-opioid analgesia. Such pain in the context of gynecological malignancy may arise for sacral plexus infiltration in cervical or ovarian cancer, radiculopathy secondary to spinal cord compression or as a side effect from platinum based cytotoxic chemotherapy. A number of drugs, which are not conventional analgesics, may be helpful and are classed as adjuvant analgesics. Adjuvant analgesic drugs include tricyclic antidepressants such as Amitriptyline, which is thought to act by increasing Serotonin levels in the central nervous system and therefore enhancing central inhibition of nociception. Other drugs such as Sodium valproate (an anticonvulsant) or Mexiletene (a cardiac antiarrhythmic) act by reducing neuronal excitability, while corticosteroids such as dexamethasone act through reduction of peritumor edema.

Invasive Techniques for Pain Control

These include nerve blocks, epidural/intrathecal administration of drugs along with neurodestructive procedures but are all the remit of specialists in pain management.

Alternative Therapies

Transcutaneous nerve stimulation (TENS), Acupuncture, aromatherapy, hypnotherapy and psychological therapies may be helpful in the management pain.

Nausea and Vomiting

Effective treatment of nausea and vomiting has a major impact on improving the quality of life of the patient. A logical approach is to determine the causes of nausea and vomiting in an individual patient as the cornerstone of effective management of the condition. The emotional/psychological morbidity associated with a diagnosis of cancer and in particular palliative nature of any treatment may exacerbate nausea and vomiting and should also be addressed. Nausea and vomiting may be secondary to biochemical disturbance (hypercalcemia, uremia), chemotherapy or drug induced, secondary to GI involvement in the malignant process (tumor infiltration, obstruction, gastric stasis), raised intracranial pressure or may be of unclear origin. Management of nausea and vomiting should be a multifaceted approach simultaneously treating any underlying treatable or preventable cause while also providing symptom relief. Route of administration needs to be given some thought as in many patients with nausea, gastric stasis is coexistent and results in poor absorption and bioavailablity of the drug. Drugs such as Haloperidol and Prochloperazine (stemetil) are antidopaminergic agents and effective against biochemical and drug induced nausea. Metoclopramide (maxolon) and Domperidone, also antidopaminergic agents, have a prokinetic effect so are also suitable with gastric stasis. Cyclizine has an antihistamine and anticholinergic effect and is useful as a broad spectrum agent along with particular value in cases of nausea due to raised intracranial pressure and movement related nausea. Movement associated nausea also benefits from anticholinergic agents such as hyoscine hydrobromide. The antiserotonergic agents Ondansetron and Granisetron, are particularly valuable with chemotherapy associated emesis and their effects can sometimes be enhanced by co administration of corticosteroids such as dexamethasone. Other broad spectrum antiemetics include methotrimeprazine. Often more than one agent with differing mechanisms of action may be required for effective symptom control.

Dry Mouth/Oropharynx

Dry mouth/oropharynx as a result of cancer or treatment for cancer can cause much discomfort. Useful measures include sucking ice or acid sweets, chewing gum or pineapple pieces. Oral hygiene is essential, as is prompt diagnosis and treatment of oral *Candida*.

Constipation

Generally a side effect of opioid analgesia and therefore predictable and to some extent preventable. Patients on weak or strong opioids should have laxatives prescribed and the dose of the latter increased in tandem with increases in the medication causing the adverse effect of constipation. Stimulant laxatives include senna and bisacodyl, whereas codunthrusate and codanthramer combine stimulant and softening properties.

Diarrhea

In advanced cancer when diarrhea occurs it is essential to exclude fecal impaction with overflow. A rectal examination is mandatory and a plain abdominal X-ray may help. Other common causes of diarrhea in advanced cancer include tumor infiltration of the bowel wall or the effect of treatment such as radiotherapy (radiation colitis) or antibiotic treatment leading to Clostridium Difficile infection. Loperamide and adequate fluid replacement would deal with non-specific diarrhea while oral metronidazole or oral vancomycin will be required for Cl. difficile diarrhea.

Intestinal Obstruction

This occurs not uncommonly in ovarian cancer. Management may be conservative or surgical. Surgery aims at relieving the mechanical obstruction to improve quality of life and provide symptom alleviation but may be associated with a significant postoperative morbidity and mortality. It is best reserved where a single site obstruction is suspected with localised intra-abdominal disease and in patients with otherwise good nutritional and physical status. Conservative treatment aims to deal with the pain due to colic and distention, the nausea and reduce the sensation of thirst. Hyoscine hydrobromide may help by reducing colic while a review of current medication to stop prokinetic agents and laxatives may also prove helpful. The nausea may be best controlled by a subcutaneous infusion of cyclizine and haloperidol while intravenous fluids, ice, drinks and mouth care may help to deal with sensation of thirst and prevent dehydration. Nasogastric tube and intravenous fluids may help to rest the bowel and aid resolution. Any medication should preferably be administered subcutaneously or intravenously avoiding the oral route.

Ascites

Ascites is the accumulation of fluid in the peritoneal cavity and is commonly seen with advanced ovarian, endometrial and cervical cancer. The accumulation of fluid although not painful does cause discomfort and may also cause dyspnea, indigestion, poor mobility, nausea and vomiting and even obstruct ureters in severe cases. Palliative treatment such as chemotherapy or radiotherapy may help, but usually these alternatives have already been exhausted. The simplest and most frequent treatment involves repeated paracenteses to drain fluid. In some cases Spironolactone may slow down reaccumulation and is worth considering. Where there has been extensive abdominopelvic surgery with risk of adhesions or where fluid is loculated, an ultrasound guided procedure is recommended. Care should be taken to avoid large fluid shifts in elderly or frail patients, slow drainage over several days should be aimed for to avoid the risk of depletion of intravascular volume with resultant renal failure and cardiovascular collapse.

Fistulae

Enterocutaneous or enterovaginal fistulae may occur with advanced malignancy resulting in severe ulceration and irritation of the skin surrounding the fistula. Surgical diversion is the best option, although this may not always be possible or appropriate. Conservative measures aim to reduce the production of the proteolytic enteral secretions using somatostatin or octreotide and protect surrounding skin by use of stomal bags and barrier creams such as 1% silver sulphadiazine. With rectovaginal fistulae the preferred option is an end colostomy or a loop colostomy (next best option). If neither are possible, barrier creams and attention to hygiene are essential. Fistulae are often associated with large amounts of necrotic tumor and even if surgical diversion has been possible, large amount of foul smelling discharge may still persist. Regular douching with betadine or saline combined with oral and/or topical metronidazole may help reduce the smell of anerobic organisms. Similarly, topical or oral metronidazole may have a role in managing fungating necrotic tumors.

Obstructive Uropathy

The route of the ureter as it enters the pelvis and course forward in close proximity to the uterus makes it particularly susceptible of obstruction in pelvic malignancies. Ureteric obstruction may however, pose a management dilemma. It can easily be relieved by percutaneous nephrostomy decompressing the kidney and preserving its function thus, prolonging the patient's life. In general if obstructive uropathy is for example, the presenting symptom in cervical cancer, denoting stage 3b disease, then a nephrostomy and palliative radiotherapy may be of value in providing the patient with time to come to terms with the diagnosis and to sort out her affairs whilst providing a good quality of life. On the other hand, obstructive uropathy may be a terminal event, enabling the patient to gradually drift in to unconsciousness and death. It is therefore important to determine whether relieving the obstruction and prolonging the patient's life is indeed in her best interest. Although discussion and informed consent is crucial, in reality this may be very difficult when urgent need for treatment arises.

Hypercalcemia

This may be the cause of a variety of symptoms in advanced malignancy. Hypercalcemia may present with lethargy, weakness, confusion, psychiatric disturbances, nausea, vomiting and constipation. In the context of gynecological cancers, it may be a result of bony metastases or occur with clear cell and small cell ovarian carcinomas. The most effective means of dealing with the condition is removal of the cause which in advanced disease is not an option. Furthermore, hypercalcemia indicates short life expectancy and in some situations treatment may not be warranted. Intravenous rehydration and administration of frusemide may be all that is required in the mildest cases, but usually bisphosphonates such as pamidronate are required and in resistant cases subcutaneous calcitonin may also have to be added.

Lymphedema

This is the accumulation of lymphatic fluid in the subcutaneous tissues. It is usually a result of damage to the lymphatic system through surgery, radiotherapy, compression by or tumor involvement of the lymphatic system. In the initial stages of developing lymphoedema the swelling is soft and pitting. With progressive protein deposition and resulting fibrosis of the subcutaneous tissues, the swelling becomes tense and less pitting and is associated with hyperkeratosis. From the natural history of the condition it is obvious that the earlier treatment is instigated the better the results are and therefore preventative advice is paramount. Management of lymphoedema involves prevention of infection, along with early treatment of cellulitis and maintaining limb function and lymph drainage through exercise. Swelling can be reduced by external compression bandaging, manual drainage and exercises or the use of intermittent positive pressure boots for 1-2 hours a day, while an ongoing use of containment hosiery and massage/exercise are required to maintain optimum lymphoedema control. Physical treatment should be complemented by appropriate psychological support as well, as the impact of lymphoedema on body image, sexual relationships and mobility should not be forgotten.

Terminal Care

Continued involvement of the medical team is essential in the care of the dying patient. It is important that such patients do not feel abandoned and there is continuing re-evaluation of problems as they arise. Agitation and confusion may be due to a variety of reasons including hypoxia, hypotension, biochemical abnormalities to name a few. The patient and the family are in need of reassurance that all efforts are being made and will continue to be made to control symptoms and alleviate any suffering. Excess respiratory secretions (death rattle) can be dealt with effectively with anticholinergics. Mouth care and appropriate repositioning may need to be performed fairly frequently as the patient becomes weaker. If the patient is very distressed then sedation is appropriate via the subcutaneous or rectal route. It is essential also to continue supporting the family at this emotionally distressing time

CONCLUSION

Palliative care spans the time period from when treatment with the aim of cure is no longer possible through to terminal care and death. Clearly its duration is very variable as is the patient's outlook and needs. The emphasis is to maintain the best quality of life achievable for the patient allowing them dignity and providing reassurance that all efforts will be made to provide symptom control. Optimum palliative care requires multidisciplinary input to make best use of all available resources and expertise.